I0982761

THE LIFE EXTENSION
WEIGHT LOSS PROGRAM

THE
LIFE EXTENSION
WEIGHT LOSS
PROGRAM

by Durk Pearson and Sandy Shaw

WITH A FOREWORD BY DR. RONALD KLATZ

DOUBLEDAY & COMPANY, INC.
GARDEN CITY, NEW YORK   1986

Library of Congress Cataloging-in-Publication Data
Pearson, Durk.
    The life extension weight loss program.
    1. Reducing diets. I. Shaw, Sandy. II. Title.
RM222.2.P425   1986   613.2′5   85-29909
ISBN 0-385-23365-5

This book is dedicated to:

The many scientists and physicians whose research has made this book possible,

And to

You, the purchaser of this book, whose support makes more of our own research possible.

And our special thanks to

Those scientists who generously provided information when we asked about their research.

Contents

Foreword to a Physician's Foreword

Weight and fat loss is a medical subject, and anyone about to read a popular book on this subject should have some guidance from an experienced physician. We selected Dr. Ronald M. Klatz to write a foreword to *The Life Extension Weight Loss Program* for several reasons.

Dr. Klatz is a physician whose patients come in for office visits. Only a few of them are hospitalized. Diets that work on hospitalized research subjects may not work outside of the institutional hospital setting because the hospital can completely control exactly what, when, and how much hospitalized patients eat. You don't need willpower in a hospital.

In addition to helping his patients with their obesity problems, Dr. Klatz works in sports medicine, preventive medicine, and family practice. He frequently works with people in good health who want to maintain and further enhance their health. His sports medicine practice has made him experienced in judging reasonable uses versus dangerous abuses of substances. Dr. Klatz is coauthor of *Death in the Locker Room,* a book about the abuse of anabolic steroids in athletics and bodybuilding. He brings this perspective to the use of nutrient supplements in a program of metabolic modification to achieve fat loss without the conventional hunger, dieting, and lengthy exercise. The nutrient supplements described in this book are recognized only as foods by the U.S. Food and Drug Administration. Their use as aids in fat loss or muscle building is still legally experimental, even though hundreds of thousands of people have used these nutrients safely for athletics and for other purposes in accord with our instructions in *Life Extension: A Practical Scientific Approach* and in *The Life Extension Companion.*

Dr. Klatz is experienced and well qualified to comment on both nutritional and behavioral therapies, and we are grateful for his having written part of Chapter 13, on behavioral therapy.

A Physician's Foreword

American medicine is on the verge of a great transformation, which will impact positively on the life of every man, woman, and child on the face of the planet . . . today and forever.

Until now, American health care has meant illness care. People saw their doctor when they were sick, not well. Doctors and medical researchers concentrated on disease and its treatment but almost never on its prevention. It is a sad fact that America, possessing the most affluent and advanced medical system in the history of the world, spends less than 5 percent of its health budget on preventive medicine. Fortunately, this situation is changing, a new era is dawning on modern medicine, the era of MAXIMUM HUMAN PERFORMANCE Health Care.

Breakthrough medical technologies are now making it possible for everyone to expect a longer, more productive, and healthier life span. Daily, we are making fantastic discoveries in the understanding of immunology, metabolism, and the mechanisms of human aging itself. Life extension physicians and researchers are developing new instruments and drugs that can detect cancer, heart disease, and other metabolic disorders at the earliest and most treatable stage; today we can regrow hair on persons who have been bald for four years and longer, improve athletic performance, end panic attacks and depression, improve memory and intelligence, reverse impotence, and enhance sexual performance.

Things are changing, thanks to the efforts and success of visionaries such as Durk Pearson and Sandy Shaw. Their book *Life Extension* has seemingly overnight sparked a grass-roots movement in America, of over 2 million private citizens who realize that modern biotechnology can perform the same level of high-tech miracles in the human body that computers have performed for electronics. Durk and Sandy, who have shown us the possibilities of living a longer and healthier life, now show the way to more effective methods of *permanent* weight loss.

We are at the forefront of a revolution in modern medical care. Soon doctors will spend more time preventing than treating disease. As testimony to the value of prevention, the 1980s have seen a 40 percent decrease in strokes and a 15 percent decrease in fatal heart attacks, thanks to better control of hypertension, improved nutrition, and an increase in physical fitness on the part of the general public. In the 1950s the diagnosis of cancer meant almost certain death, while today over 50 percent of all cancers are curable and greater than 75 percent are preventable with proper nutrition and life extension therapies.

The diseases of aging—senile dementia, hearing loss, heart disease, and arthritis—are generally accepted as the normal consequences of a long life. Today, as we shift our perspective in medicine to a *health* rather than a disease orientation, we are no longer satisfied to sit back and passively wait for the diseases of age to creep up. A closer look at the infirmities of aging reveals that what we called the chronic diseases (associated with aging) may instead be the process of aging itself. If this be the case, then shouldn't age be treated as a disease and a cure be sought?

As the average life span in America is now approaching seventy-six years (up from forty-six years in the early 1900s), wellness care and the prevention of disease are of intimate importance to us all. Life science researchers believe that the average human life span will continue to increase by three days for each week, as it has over the past eighty-five years. The U.S. Census Bureau predicts that 50 out of every 100 people will live to be 84 years and beyond early in the next century.

Scientific study has confirmed the popular wisdom that obesity (greater than 20 percent above the ideal body weight) can contribute to a significantly increased risk of diabetes, heart disease, cancer, arthritis, metabolic disorders, and premature death. *The Journal of the American Medical Association,* in July 1985, reported new evidence indicating that obese children have higher blood fat levels than normal children, and thus get an unfortunate head start on heart disease.

As you read this, 20 million Americans are actively involved in a weight loss program. Hundreds of books have been published on this topic, but, as the innovators they most certainly are, Durk Pearson and Sandy Shaw have taken a radically different approach to this disorder. *If weight loss were simply a matter of inadequate exercise or excessive caloric intake, dieting would not have a failure rate of greater than 95 percent.* In fact we're now learning that obesity is a multifactorial disorder with a basis in neurochemistry, metabolism, genetics, and psychology, as well as environmental origins.

Statistics tell us that the U.S. population is 2.4 trillion pounds overweight, with more than 25 percent of women and 15 percent of men obese. In an effort to reverse these grim statistics, we spend in excess of $10 billion each year fighting flab. Yet, despite this, the Battle of the Bulge has been for most a bitter defeat. *The odds of beating cancer are better than those for losing weight and keeping it off!*

In the past, medicine and physicians have concentrated on psychological and behavioral analysis to explain the obese person's condition; we mistakenly believed that the obese were weak of will, or sedentary, or that their fat was a defensive shield against a hostile world. Food was their comfort, so we thought. Yet, because of new information, the experts of yesterday may be regarded as the fools of today. Many obese individuals do not eat any more and, in some cases, consume less than their thinner counterparts. In fact, our nation is eating approximately 400 fewer calories per day than we were thirty years ago. Medicine is learning that overweight is much more a question of metabolism than just id and ego.

Weight loss is taking on greater importance in light of the promising research on diet and longevity. Controlled scientific studies have reportedly shown that aging of nonhuman primates (the closest research animal to man) can be slowed and longevity increased by 20 percent with the use of caloric restriction and nutrient antioxidant supplementation.

In Japan, Mr. Yasuhisa Uemura, the world's oldest man, at age 120, stated that he attributed his longevity to a simple diet of natural foods, a 60-proof sake, frequent naps, walks after every meal, and a low-stress life-style. Genetics, of course, had an important role in this man's amazing life span, but we are increasingly coming to realize that life-style and behavior are as important as genes in determining one's health and longevity.

Studies of centenarians indicate that habits for a long and healthy life can be adopted late in adulthood with excellent results. Many 100-year-old people living today admit to poor health habits during their youth. Most, in fact, have survived serious diseases, including cancer and heart attacks. A majority report modifying their diets and achieving a proper body weight, usually after a confrontation with a life-threatening disease.

Chronic disabling illness such as heart disease, arthritis, and diabetes often responds dramatically to weight loss. The Pritikin Program and the American Heart Association's Prudent Diet are testimony to the importance of nutrition and weight loss in the rehabilitation of heart disease victims. Patients with arthritis of the knees, hips, and ankles improve greatly with a loss of body weight along with a muscle fitness training program, and over 50 percent of all diabetes can be controlled by diet alone.

While blood and sweat, willpower, fasting, diet foods, enemas, and hunger have a 5 percent overall long-term weight loss success rate, the true hope for permanent weight loss lies in a better understanding of metabolism and methods of altering it. The breakthrough technologies and advanced medical research examined in this book bring new hope to the 30 million Americans whose lives are blemished by the handicap of obesity, and to the millions more who are coming to realize that it is now possible, through modification of body weight and metabolism, to gain ultimate control of the vitality of their own minds and bodies and, perhaps, even the aging process itself.

WARNING: The new dietary, nutritional, and drug therapies discussed in this text, though extremely promising, are experimental, *and some could be potentially hazardous.* No individual should embark on a self-medication or self-treatment program without the direct supervision of a licensed medical physician knowledgeable in these therapies.

Dr. Ronald Klatz
Medical Director
Pain Clinic of Racine, Wisconsin
Human Performance Center, Niles, Illinois

THE LIFE EXTENSION
WEIGHT LOSS PROGRAM

1

Why You Can Benefit from Our New Natural High-tech Approach

Don't ever confuse hard work with hard thinking.
Dr. James Watson, Nobel laureate

We are two sedentary scientists. We hate diets and exercise. We want to have healthy, lean, muscular bodies without giving up our gourmet food, swivel chairs, and water beds. Of course, we always have something more interesting to do than exercise. We have taken seven years of our own original research and hard thinking, and literally thousands of man-years of research and hard thinking from hundreds of other scientists, and have developed a system that you are going to love, because *all this hard thinking is going to replace your hard work.*

We believe that you have been working far too hard to lose weight or to maintain your desired figure if you have been following conventional diet and exercise programs. Sweat is a poor substitute for knowledge.

There is a much better way. You will have to think a little harder, but you will be rewarded by getting what you want with a lot less work.

The Life Extension Weight Loss Program can help you create and maintain the figure that you want *without restrictive diets, hunger, or time-consuming exercise.*

This is going to be far easier than you ever dreamed. . . .

Are you someone who:

Wants to improve his or her appearance?

Wants to maintain his or her figure?

Wants to be physically fit?

Hates diets and boring time-consuming exercise?

Loves lots of fine food and yummy desserts?

Has lost weight and put it right back on?

Has lost weight and then reached an impassable plateau?

Wants lots more muscles—with 5 minutes per day of exercise?

Has a cellulite problem?

Wants to lose fat without shrunken breasts?

Wants to improve health by losing unhealthy fat?

Wants to improve cardiovascular conditioning?

Is a dancer or an athlete?

Wants to lose 10 to 30 pounds easily?

Wants to lose up to 150 pounds?

If you have answered "yes" to any of these questions, our program can probably help you to achieve your goals without deprivation and without a lot of hard work.

The Life Extension Weight Loss Program is very different from any book on diet or exercise that you have ever read. That is because we are very different from the authors of these other books.

We are scientists; we have studied the fundamental biochemical mechanisms that govern fat storage and metabolism. Very few books on weight loss are written by scientists, and most of these are written for other scientists, not intelligent laypersons. We have our own biomedical research library, and we currently subscribe to well over one hundred scientific research journals. Our library is large enough to qualify as the research library for an accredited Ph.D. granting university; it fills one and a half houses. In addition, we make frequent use of the National Library of Medicine's computerized literature search services, and the immense regional UCLA Biomedical Research Library.

To repeat, we are extremely sedentary. Sure, it might be better if we walked ten miles per day, but we always have something more urgent to do. We love our work, but that work is primarily reading, thinking, and writing. Sandy spends almost all of her waking time in a swivel chair. The rest of her time is spent on a water bed. Durk spends most of his waking time lying in great sedentary comfort on his water bed. One of our computer work stations rolls up to his bed, a computer terminal on an arm swings out to float over his hips, and all that moves is his eyes and his fingers. It is the ultimate in ergonomic work stations. He can work twelve hours a day seven days a week without a backache. When he isn't floating, he spends the rest of his time in a swivel chair. Then he sleeps on the water bed. Our laboratory work isn't much exercise, either.

We are gourmets. We eat lots of red meat, eggs, dairy products, gourmet sauces, and other delicious, fattening high-calorie foods. When Durk eats at a gourmet restaurant, he usually eats two appetizers, soup, salad, main course(s), and two to three desserts. Sandy is smaller, so she can hold a little less, but she, too, is a very eager eater. At home we always have lots of yummy goodies around, and Sandy is a gourmet cook. We eat very well, and plenty. This is normally a great recipe for growing fat and suffering from cardiovascular disease. . . .

We know that an extremely sedentary life-style is normally unhealthy, and a rich gourmet diet is bound to make it worse. Instead of going on a boring and restrictive diet and investing a couple of hours per day in exercise, we invested that time in finding out *why* a sedentary gourmet life-style can be unhealthy, and *how* to stay slim and in good health *without significant changes in either diet or life-style!*

Our program works naturally. We have studied the work of many scientists on how the body's biochemistry deals with fats, carbohydrates, and proteins, and have found ways to augment those biochemical routes that reduce the percentage of the body that is fat.

There are ways of using nutrient supplements that actually alter the way that the human body metabolizes food: whether you burn it off, or whether you grow muscles or fat; they affect what foods you crave when you are hungry, and even whether you feel hungry or full and satisfied.

This program will *require that you add certain nutrient supplements to your diet, in the right amounts, at the proper times, and under the appropriate conditions.* We will explain those considerations in detail so that you will not have to guess what to do. These supplements will alter your metabolism to help you achieve your goals far more easily than you ever imagined.

This program will not *tell you that you must remove favorite foods from your diet or that you must ever go hungry. You love ice cream? Enjoy! Enjoy!*

This program will not *require time-consuming exercise. Our exercise program is* optional *and requires only* 5 minutes *of exercise per day, plus certain nutrient supplements, to improve your figure and build your muscles with better results than an hour or more of jogging per day.*

This program is multiphasic. Excess weight is rarely due to "a lack of willpower." It is a problem that involves many different biochemical reactions in your body and brain. A problem with multiple causes requires multiple solutions. We have selected seventeen of the most effective techniques from our seven years of study in the field, and will describe how they work, and precisely how you can use them together in an integrated, personalized program, designed around your own personal problems, goals, and life-style. There are many millions of possible programs using some combination of these seventeen techniques, so your chosen program may be unique, and will certainly be a far closer fit to your personal needs and desires than a conventional everyone-does-the-same-thing diet.

This program is suitable both for losing fat and for helping you maintain your new leaner figure afterward. Even if you were willing to lose that excess fat with a conventional program of severe caloric restriction plus lengthy hard exercise (Bray, 1983), you wouldn't want to live that way for the remainder of your life. That is why nearly all dieters lose weight and then put it right back on. (Bray, 1970; Rosenblatt, 1982; Wooley, 1984) This program offers a far more palatable way to lose fat, and the continued use of some of our seventeen techniques in your program will help you stay slim without the continual unrealistic lifelong deprivation and hunger required by conventional diet programs.

Our program requires little or no change of life-style! The word "diet" is derived from the Greek word *diaita,* which means "manner of living." Most diets are a way of life, and it is never your desired way. Diets require major changes both in what you eat and in other aspects of your life-style. How often can a businessperson obtain a real Pritikin-type meal at a business luncheon in a typical restaurant? How often does the dieter's family have to pay part of the cost for the dieter by having to change their diet, too, to avoid cooking different meals for different family members?

Our program requires little or no caloric restriction! This is not *another diet book.* The word "diet" is defined in the dictionary as "restriction." For most people, caloric restriction by food deprivation means looking forward to a life of gnawing hunger, boredom, eating food that you hate, passing over food that you love, constantly thinking about food, fatigue, irritability, and just plain feeling lousy.

One way that our program attacks excess body fat is caloric reduction *by appetite* modification. You will use nutrient supplements to alter your metabolism to reduce your appetite, to make you feel full and satisfied on fewer calories, and to actually biochemically change your food preferences from relatively fattening carbohydrates to protein. Appetite modification (instead of restriction) means no gnawing hunger, almost no no-nos, eating what you want, and eating added metabolism-modifying nutrient supplements, instead of depriving yourself of your favorite foods.

Our program requires little or no exercise! This is not another exercise book. Exercise is optional but very desirable for improved cardiovascular health, for better athletic ability, and for building muscles. We offer different techniques to suit different goals.

We have variations of our program for:

Fat loss with no exercise.

And for:

Fat loss combined with muscle growth requiring only five minutes of exercise per day.

This latter variation also provides rapid cardiovascular conditioning. Using nutrient supplements to change your muscle and fat metabolism, five minutes of peak output exercise per day can probably do more to improve your figure and build your muscles than an hour or more of jogging. This very rapid progress encourages continued exercise, unlike the usual hard work (instead of hard thinking), which may require months before you can see any results.

This is a do-it-yourself biomedical fat loss handbook. Diet book authors generally expect you to take what they say on faith. You have no way of knowing whether their statements are correct or utter nonsense unless you are a scientist or health professional who is personally familiar with the relevant research. If the authors have not surveyed the scientific research literature, why should you think that they know what they are talking about? There is a great deal of bad advice in popular diet books. (Fisher, 1985; Itallie, 1978) Even if they have studied the literature, if they do not cite research references, how do you know if what they write is correct? *Do not buy health books unless they have a bibliography of scientific references.*

We do not ask anyone to simply believe *what we have to say.* Throughout this book, we have included hundreds of references to the published scientific work of hundreds of scientists so that you can check our facts, and so that you can find out more about any scientific experiment or subject that interests you. As you read, you will see references reported like "(Bray, 1970)." If you want to find that scientific paper or book, turn to Appendix 3, "Further Sources of Information," go to the section on the chapter that you are reading, and you will find Dr. Bray's paper referenced in a list alphabetized by author. In this case, the reference is: "Bray, 'The Myth of Diet in the Management of Obesity,' *Am. J. Clin. Nutr.* 23(9):1141–1148 (1970)." This means that Dr. Bray's paper was in a scientific journal called the *American Journal of Clinical Nutrition,* volume 23, issue number 9, pages 1141 to 1148, in 1970.

If there is more than one author, only the senior one is given in the citation in parentheses in the text unless there is more than one paper by that author in a particular year. All the authors are given in Appendix 3, however. Appendix 3 also tells you where you can find a library that will have these papers. The librarian at any biomedical library will know the standard scientific journal name abbreviations.

We have sometimes put citations in the bibliography that are not keyed to specific statements in the text; these are generally reviews and background information.

Most people will probably never want to look at any of these scientific references, but it is reassuring to know that they are there, and that this book is based on the work of hundreds of scientists and physicians. They, rather than we, deserve credit for most of the research that we report in *The Life Extension Weight Loss Program*. For those scientists and clinicians whose continuing research will go beyond what we report here, we hope that our bibliography may direct you to some new and interesting knowledge and help you in your exploration of how life works.

2

Why Nature Makes You Fat

When you are having difficulty losing weight, does it sometimes seem that nature is conspiring against you? Does it seem that there is some terrible secret power lurking within you, making you fat? Well, it is not just your imagination. Nature does tend to make many people fat, especially after their teens. It was originally for your own good. *Body fat is nature's life insurance, Ice Age style. Most people have a genetically programmed tendency to increase fat stores as they get older.* After the teens or early twenties, it's fat hips for most women and a roll of fat around the waist for most men. This is a survival trait left over from the Ice Age.

Back in the bad old days when our species evolved, we had not yet invented mechanized agriculture and the supermarket. Body fat was food storage for famines, and famine was a major cause of death, whether or not your ancestors came from Ice Age Europe. You either lived off your fat stores or you died.

Fat stores three times as much energy per pound as muscle, and you can burn it more easily, so it is a much better energy storage medium. In Ice Age hunting and gathering tribes, young adult hunters were generally the first to get the food. Since Ice Age Europe had a growing season of about forty days, meat was the major food source most of the year. If you hunt mammoths with a pointed stick you had better be fast or you won't survive to pass on your genes, which means that you had better have lots of muscle and relatively little dead weight fat. If you were over twenty-five or so, you were old and run down by Ice Age standards and would not have food priority in times of famine, so old folks over about twenty-five had to store lots of food as body fat. (Beller, 1977)

In addition to its being the best form of energy storage, fat was excellent insulation against the Ice Age cold. Just ask a whale, seal, or polar bear about the merits of a thick layer of blubber in an arctic climate. Back in the bad old days, cold was a major cause of death. Cold greatly increases caloric requirements, and muscles are very poor insulation as well as a poor means of storing energy.

Note that many people whose ancestors came from relatively cold climates have their fat layer spread over most of their body. They needed a layer of blubber as insulation against the pervasive cold. On the other hand, people whose ancestors came from warmer climates usually have their fat arranged quite differently. They didn't need too much insulation because overheating during heavy labor could be a problem, and fat storage around the hips and stomach doesn't impair athletic agility as much as fat that is farther away from one's center of gravity. Nevertheless, as they grew older, they still needed to store plenty of fat as insurance against famines, particularly if the area was semiarid with a rainfall that varied greatly from year to year.

Of course, there is a health cost to being fat. Excess fat increases your chances of cardiovascular disease and cancer. Ice Age humans simply didn't live long enough for cardiovascular disease or cancer to kill enough of them to provide an evolutionary selection process to mitigate the problem.

There is some controversy, however, over the question of exactly how much being moderately overweight increases health risks. A number of studies seem to suggest that risk of early death is increased only for those at the extremes of under- or overweight. (Wooley, 1984) Overweight seems particularly to be less risky for women, where there is no relationship between fatness and mortality for those women who are so heavy for their height that only 10 to 20 percent of all American women are fatter.

Genetic factors also play a major role in determining the risk of excess fat. The Pima Indians of Arizona have particularly high rates of both obesity and diabetes. Yet their lowest mortality rate is for those whose fatness we would normally consider very obese. The least risky weight range for the Pimas was equivalent to 167 to 190 percent of the normally desirable weight for women and 145 to 176 percent of the normally desirable weight for men, based on the Society of Actuaries standards. (Wooley, 1984)

Dr. Reubin Andres, clinical director of the Gerontology Research Center of the National Institute on Aging in Baltimore, Maryland, reexamined data from a number of obesity studies and concluded that there was no excess mortality up to 30 percent overweight. (Rosenblatt, 1982; Andres, 1980)

The concept of personal beauty, particularly for women, has changed significantly in the past few hundred years as food supplies have become very reliable in the industrialized world. From the days of the wall-painting cavemen to relatively recently, the best-looking and most desirable women were fat by modern standards. Look at the women painted by Rubens; they were probably thought to be some of the most beautiful women in the world at that time. Back then, the fat stores of a well-padded wife could easily make the difference between her infant's starving or surviving on mother's milk during bad times. Today a woman could be as lean as a *Vogue* model and her infant wouldn't starve. (She might not be able to become pregnant, however; menstruation becomes irregular or ceases at about 17 percent body fat.) Today one of Rubens's models would probably rush out to buy a copy of this book as an essential career tool.

In our personal opinion, if you are in good health and have a reasonably normal genetic background, you probably do not need to lose fat for pressing medical reasons unless your body fat percentage is over about 25 percent for a man and over about 30 percent for a woman. Most people who want to lose fat do so for nonmedical reasons. Our *Life Extension Weight Loss Program* can help members of both groups.

Why don't diets work? The problem is usually genetic survival progamming to make you fat. The tendency to become fat, even in experimental rats, is made much worse by cafeteria feeding. Cafeteria feeding means having a large variety of delicious foods available in unlimited quantities. That is just the way things are in all the developed countries today. Nowadays we have a cornucopia of twenty thousand food products at the local supermarket, and the fat that once could have saved your life during famine is more likely to kill you with a heart attack, stroke, or cancer. Nature has provided you with survival instincts: eat it while you can, and eat some of everything while you are at it to make sure that you aren't deficient in some essential nutrient that is found in some foods but not others.

Nature's genetic survival programming has another lifesaver for the famine victim and another dirty trick for the well-fed modern overweight person. Nature has provided us with "thrifty genes" that can greatly increase our metabolic efficiency, making it possible to survive on a very small number of calories per day. (Coleman, 1979) These thrifty genes, which intimately involve insulin, are responsible for some people being unable to lose weight on 750 calories per day. That's great during a famine, but it can kill you, or at least make you fat, when there are restaurants and supermarkets wherever you look.

Beware of creating a pseudo-famine. Do not try to lose weight too fast! Not only does excessively fast weight loss subject you to unnecessary physiological stress, it is usually self-defeating. Rapid weight loss can switch on your thrifty genes, causing a weight plateau that even a dangerous starvation diet may not overcome. If your haste to lose weight has persuaded your body fat storage control system that there is a famine, you may actually have to eat more food, and put back on 5 or even 10 pounds before you switch back to your normal, less fat-conserving nonfamine metabolism.

How fast is too fast? We have found that almost anyone can lose 1 to 2 pounds per week without pseudo-famine problems. This is 50 to 100 pounds per year. Why make things more difficult for yourself?

When you eat a meal, insulin is released. Insulin is a natural and essential hormone in carbohydrate and fat metabolism. Insulin regulates how much blood sugar enters your cells, and thereby helps regulate how much you burn. *Insulin also helps to convert carbohydrates to stored fat and prevents you from mobilizing and burning your fat.* Your body can store very little carbohydrate, so excess carbohydrates that are not burned immediately are converted to body fat with the help of insulin. Even extra protein can be converted to sugar in your liver and then stored as more body fat with the help of your insulin. (Cahill, Jr., 1979; Larner, 1980)

Growth hormone is another natural and essential hormone. In many respects it is the functional opposite of insulin. High levels of insulin can block the effects of growth hormone, and high levels of growth hormone can block the effects of insulin. *Growth hormone promotes the conversion of dietary protein into muscle instead of body fat, promotes the mobilization and burning of body fat, and blocks the insulin-induced conversion of dietary carbohydrates to body fat.* (Christy, 1979; Murad, 1980)

You will be hearing a lot more about growth hormone and insulin in the chapters ahead. It is a respectable medical hypothesis among scientists specializing in obesity that *the ratio of growth hormone to insulin in your body has a great deal to do with your ratio of muscle to body fat.* (Bray, 1983; Ratzmann, 1978; Assimacopoulos-Jeannet, 1976) *You will learn how you can use nutrient supplements to manipulate this ratio to favor a new, naturally leaner you.*

Do not feel disgusted if you have put on excess fat since your teens, even if this occurred as early as your twenties. It's natural for most people. We know rock stars in their twenties who have had to fight a constant battle against ugly career-destroying flab, even though they are physically active and not big eaters. Since going on our fat loss program, all of our rock star experimental subjects have had to have their skintight clothes altered or new clothes made with a smaller waist and bigger chest. None of them counts calories anymore, either!

This postteen onset of enhanced fat accumulation is caused by the postteen drop in the levels of growth hormone, an important natural hormone from your brain. (Growth hormone decline with age: Bazzarre, 1975; "Muscle," 1980; Zadik, 1985)

Chapter 5 tells how to turn back your brain's fat accumulation clock to that golden teenage period when most people can stuff themselves with hamburgers and shakes, sit on their tails, and still be slim.

Our approach is not a conventional diet that fights an endless battle against your fat-promoting genes, nature's life insurance of days gone by. Instead of a diet, we teach you to take command of your natural body fat and muscle control systems! You will work with nature, not against it.

3

Fat Loss Versus Weight Loss: The Vital Difference, or How a Ubiquitous Fallacy Makes Most Diet Books Useless or Even Dangerous

No matter how much you weigh, you should not be on a weight loss program! If you are fat, you should be on a fat loss program. There is a vital difference.

A body builder like Arnold Schwarzenegger may be 50 pounds overweight according to the "ideal" height-versus-weight tables. But is it really reasonable to say that he is overweight? Of course not. It is excess fat, not muscle, that looks ugly. It is excess fat, not muscle, that increases your risk of cardiovascular disease and cancer. You want to lose fat, not something else. Unfortunately, most diets cause *weight* loss rather than just the desired *fat* loss.

What, other than fat, do most diets make you lose? Why should you care?

Many diets cause a very impressive and rapid initial loss of weight, yet there is relatively little fat loss compared to the electrolyte loss. *You want to lose fat, not vital mineral salts and water, which are called electrolytes. This weight loss is fast but very temporary.* As soon as you go back to drinking normal amounts of fluids and getting normal amounts of the essential mineral salts and calories, most of the lost weight is regained. You can lose five pounds in a day this way, but it is almost entirely five pounds of electrolytes, not five pounds of fat. (Bray, 1983)

Diets that cause rapid weight loss by causing loss of electrolytes are worse than just temporary; they can kill you. They can cause serious cardiac and kidney hazards, and even sudden death by heart failure in otherwise healthy young adults. The liquid protein diet fad killed scores of dieters!

Several years ago one of Durk's co-workers, an aerospace engineer, had a close call with one of these diets. Fortunately for him, he asked Durk what he thought of the latest diet fad, the liquid protein diet.

Durk said, "Let's see the formula," and the engineer passed him the bottle. Durk looked at it for a moment and said, "Are you really following these instructions? Is this all that you are eating?"

The answer came back, "Yes."

Durk said, "For how long?"

His friend answered, "Five days now, and I've already lost a lot of weight. It's the best diet I've ever been on."

Durk replied, "If you continue to follow those instructions, you are likely to die of heart failure in about two more weeks. This is a lethally bad formulation. It has many defects, but the one that will kill you first is the potassium. There isn't any potassium at all! You will continue to lose some potassium every day in your urine. When your tissue potassium gets too low, your heart will fibrillate, that is, stop beating regularly and just sort of vibrate without pumping blood. Fibrillation is usually how electrocution kills. It is how many sudden heart failures kill. I would prefer that you discontinue this diet, but if you must persist, be sure to either take a 100 percent RDA [Food and Drug Administration's U.S. Recommended Daily Allowance] potassium supplement or drink at least two quarts of tomato or fruit juice per day. These juices are rich in potassium."

Durk's friend followed his advice by adding potassium to his diet. It is a good thing that he did. This particular formula killed scores of dieters by sudden death from cardiac dysrhythmias.

Diets that are low in both calories and carbohydrates, such as the one used by Durk's engineer friend, cause a condition known as ketosis. This helps reduce appetite and causes an especially rapid early weight loss. This rapid early loss is only a little fat; it is mostly electrolyte loss due to less water being bound with your glycogen (your body's principal carbohydrate energy store), and to a ketosis-induced increase in urination. Moreover, animal experiments have shown that prolonged consumption of low-carbohydrate diets can lead to a rebound effect; after dieting, carbohydrate craving and consumption are increased beyond their prediet level. (Wurtman, 1983)

Do not make the mistake of thinking that potassium loss is the only cause of sudden death on extreme caloric restriction diets. Diets that contain only 300 to 400 calories per day, mostly or entirely protein, do cause the expected rapid initial weight loss comprised primarily of electrolytes. After a few months, they can also cause death by heart failure, even if the dieter is taking potassium supplements, and even if the dieter is under continuous medical supervision. (Sours, 1981)

Hair loss was frequently reported before death, so we suspect that the diet may have caused serious deficiencies of essential antioxidant nutrients such as selenium. These dieters were taking a multivitamin supplement, but the stress of this extreme diet could plausibly increase their body's antioxidant demand above the meager supply in a typical multivitamin.

Moreover, the popular multivitamins at that time did not contain selenium. Selenium is essential for cardiac health, and selenium deficiency leads to heart muscle atrophy and damage, which was also found in autopsies of the diet victims. In fact, selenium deficiency was a major cause of death in children (heart failure) in a selenium-deficient area of China. The problem has been completely abolished by selenium supplements. It is interesting to note that Americans get most of their dietary selenium from grains, and that this lethal diet did not contain either grain products or a selenium supplement. (See our *Life Extension: A Practical Scientific Approach* [Warner Books, 1982] and our *The Life Extension Companion* [Warner Books, 1984] for more information on the connection between lack of antioxidant nutrients and cardiovascular disease.)

Avoid this extremely restrictive under-700-calorie-per-day type of diet like the plague or you will lose more than fat, possibly with deadly results.

Most diets cause a serious loss of several essential nutrients, unless the dieter is taking a properly formulated nutritional supplement. Indeed, according to the U.S. Department of Agriculture, 60 percent of Americans are deficient in one or more essential nutrients, even by the standards of the FDA Recommended Daily Allowances. If you eat a lot less, you are apt to get a lot less of the essential vitamins and minerals, too. This problem is particularly severe with popular fad diets. (Fisher, 1985; Itallie, 1978) Medically supervised weight reduction clinics provide their clients with nutritional supplements to correct for this problem, but many diet book authors simply ignore it. The results of these diet-induced deficiencies do not have to be as dramatic as a heart failure; you may merely become less resistant to disease and become ill more frequently. (Phillips, 1981)

Most diets cause muscle loss as well as fat loss. You want to lose fat, not precious muscle. Twenty-five percent of conventional diet weight loss without heavy exercise is muscle. Only 5 percent of conventional diet weight loss with heavy exercise is muscle. (Brownell, 1983)

According to studies by the National Institute on Aging, people usually have considerable difficulty gaining or regaining muscle if they are over thirty years old, even with heavy exercise. This is because GH (growth hormone, a natural hormone released by the pituitary gland in your brain) is needed to build muscle, and as people age, their GH release drops considerably, and their exercise-induced GH pulses become much smaller or disappear entirely. (Bazzarre, 1975; "Muscle," 1980; Zadik, 1985) We have a nutritional supplement solution to this problem, which you will read about in Chapter 5, "Growth Hormone Releasers and Your Muscle-to-Fat Ratio."

Nearly all diets do cause some fat loss. Fat is *all* that you should lose, but only 75 percent of conventional diet weight loss without heavy exercise is fat, and 95 percent of conventional diet weight loss with heavy exercise is fat. At first glance, things look pretty good if you are willing to do *regular heavy exercise.* Jogging is *not* heavy exercise. If you do not engage in heavy exercise, you will definitely have a serious cumulative muscle loss problem.

Almost all dieters undergo repeated diet-induced weight loss/ weight regain cycles. The nonelectrolyte portion of the regained weight is usually 100 percent fat. Each time you diet, you lose some muscle. Heavy exercise slows the muscle loss by a factor of 5, but muscle loss still occurs with conventional diets, and very high-protein diets do not help. So each time you diet you lose some muscle, and each time you regain weight, you regain fat instead of muscle. If a man loses 20 pounds on a diet that does not involve lots of vigorous exercise, he will lose about 5 pounds of muscle. Without GH releasers, he will have to spend about one year doing daily heavy exercise to regain that lost 5 pounds of muscle. This is why regular sustained heavy exercise is essential in conventional diet weight loss programs.

The result of conventional weight loss/weight regain diet cycles is inevitable; the more often you diet, the higher your body fat percentage can become! With great discomfort, you may weigh the same as you did ten years ago, but that same weight may be comprised of a lot more fat and a lot less muscle. You can even lose weight while gaining fat! Our GH-releaser *fat* loss technique solves this problem. Using GH-releasing nutrients, you can actually *gain* muscle while *losing* fat!

Fat loss is the only desirable form of weight loss. This book is not really a weight *loss book. This book is a* fat *loss book.* (Our publisher wanted to call it a weight loss book or a diet book so that bookstore buyers wouldn't miss it. We couldn't honestly call it a diet book since caloric restriction is usually unnecessary with our program.)

Our program causes people to lose body fat, not necessarily body weight. Some people on the program even put on some weight, but it is muscle, *not* fat.

How can you be certain that you are losing fat rather than muscle, or that you are losing fat if your weight is unchanged or even increasing? We will tell you how to do that in Chapter 16, "Measuring Your Own Progress."

Now that you understand the vital difference between fat loss and weight loss, it is time for you to learn how you can use our program.

4

How You Can Use Our Program

Before you begin your own fat loss program, you should determine your own goals. There are many valid reasons for going on a fat loss program, including improving and maintaining your figure, improving your health and fitness, increasing your muscle size and definition, and eliminating excess fat. Your health can be improved by discarding excess fat because too much fat is associated with an increased cardiovascular risk, increased cancer risk, and a depressed immune system (the system that protects you against cancer and infectious diseases).

How much fat do you want to lose? Do you really want to be as lean as an Olympic athlete or a high fashion model? These extremes are hardly necessary for good health and good looks. You will have to decide what you want to do with your body.

Olympic athletes have body fat percentages of about 7 percent to about 27 percent for females and about 5 percent to about 15 percent for males, depending on the sport involved. (Fleck, 1981) Male bodybuilders may have body fat percentages as low as 3 or 4 percent.

There are disadvantages to having very low body fat percentages. If a woman's body fat percentage drops below about 17 percent, menstruation may become irregular or entirely cease. Very lean people have little insulation from the cold. They may respond differently to some prescription drugs that are especially soluble in fatty portions of the body. A very lean person may be overdosed by a fat-soluble drug in quantities that would be appropriate for someone of the same weight with a normal body fat percentage. Since the very lean have small fat stores, their liver is less willing to release its stored carbohydrate, glycogen, when their blood sugar drops, so they will have to be more careful to eat regularly.

On the other hand, if you are a competitive athlete or bodybuilder, the techniques that we describe in this book will blow away your competition—unless they have been using this book, too. You can build muscles faster than you have ever dreamed possible while simultaneously burning off all but a few percentage points' worth of body fat. You will no longer have to sacrifice some of your muscle mass to lose subcutaneous fat for superb muscular definition. How do we know? Some of our earliest experimental subjects were bodybuilders. One won a national championship with only two years of part-time workouts, and credits our techniques for the win.

In our personal opinion, a reasonable body fat percentage for a healthy nonathlete without serious genetic obesity is 20 to 25 percent for a female and 15 to 18 percent for a male. These percentages are significantly less than average, so you will look noticeably fitter than average, yet they are high enough so that most people should have no problems due to extreme leanness.

See Chapter 15, "Designing Your Own Personal Program," for more information to help you decide your fat loss target. This chapter includes quantitative data on average height and weight relations, and on the relation of excess weight to increased risk of death.

Scientific studies show that most dieters go from one diet to another, and that in the long run they are rarely satisfied with their results. About 95 percent of those who lose weight on a diet quickly regain it. As Dr. Klatz said in his foreword, your chances of beating cancer are better than your chances of successfully controlling your weight by dieting! Don't try to fight the genes that evolved to protect you from starvation by starving yourself. It won't work unless you want to make starvation a way of life, and even then it still may not work.

Losing fat very rapidly is not the best way to get rid of body fat! Most people who lose fat rapidly run into an intractable weight plateau problem. No matter how little they eat, they can't lose any more fat. The hypothalamus gland in the brain, which ultimately controls eating behavior and fat storage, detects a low-calorie diet and subsequent rapid fat loss. It then activates metabolic pathways that tend to conserve body energy stores, especially fat. You may stop losing fat (but might continue to lose muscle) even if you're on a 750-calorie-per-day semistarvation diet. This is a survival mechanism that allows one's body to conserve energy during times of famine.

To avoid triggering this biochemical fat conservation mechanism, you must not lose fat too fast. *We usually recommend losses of no more than 1 or 2 pounds of fat per week.* If you are planning to lose less than 5 percent of your body weight, most people can do it more rapidly. But remember, even at the rate of 1 or 2 pounds a week, that is 50 to 100 pounds of fat lost per year.

If, against our advice, you insist on losing fat rapidly, you must recognize that you are putting a severe physiological stress on your body. It is especially important that you do not attempt to lose fat rapidly if you are also under a lot of stress from other sources, such as an illness or depression. *NEVER attempt to lose more than 5 percent of your weight rapidly without a doctor's supervision.*

Monitor your progress with a tape measure and, optionally, with a skin-fold caliper, as well as with a good scale. Remember that this is a fat loss program, not a weight loss program. You want to know your total body weight. You also need to know how much of that weight is fat. It is the fat that you want to lose. You can't know how much fat you have with just a scale. A tape measure will monitor your fat far better than a scale alone. Use your tape to measure your fat-prone areas daily. Remember that part of the day-to-day variation will be due to changes in your water content; this effect will be especially prominent around a woman's menstrual period. The optional use of a skin-fold caliper will tell you your actual body fat percentage. It is good practice to record the tape measurements, weight, and skin-fold measurements that you take. Tape-measure and weigh yourself at the same time each day and optionally take a skin-fold measurement at least once a week. You learn how to perform these measurements in Chapter 16, "Measuring Your Own Progress," and how to keep and use this data in Appendix 1, "Your Own Case History."

Men using growth hormone releasers may not lose weight even though they do lose body fat. This has happened fairly frequently. Men have considerable amounts of testosterone, the male sex hormone, circulating in their bloodstream. Testosterone is a natural anabolic steroid that works synergistically with growth hormone to increase muscle mass, and it can also enhance the amount of GH released. (Drop, 1982; Illig, 1970; Job, 1983; Kaplan, 1972; Zachmann, 1970) This muscle mass increase will generally be very large and very rapid if peak output exercise is used. (See Chapter 14, "Peak Output Exercise: The Astronauts' Fast Exercise Method.") Males who have increased their growth hormone may gain as much, or even more, muscle and lean body mass as they lose in body fat, so body weight may stay the same or even increase. (Tanner, 1971; Tanner, 1972; Tanner, Whitehouse, 1972; Prader, 1972) That is why it is so important to measure your body fat with a skin-fold caliper or a tape measure.

Avoid repeated weight loss/weight regain cycles. With most diets, the weight you lose is about 25 percent lean body mass, while the weight you gain back is nearly all fat. If you repeatedly cycle from one diet to another, you can actually end up with more body fat at the same overall body weight than when you started! But by using growth hormone releasers, you can eliminate this loss of lean body mass, even if you don't exercise at all. Lengthy heavy exercise without GH releasers limits this loss to about 5 percent. An effective way to avoid weight cycling is to continue to incorporate some of our techniques into your normal nutritional practices once you have used our full program to achieve your body fat percentage goal.

Most low-calorie diets induce vitamin and mineral deficiencies. (Fisher and Lachance, 1985) When you eat less, you are apt to eat fewer vitamins and minerals, too, unless you are wise enough to take a properly formulated nutrient supplement. The U.S. Department of Agriculture has said that 60 percent of Americans are deficient in one or more essential vitamins or minerals, even by the minimal U.S. Food and Drug Administration RDA (Recommended Daily Allowance) standards.

These deficiencies can lead to reduced resistance to disease (Phillips, 1981), increased susceptibility to cancer and cardiovascular disease, and more damage from sunlight, tobacco, and alcohol (the three biggest causes of human cancer). These diet-induced nutrient deficiencies can also cause lack of energy, feeling the blahs, and irritability. Many diets do more harm to your health than good.

Diet books usually recommend that you just take a simple RDA multivitamin once a day, in the unlikely event that they suggest anything at all. In our opinion this is inadequate because of the increased free radical stress of losing a lot of fat. (Free radicals are highly reactive chemical entities created during normal metabolism and during the oxidation [burning] of fats. Free radical processes have been implicated in the causation of cancer, heart attacks, strokes, and even aging itself.) See the Safety Appendix for our suggested vitamin and mineral supplement. (For more on free radical pathology and the effects of vitamins and minerals and their deficiencies, see our *Life Extension: A Practical Scientific Approach* and *The Life Extension Companion.*)

We strongly suggest that you see your doctor for a physical exam every year. If you haven't had one in a year, be sure to get one before starting our fat loss program!

This examination should include blood pressure, a comprehensive serum lipid panel (HDL, LDL, and VLDL cholesterol and triglyceride measurements), a complete differential blood count, a comprehensive liver function panel, a test for traces of blood in the feces, a urine analysis panel, a test for possible hypothyroidism, and a glucose tolerance test to detect possible borderline adult-onset diabetes. If any of your relatives have had cardiovascular disease, an electrocardiogram is good insurance; every day, lots of people in their thirties or even twenties die of heart failure. It is not safe to assume that your excess fat is merely due to overeating; you might have a medical problem. Excess weight can be caused by a number of serious diseases, such as hypothyroidism (which is usually easily corrected) and diabetes. You should be checked for these before beginning your fat loss program. Unfortunately, you could be seriously ill and still feel good, so play it safe.

If you have had a large sudden weight gain, particularly if your weight has been stable in the past, see your physician at once. You may have a medical problem.

For safety's sake, you should have medical supervision if you plan to lose more than 10 percent of your body weight. If you can afford it, continuing medical supervision after your comprehensive initial physical exam is prudent and desirable for 5 to 10 percent weight loss objective programs. Losing large amounts of fat is quite stressful even at a moderate loss rate. *Never* attempt to lose more than 10 percent of your body weight without a thorough physical exam and medical supervision.

NEVER attempt to lose more than 15 percent of your body weight without a doctor's CONTINUING AND REGULAR supervision. Our techniques have helped people lose as much as 35 or 40 percent of their weight, but these extremely large losses *must* be done under close professional supervision!

Regular medical monitoring and supervision is always necessary if you are diabetic or hyperobese, or if you have cardiovascular, kidney, liver, or blood disease, cancer, a psychosis, or other serious medical problem.

Our program is definitely NOT for pregnant women, children, adolescents, or those with psychiatric eating disorders.

This is an experimental program. Although the nutrients we use in this program are recognized by the Food and Drug Administration as foods, they are NOT approved as fat loss aids.

In evaluating diets for your own personal use, be very careful not to confuse cause and effect. For example, one very well-known diet formula tells people to eat the special formula in place of two meals a day. Then when people lose weight, the product's manufacturer proclaims that it is the special secret herbal formula that is responsible. But if you look at the total calories that are supposed to be consumed by persons using the formula you will see that this is a semistarvation diet. The formula involves no miracle fat loss mechanisms. Going on a one-small-meal-a-day diet is what is causing weight loss. Rather than buy an expensive formula, these people would have been better off just going on the low-calorie diet using calorie-controlled microwave convenience meals purchased at their local supermarket and taking a good high-potency vitamin and mineral supplement.

Although we refer frequently to anecdotes about our personal experiences and those of our experimental subjects, such case history material never proves anything by itself! We use these concrete examples to illustrate the results to be expected from applying certain principles. It is best to use diets or fat loss metabolic modifications where the principles have been tested scientifically at least in animals, and preferably in people.

Whenever a new diet book comes out, there are soon eager followers (no matter how ridiculous the program is) who swear that it is the greatest thing ever invented. Then why are they out buying another diet book the next spring? They are not mentally retarded. They have been tricked by the placebo effect.

The placebo effect may make any diet seem to work for a little while. If you think that an inactive substance, the placebo, is really an active drug, your mind may make that placebo seem to work like an active drug . . . at least temporarily. This is true for programs as well as for drugs. It is your expectations that cause the response, not the inert substance or the ineffective program. About 40 percent of the population will respond to an inert placebo as if it had the pain-killing effects of morphine, but only if they believe that they received morphine. The placebo effect wears off rapidly, however. After a week's use, only about 10 to 20 percent respond to the inert placebo that is labeled morphine with effective pain relief. After a year of regular use, less than 1 percent still respond positively. Just because someone loses weight on a diet doesn't mean that the diet is really effective in the long run. It may just be the temporary placebo effect.

Animal experiments and the double-blind placebo-controlled study technique are used by scientists to be sure that what they have found is not just another placebo effect. Laboratory animals do not expect a candidate diet pill to make them lose weight, hence their weight loss is due to the drug, not the placebo effect. This is one reason why we have referenced so many animal studies in the bibliography in Appendix 3.

In the human subject double-blind placebo-controlled study, neither the doctors nor the patients know which colored pill is the real drug and which is the placebo until after the study is over. It is called double-blind because neither the doctors nor the subjects know which pill is which during the experiment. That way, no one's expectations can affect the experiment's outcome. The random positive results that occur by chance with the placebo are subtracted from the results obtained by the test drug; this is called placebo-controlled. If the real drug works at all, it should show better results than the placebo.

We have one substantial advantage over most of our scientific colleagues: we fund our own research. This means that we do not have to depend on a federal government committee to pay for our work, nor do we have to obtain federal permission to experiment on consenting informed adult human subjects. This also means that most of our after-tax income from this book will go into further biomedical research. Thank you for your support!

We also have some substantial disadvantages, too. One obvious one is that we cannot afford a megabuck laboratory, especially after donating about half of our earnings to nonprofit biomedical research foundations and paying out about half of what was left in taxes and associated accounting and tax lawyer fees.

More frustrating, however, is the difficulty that we have in performing double-blind placebo-controlled studies. Our academic and government laboratory colleagues have access to a population of rigidly controlled hospitalized patients. If a patient wants to try a new drug, he or she has to try it under conditions defined by the experimenter. If the experimenter says that the patient will be randomly given either the new drug or an inactive placebo, the patient has to accept the chance of getting the worthless placebo if he wants a chance to try the new drug.

Our subjects are free agents; they are not hospitalized, and we have no real control over their behavior. When we suggest a double-blind test of a nutrient versus a placebo to a subject, we ethically must inform the subject about that nutrient. The subject then typically just goes to a health food store and buys the nutrient for himself, eliminating the chance that he will receive an inactive placebo, and also eliminating our chance to do a double-blind placebo-controlled experiment. We consider ourselves fortunate when we can persuade our subjects to take clinical laboratory tests (administered by a physician and processed at a commercial clinical testing laboratory) and give us copies of the results. We have been able to accumulate a substantial amount of lab test data in this way, a considerable amount of it on famous TV, movie, and rock stars, race car drivers, and athletes. One real advantage of working with these persons is that they can readily afford to pay for their own lab tests!

Remember the placebo effect. Almost any diet can work for a while in about half of those who try it if they believe that it will. An animal does not have these expectations, and a double-blind test procedure with people will prevent human expectations from influencing the result of the experiment. The double-blind test procedure is easy to use when evaluating the effects of drugs on human eating behavior because the identity of the pills can be easily disguised. However, it is much more difficult to do a double-blind study of humans eating a low-calorie diet or certain types of foods because the people will know what they are eating.

Please note that there has been no double-blind placebo-controlled test of the particular combination *of the up to seventeen methods that you will eventually select for your personal fat loss and control program because there are millions of different combinations possible.* The principles on which these seventeen methods are founded have been the subject of scientific study on an individual basis, however. These animal experiments and the double-blind placebo-controlled human experiments that we reference are your assurance that this book is not just another big expensive placebo that will leave you looking for another diet book every year. Just think of all the time and money that you will save.

ORGANIZATION OF THIS BOOK AND HOW TO USE IT

This book includes a foreword by a physician, sixteen short chapters, and six appendixes. You will find them easier to understand if you read the book from the start. However, if a particular subject is of special interest to you, feel free to go directly to that chapter. You may then wish to read some of the earlier material, which will explain what you might not have entirely understood.

Diet books and their ill-designed programs have killed a shocking number of their users. Few diet books ever warn you of the risks of their techniques. Unlike our book, they do not contain a Safety Appendix. This may seem to make them appear simple and safe, but in matters of safety, ignorance is not bliss.

This book is a practical how-to-do-it-to-yourself biomedical fat loss handbook. It gives you many methods by which you can actually modify your metabolism. For that reason, you must read the Safety Appendix before you take any of the nutrients, food constituents, or drugs described. This appendix deals with substances that you might want to ingest; it does not have listings for everything mentioned in this book. To make sure that even our most reckless readers read this important information, we have put nearly all dosage information in this alphabetized appendix! Just because a substance is a natural nutrient does *not* mean that it cannot be dangerous under certain circumstances. *Nothing is perfectly safe. So read the Safety Appendix precautions and warnings before you take anything!*

The appendixes also contain a section on "Further Sources of Information" which describes data sources for both laypersons and scientists and physicians. We have provided scientific references so that you can check our information sources.

The lack of scientific literature citations in almost all diet books should be a real warning. First, if the authors haven't read any of the scientific literature, they do not have a very good chance of being right. And if they don't cite it, you cannot tell if they've read it. Second, even if the diet book authors are right, how can you check up on them? How will you ever know for sure? Most laypersons will not bother to look up the original scientific papers that we cite, but it is nice to know that those references are there, and health professionals will find them invaluable.

The "Your Own Case History" appendix contains convenient record forms for documenting your program's progress.

"How to Join Our Research Program" in the appendixes tells you how to do just that. We want to learn from your experiences! You can also reach us at the address therein to get certain supplementary information that was not available in time for the publication deadline of this book.

The "Suppliers' Appendix" tells you how you can locate competitively priced sources for all the nutrients and equipment we mention in the book. We have also included a convenient postcard printed on the endpaper of the book that you can cut out, fill in your name and address, and drop in the mail to receive catalogs from several different reputable competitive suppliers.

The "Supermarket Shopping Guide" appendix contains data charts that you can take with you to the supermarket to help guide your food purchases, especially with respect to the glycemic indexes (which you will soon read about) of various foods. It also contains some recipes for foods and snacks that aid fat loss.

Now it's time for you to go on to the next chapter and do some of that hard thinking that is going to save you so much hard work.

5

Growth Hormone Releasers and Your Muscle-to-Fat Ratio, or Sandy's Lucky Break: A Broken Foot Leads to a Breakthrough

In this chapter we will tell you how most overweight adults can take the first step to becoming as lean and muscular as most teenagers by reactivating some of the same natural biochemical mechanisms that most teenagers have.

Your brain's pituitary gland produces and releases an important natural nonsteroid hormone, *GH, or growth hormone.* Using natural nutrients that release growth hormone, it is possible to build GH levels back up to those found in healthy teenagers. This growth hormone will not make an adult grow taller, but under the proper conditions, it can dramatically promote fat loss and muscle growth.

We think that your growth hormone level and growth-hormone-to-insulin ratio are major factors in controlling your body's muscle-to-fat ratio. Although we arrived at this concept independently around 1980, we are not alone in this conclusion; it is a respectable hypothesis in baryology (the study of weight disorders), and the work of other scientists supports it. (Bray, 1983; Ratzmann, 1978) Low levels of GH and high levels of insulin are both associated with obesity, at least in nondiabetics. (Assimacopoulos-Jeannet, 1976; El-Khodary, 1972; Quabbe, 1971) For example, in one experiment the average

GH levels in normal humans were about 5 times higher than in the very obese (153 to 203 percent of "ideal" weight) subjects, and about 4 times higher in normals than in the obese (over 120 percent of "ideal" weight) in another study. (Irie, 1970; Ratzmann, 1978)

You naturally have high levels of growth hormone during childhood and adolescence. Most teenagers can eat amazing amounts of food, even junk food, without becoming fat. For most teens, this is true even if they don't exercise. For most older people, however, the same diet and same amount of exercise lead to a considerable fat buildup, usually starting sometime in the twenties. GH levels, particularly peak levels, drop as you get older, and the amount of GH released during sleep decreases as you age. The GH released by exercise becomes much less. The rate of decline is especially rapid during your twenties and thirties, a time when the accumulation of excess fat often becomes a problem. (Bazzarre, 1975; "Muscle," 1980; Prinz, 1976; Zadik, 1985)

If your GH remained at a relatively high late-teenage level, it would not cause you to continue to grow taller after puberty, but it would cause your body to devote food resources to building muscles, tendons, and other tissues, and it would reduce your ability to accumulate and store excess food as body fat insurance against a famine. You want enough growth hormone, but not too much. Too much growth hormone can cause too much blocking of needed insulin activity, as well as other problems that we will discuss in the Safety Appendix. *How much GH is enough, but not too much? We think that nature has provided a good guide; we are trying to emulate the growth hormone levels and pattern of GH release pulses found in healthy lean athletic humans in their late teens to early twenties.*

The successful use of growth hormone releasers requires a little more thinking than simply taking some nutrient supplements, however. There are factors that can interfere with GH releaser effects, such as eating many, but not all, types of sugars and starches at around the same time as you take your growth hormone releasers. For example, ice cream is OK at any time. Potatoes and carrots are a no-no—but they are no-nos only around the time that you take your GH releasers. *Since you take the GH releasers only at bedtime or ninety minutes before an optional five minutes of peak output exercise, this is not much of a restriction on eating.* There are plenty of sweet, tasty things that you can eat even around the time that you take GH releasers. You won't have to go hungry.

This is the most difficult and complex chapter in our book; you will not have to do nearly as much hard thinking to understand and use the other chapters. This chapter is complex both because the subject is unusually complex and because we have to document carefully what we say. Without this documentation and detailed exposition, health professionals would have no reason to investigate this remarkable new technique for controlling body-fat-to-muscle ratio.

You may want to take a quick look at the case histories and the short summary that we have written for this chapter. The summary is near the end of the chapter, just before a long optional technical note that will be of interest primarily to health professionals. Remember that case histories never prove anything; they are given to illustrate the application of these techniques and the results that can be obtained. The evidence is to be found in the referenced scientific papers.

You do not have to read this chapter to understand and use the sixteen other fat loss methods in our program, so if you wish, you can simply skip to Chapter 8, "Sweets: How to Have a Sweet Tooth Without Putting On Fat."

This chapter will be of special interest to those who wish to build their muscles with minimal amounts of exercise.

THE AMAZING CASE OF SANDY'S LUCKY BREAK

Sometimes a scientific quest takes you somewhere totally unexpected, as in the discovery of penicillin. Here is how we made the discovery that growth-hormone-releasing nutrients can be spectacularly useful in a properly designed program for losing fat and building muscle.

We have been studying aging mechanisms and methods for slowing or reversing them since 1968. (See our *Life Extension: A Practical Scientific Approach,* and our *Life Extension Companion.*) Slowed tissue damage repair and reduced immune system competence are two serious aging problems. It is known that growth hormone and agents that release growth hormone speed healing and stimulate the T-cell immune system, which protects one from infectious disease and cancer. (Barbul, 1977; Barbul, 1978; Beard, 1943; Catt, 1970; Larner, 1980; Levy, 1954; Milner, 1978; Milner, 1979; Prudden, 1958; Rettura, 1978; Rettura, 1981; Seifter, 1978; Sorkin, 1972; Takeda, 1975; Weisburger, 1969) It is also known that growth hormone release decreases very significantly with age. Compared to late-teenage levels, GH levels typically drop about 40 percent for the 20-to-30-year-old decade, and then drop about another 40 percent for the 30-to-40-year-old decade, with further drops with continued aging. (Bazzarre, 1975; "Muscle," 1980; Prinz, 1976; Zadik, 1985)

In 1976 Durk hypothesized that increasing the growth hormone output of an adult to that of a healthy teenager might partially reverse these aging problems. We submitted a small research grant proposal to a private biomedical foundation; it had an eminent scientist who is an expert in human growth hormone judge it, and awarded us the grant. We started work by doing computerized literature searches on the National Library of Medicine data base for substances that release growth hormone. (We subsequently discovered that Durk wasn't the only scientist to have this idea. See Sonntag, 1982)

By the spring of 1979 we knew enough about the subject (and its safety considerations) to be ready to start cautious experimental trials on our favorite human guinea pigs, ourselves. Then Sandy had her lucky break! She broke her foot at the Gordon Research Conference on the Biology of Aging. She soon discovered that having a broken foot was very inconvenient. For example, we suddenly noticed that women's rest rooms at biomedical research libraries often seemed to be at the top of a very long, steep flight of stairs. Going up a long flight of stairs on crutches is difficult. Going down them again is scary!

Scientists have known for years that the nutrient amino acid arginine caused growth hormone release in experimental animals when given either orally or intravenously. We also knew that an intravenous injection of 30 grams of arginine is a standard human medical test for normal ability to release growth hormone. (Barbul, 1977; Christy, 1979; D'Alessandro, 1974; Holvey, 1972; Isidori, 1981; Jacoby, 1974; Job, 1983; Josefsberg, 1983; Kenny, 1972; Knopf, 1965;

Laron, 1972; Martin, 1983; Merimee, 1969; Murad, 1980) Sandy started taking 10 grams of arginine per day, orally. She took it on an empty stomach because we knew that certain other amino acids (either as amino acid supplements or from the digestion of protein) could interfere with the arginine's getting into her brain, which was necessary for the pituitary gland in her brain to release its growth hormone. (She also took some other nutritional supplements, which we will describe and discuss later.)

In order to give it time to work, Sandy took the GH-releasing nutrient arginine as a powder 1 hour before a daily total of 2 or 3 minutes of peak output bench press and curls weight-lifting exercise. (See Chapter 14, "Peak Output Exercise: The Astronauts' Fast Exercise Method.")

In 6 weeks of using the GH-releasing nutrient with 2 or 3 minutes per day of exercise, Sandy lost 25 pounds of fat and put on about 5 pounds of muscle! She had not reduced her caloric intake but ate normally.

Oh, by the way, her foot did heal twice as fast as the doctors said it would, and we have the dated series of X rays to prove it. This doubling of healing rate was exactly what we had expected from the rat injury experiments. But we had discovered something far more interesting! This remarkable fat loss and muscle-building effect hadn't come as a complete surprise to us; we knew that GH promoted muscle building and fat burning, but we had not expected this astoundingly dramatic response.

To put Sandy's accomplishment into context, world champion bodybuilder Arnold Schwarzenegger said in his *Arnold's Bodybuilding for Men* that it is difficult for a male bodybuilder to put on 5 pounds of muscle per *year!*

Sandy's fat loss was as astounding as her muscle gain. We knew how much weight Sandy was lifting, how far she lifted it, and how many times she lifted it. That allowed us to calculate the amount of mechanical work she had done. That, in turn, allowed us to calculate how many calories she had *worked* off during those 6 weeks. We then knew how many calories of her daily food or body fat would be consumed to produce this work, correcting for the efficiency of her muscles. *Sandy should have lost 1 to 2 ounces of fat doing those 2 to 3 minutes per day of exercise. Instead, she lost 25 pounds of fat!*

THE CASE OF THE ACHING ARM:
SANDY STRONG-ARMS DURK
INTO TAKING GH RELEASERS

Sandy was so proud of her big new muscles that she challenged Durk to an arm-wrestling match. Durk figured that she didn't have a chance; he is over a foot taller and 50 pounds heavier. He got a very big surprise; she nearly beat him! That's when Durk started taking his arginine. Six weeks of 3 minutes per day GH-releaser-augmented pumping iron and Durk was much stronger. Sandy was still no pushover, but it wasn't embarrassingly difficult to beat her anymore. At this point, Durk reverted to his former sedentary ways and stopped working out—but he didn't stop taking his arginine. Sandy continues taking GH releasers, too, so Durk had better not let up. Durk's weight did not change, but his proportions did. He had to have his pants taken in at the waist and his shirts and jackets let out at the chest, shoulders, arms, and neck.

We suspected that we were onto something really interesting, but we had to make sure that this technique was reasonably safe before asking anyone else to try it. For the next two years we experimented on ourselves. Our clinical laboratory test results remained excellent, and there were no indications of the pathologically high GH levels that occur in the condition acromegaly (gigantism due to the pituitary gland's abnormal release of huge amounts of GH).

We then told a few selected friends about our technique, its potential benefits and possible risks. These people were chosen for their willingness to be medically tested to make sure that this new experimental technique wasn't harming them.

THE "MERV GRIFFIN SHOW" CASE:
THE PLUMP BODYBUILDER
WHO COULDN'T BUILD

Three of our relatively early experimental subjects were would-be bodybuilders, one of them an employee at "The Merv Griffin Show." He had been working out at the famed Gold's Gym in Venice under the supervision of a bodybuilding champion for a couple of hours per day, nearly every day for over a year, and his body still looked the same. He said that both of his parents had been on the plump side, and that he apparently just didn't have the genes needed to develop big muscles, no matter how hard he worked. After a discussion of possible risks and benefits, Durk told him how he could take 12 grams of arginine per day on an empty stomach an hour before his workout. (He weighed more than Sandy, hence the higher dose.)

About four months later, Durk came back to do another "Merv Griffin Show." *The results had been so spectacular that Durk didn't even recognize the experimental subject until he reintroduced himself! He now had huge shoulders, biceps, and bulging muscles everywhere. He was ecstatic!* His friends at Gold's Gym kept asking him what sort of new experimental anabolic steroid he was taking, since they couldn't believe that a mere *nutrient supplement* could have accomplished this miraculous transformation. (He was not using anabolic steroids since he was familiar with their very substantial dangers.) Soon a lot of bodybuilders at Gold's Gym were carrying around copies of our *Life Extension: A Practical Scientific Approach,* and arginine started appearing in health food stores.

THE CASE OF THE SECOND PLUMP WOULD-BE BODYBUILDER

There was no doubt that something very unusual had happened to Sandy, Durk, and the previously plump bodybuilder from "The Merv Griffin Show," but would the GH releasers work this well for everyone? Of course, what had happened to these three individuals was comprehensible in light of the published scientific papers, but we still needed more experience in the long-term application of these techniques to human subjects.

The second would-be bodybuilder was the young adult son of a *Fortune* 50 division president for whom we did scientific consulting work. He had identical problems. His parents were plump, as were the entire families on both sides. He worked out a couple of hours per day in a professional gym, receiving weight training from a famous world championship bodybuilder. After over a year of hard work he had gotten nowhere. He looked just the same. His genes were set up to protect him from an Ice Age famine, and in spite of all his sweat and dedicated hard work, they resolutely insisted on allocating his food to building energy-storing fat rather than muscle. When Sandy did a double biceps muscle pose for him, he blushed, became embarrassed, and refused to show her his muscles. Why? Because Sandy's 3-minutes-a-day-exercise-for-6-weeks GH-releaser-augmented high-tech muscles were so much more impressive than his! And Sandy was a girl!

After a discussion of possible risks and benefits, he decided to try 12 grams per day of arginine an hour before his heavy exercise. The results were equally wonderful: lots of muscles fast, and the fat melted right away. He thought that he could see the results in a week. Within two or three weeks everyone at the gym wanted to know what he was taking. Within a few months he had the big muscles he had always dreamed about, without using potentially dangerous anabolic steroids.

THE CASE OF THE WOMAN BODYBUILDER

A woman bodybuilder was another one of our early experimental subjects. She was an amateur who worked out about two and a half hours a day most days, well below the level required for success in serious competition. We told her how to use GH-releasing nutrients, and about their potential hazards. She followed our instructions. In two years, without increasing her workout time, she became women's national champion in her class! She didn't use anabolic steroids, either. She credits her phenomenal improvement (which she said would normally have required five to ten years of full-time work) to the GH releasers.

It is important to note that these GH-releaser experimental subjects were eating low-glycemic-index *diets.* Bodybuilders have learned over the years that certain diets and foods promote fat storage; by long experience and tradition, they already knew how to avoid high-glycemic-index foods, even though they had never heard of a glycemic index and did not understand its scientific basis. (See later in this chapter for information on glycemic indexes.)

In these cases the effects were much more dramatic than if there had just been a buildup of muscles. The dramatic impact of one's muscles depends on muscular definition, which is affected by the amount of subcutaneous fat (fat under your skin) that hides your muscles and sinews. These bodybuilders put on a lot of muscle and burned off a lot of fat—fat that their genes had heretofore doomed them to carry as famine insurance no matter what diet they ate (both of the male subjects had tried several diets without avail) or how long and hard they exercised.

The use of GH releasers has become widespread in bodybuilding since 1982 with the publication of some of our early work on the subject in our book *Life Extension: A Practical Scientific Approach.*

GH releasers are not just for bodybuilders. Sandy's broken foot made her even more sedentary than usual, and she exercised for only 2 to 3 minutes per day. Toward the end of this chapter you will read about "The Case of the Determined Fashion Designer" who did no exercise at all while her GH levels were elevated, and this fat loss technique worked for her, too, though she did not develop bulging muscles.

Even though we said relatively little in our first book about the fat loss and muscle gain benefits of GH releasers such as the nutrients arginine and the related ornithine, it was enough to cause a world-wide shortage of arginine that lasted for about six months and a worldwide shortage of ornithine that lasted one and a half years! The shortages ended only when the Japanese put new production on line.

We didn't give many details for the use of GH releasers in our first book because we had not yet had enough experience with their use for fat loss by a large enough number of people with a variety of weight problems, life-styles, and personal dietary preferences. In retrospect, this was a mistake.

Even though we didn't know everything, we knew far more than the people running the commercial operations that were soon cashing in on our book by selling so-called GH releasers. As a result, over half of the so-called GH releasers being sold today are ineffective, because of either improper formulation or incorrect instructions. It has been reported that last year alone over $100 million worth of these products were sold, and many completely unjustified claims were made to sell them.

Some full-page newspaper and magazine ads quoted us out of context and in such a way as to make people think that we were associated with these businesses. We were not. We had to spend a lot of money on attorney fees to combat this misuse of our names, but for every cease-and-desist order issued, two new companies seemed to spring up. This book will probably be responsible for selling hundreds of millions of dollars of these products in years to come. Let us hope that more of the manufacturers get it right this time. We are getting sick and tired of improperly formulated products with incorrect instructions and no safety warnings!

Why can the increased release of growth hormone have a spectacular effect on reducing your body fat and increasing your muscle mass?
Growth hormone and insulin are very closely related hormones. Hormones act by triggering specific biochemical reactions when they fit like a key into a lock-like receptor site on a cell. Parts of these two hormones—GH and insulin—are shaped so much like each other that they can partially block some of each other's effects, since each will fit into the other's active receptor site, like two slightly different keys that can fit into the same keyhole. But only the right key works in each lock, and the wrong key can block the lock by preventing the other key from entering it. Growth hormone can block insulin receptors and hence block many of the effects of the hormone insulin, and insulin can block growth hormone receptors, thereby blocking the effects of growth hormone. (Manchester, 1972)
In many (but not all) respects, the effects of these two closely related hormones are opposite. (Murad, 1980)
Growth hormone alters your body's biochemistry so that it tends to use protein to build muscle, rather than converting some of the calories in the protein to sugar and then converting that sugar to stored body fat. Growth hormone mobilizes stored body fat and makes it available to be burned for energy. Growth hormone discourages your body from converting food that you eat to stored fat. (Christy, 1979; Murad, 1980)
Insulin is a hormone that is essential to the metabolism of sugar.

Without insulin, most of your body's cells cannot use the sugar in your blood for energy. Insulin has been called the hunger hormone, too; when it uses up your blood sugar, it makes you hungry for more carbohydrates, from which more sugar is made. (Lotter, 1977; Mac-Kay, 1940; Rodin, 1983; Rodin, 1984) Insulin is also a hormone that is responsible for long-term energy storage. It helps make sure that you are going to have a chance of surviving that Ice Age famine. If you eat more calories than you immediately need, insulin promotes their conversion into stored body fat. (Assimacopoulos-Jeannet, 1976; Cahill, Jr., 1979; Larner, 1980; Lotter, 1977; MacKay, 1940)

Both growth hormone and insulin can stimulate muscle growth. They are similar in this respect, but insulin is a very strong stimulus to fat storage and a relatively weak one to muscle growth, whereas growth hormone blocks the fat storage effects of insulin and is a strong stimulus to muscle growth. Muscle growth does require some insulin, but unless you are an insulin-dependent diabetic you will normally have enough for this purpose. Growth hormone and insulin work together to stimulate muscle growth and the burning of blood sugar in muscles. If you have enough growth hormone relative to the amount of insulin, it can block the fat storage effects of insulin.

You must understand the difference between *growth hormone (GH) itself* and *nutrients that release GH.*

GH is produced by the pituitary gland in your brain. Experiments sponsored by the National Institute on Aging show that even in old age there is plenty of GH in the human pituitary, but with age it becomes progressively more difficult to release it into your bloodstream. Your pituitary gland releases GH when it is exposed to growth-hormone-releasing factor (GHRF), which comes from the master hormone control center in your brain, your hypothalamus. Certain nutrients and drugs cause your hypothalamus to release GHRF, which in turn makes your pituitary release GH. You already have plenty of GH in your pituitary, so you don't need any more. You just need to trigger the release of some of the GH that is already there. You can do this very effectively by taking growth-hormone-releasing nutrients orally. *It is usually easy to obtain GH levels comparable to those of a healthy postpubertal teenager or early-twenties young adult with this technique, and this is what you want, NO MORE.*

Growth hormone itself cannot be taken orally; it is a protein and would be enzymatically broken down and digested in your gut like a piece of ultraexpensive steak. GH can be taken by injection, but you should *not* do this. It is unnecessary, extremely expensive, and potentially very dangerous, and it would deprive victims of certain types of hypopituitary dwarfism of a scarce and badly needed medication.

GROWTH-HORMONE-RELEASING NUTRIENTS

Arginine and *ornithine* are two very similar amino acids. They are both natural constituents of your body, and arginine is also a building block for proteins, which are very large molecules made from many amino acids. Arginine is an essential nutrient amino acid in many young animals; without it, they would die. Since ornithine can be made from arginine in your body, ornithine is classed as a nonessential amino acid. These two amino acids are usually effective GH releasers, when taken either orally or by injection. (Barbul, 1977; Christy, 1979; D'Alessandro, 1974; Holvey, 1972; Isidori, 1981; Jacoby, 1974; Job, 1983; Josefsberg, 1983; Kenny, 1972; Knopf, 1965; Laron, 1972; Martin, 1983; Merimee, 1969; Murad, 1980) One gram of ornithine releases twice as much GH as a gram of arginine. (Even though your body can make ornithine from arginine, the process is neither instant nor one hundred percent efficient, nor is it known how much of the GH release is due to the arginine itself.) (Handwerger, 1981; Job, 1983)

In a typical experiment on healthy young adults, 30 grams of arginine given intravenously caused peak GH levels at least 20 times as high as the prior unstimulated GH levels in 4 out of 5 subjects. The stimulated GH peak was similar in strength and duration to the GH peak that could be released by very heavy prolonged exercise in healthy lean athletic persons in their late teens. There was a slight elevation of blood sugar, which lasted for 1 hour after the injection, but blood sugar did not rise above normal human fasted levels in these subjects, who had fasted overnight. (Knopf, 1965) An experiment using intravenous ornithine as a GH releaser in hundreds of patients reported that there was a similar strong GH release in about 85 percent of the physiologically normal cases, and no significant change in their blood sugar levels. Their subjects had fasted overnight, too. (Job, 1983)

Certain food sources are relatively rich in arginine, though such foods will be much less effective than the pure nutrient supplements. Although nuts are usually high in arginine, they are also high in calories because of their large fat content. Dairy products are a good source of arginine, and bodybuilders say that they have found dairy products to be especially useful. Chicken, turkey, and other fowl are very rich in arginine. Instead of another old wives' tale, here is an old bodybuilders' tale: for many years, bodybuilders have said that one should eat lots of chicken and turkey rather than beef or other protein for building maximum muscles with minimum fat. Now that we understand the mechanism responsible for this effect, we can use the pure nutrient supplement arginine and get even better results.

Should you use arginine or ornithine? We and our experimental subjects, including athletes, bodybuilders, and the obese, have used *both* very successfully. We think that ornithine *might* be more effective in the higher dose ranges that are apt to be used by some very serious athletic competitors. Even though both of these compounds are natural amino acids with very low acute toxicity, we consider ornithine supplementation to be more experimental because this substance is *not* normally found in significant quantities in the diet. You need ornithine in your body, but your body ordinarily produces it from arginine.

We think that the use of supplemental arginine is more medically conservative than the use of supplemental ornithine, and therefore we recommend the use of arginine, especially if you are not medically monitored. Prudence suggests closer medical monitoring with ornithine use than with arginine. If you are not a medically monitored competition bodybuilder or athlete, we suggest that you use arginine rather than ornithine. It should work just as well at our recommended doses, and it is more conservative. See the Safety Appendix for dosage information and precautions.

Fructose has been reported in one paper to cause GH release in 15 normal adult humans (14 female). The fructose was administered by *intravenous injection.* Doses of 0.2 to 0.3 grams of fructose per kilogram of body weight were ineffective, whereas 0.5 grams of fructose per kilogram caused GH levels to rise by a factor of nearly 10. (Strauch, 1971) Although nothing is obviously amiss in this paper, the work has not been reproduced by anyone so far as we know. This GH release may not be due to reactive hypoglycemia. Reactive hypoglycemia is the cause of the GH release about 3 hours after a large dose of glucose. (Kenny, 1972) The fructose-induced GH release was much more prompt, and the amount of fructose required for GH release was less than that required for glucose-induced GH release.

We had intended to do some self-experiments to see if 2 ounces of oral fructose would cause GH release in us. Fructose is absorbed very slowly when taken orally, so the peak blood concentration from a reasonable oral dose might not be sufficient to cause GH release. Before we could test ourselves, we discovered a paper that had the answer. *Oral* fructose in a 100-gram dose does *not* cause GH release in humans. (Bohannon, 1980)

Why do we even mention fructose as a GH releaser if it works only intravenously? Fructose is much less expensive than other GH releasers; someone is apt to come across the 1971 Strauch paper and use it to promote the sale of their fructose product as a GH releaser. Though there are scientific papers that show that amino acid GH releasers work orally, and we know that niacin is absorbed very rapidly from the gut, so niacin is likely to work when taken orally, too, be careful when there is no data on oral effectiveness. An effective intravenous GH releaser taken orally may not work if gut absorption is slow, or if it is destroyed in the gut.

Glucose: See "Effects of hypoglycemia on GH release," below.

Lysine is an essential nutrient amino acid. The published GH release data concerning lysine exhibits certain inconsistencies. Because of the extremely widespread use of lysine in commercial products that are alleged to release GH, we discuss this matter at considerable length, but we have put this discussion in the "Technical Notes" at the end of this chapter because of the technical complexities involved.

Methionine is an essential nutrient amino acid. One paper has reported it to be a GH releaser in 4 out of 4 humans. Peak GH levels of over 30 nanograms per milliliter of blood were found in 3 of the 4 healthy normal-weight adult subjects when 15 grams of methionine were injected intravenously. This was over 15 times the pre-methionine GH levels measured in this particular experiment. The same experimenters found that 30 grams of arginine produced similar peak GH levels in 4 out of 5 subjects. No noticeable alterations of blood sugar were observed with methionine, whereas there was a slight increase with the arginine. The subjects had fasted overnight. (Knopf, 1965) Methionine does not compete with arginine, ornithine, or tryptophan for transport across the blood-brain barrier (see later in this chapter). See the Safety Appendix before taking methionine.

Niacin, a form of vitamin B-3, is a good GH releaser according to two scientific papers. In human adults of approximately normal weight, 200 milligrams of niacin increased GH levels by 8 times, with the GH peak occurring 2 hours after the dose. The GH peak average was 15 nanograms per milliliter of blood. Niacin did not release GH in very obese humans who were 153 to 203 percent of their "ideal" weight. At this dose the niacin had no effect on the blood sugar of the normal subjects, but it did slightly lower the blood sugar of obese diabetics. (Irie, 1970; Irie, 1967) Although the niacin was given intravenously in these experiments, it is absorbed very rapidly from the stomach, so it should be just as effective when taken orally. Sandy was also taking niacin when she used the arginine as a GH releaser. In later chapters we will have a lot more to say about niacin and its effects on blood sugar when it is taken in larger doses. See the Safety Appendix before taking niacin.

Tryptophan, another essential nutrient amino acid, is also a GH releaser. (Jacoby, 1974; Martin, 1980; Woolf, 1977) Your brain converts tryptophan to a neurotransmitter called serotonin with the help of vitamins B-6 and C. It is the increased release of serotonin that makes you drowsy and puts you to sleep at night. About 1½ to 2 hours after you fall asleep, the increased serotonin is responsible for releasing a big pulse of growth hormone over a period of about an hour. There is often a smaller pulse of GH released just before you wake up. If you are over thirty years old, this is most of the GH that you release, and this release decreases with age. A nutrient supplement of tryptophan (preferably with vitamins B-6 and C) taken at bedtime will help put you to sleep and can enhance your nocturnal

GH release peaks. Sandy was also taking tryptophan at bedtime when she started using arginine as a GH releaser. See the Safety Appendix for dosage and precautions.

In one experiment on 11 healthy men, 10 grams of oral tryptophan caused a significant GH release in 6 subjects. The average GH peak for the entire group was 9 nanograms per milliliter of blood, compared to the 0.5 nanograms per milliliter GH level before the tryptophan. (Woolf, 1977) These experiments were conducted in the daytime, whereas tryptophan is normally involved in sleeping GH release. We do not consider tryptophan to be a strong GH releaser during the day, but we think that it probably does better at night.

Dairy products are a relatively good source of arginine, lysine, methionine, and tryptophan, so it is not surprising that they have traditionally been popular with bodybuilders. There are two old wives' tales that are relevant:

1. A warm glass of milk will help you get to sleep at night. (Some of the tryptophan in the milk protein enters your brain and is turned into serotonin, which helps put you to sleep.)

2. If children's sleep is disturbed or inadequate, it will stunt their growth. (Sleep disturbance can abolish the normal nocturnal serotonin-triggered GH peaks, so the old wives were right again.) (Murad, 1980)

There are other nutrients that are involved in GH release, although they are *not* useful as GH releasers themselves.

Choline: Arginine and ornithine cause the release of GH via your brain's cholinergic nervous system. This is a system that uses the biochemical substance acetylcholine to send messages from one nerve cell to another. Indeed, some cholinergic stimulants (compounds that act like acetylcholine or slow its destruction) and an experimental drug rich in choline facilitate or actually cause GH release. We know of no evidence that choline itself causes GH release, but without adequate brain acetylcholine the most commonly used GH releasers—arginine, ornithine, and exercise—will not release GH.

Your brain makes acetylcholine from the nutrient *choline* with the help of *vitamin B-5*, also called *pantothenic acid* or *calcium pantothe-*

nate. As one gets older, one's level of brain cholinergic activity progressively decreases.

Make sure that you have plenty of acetylcholine in your brain. *Arginine or ornithine users should be taking supplements of choline and vitamin B-5, as we and our experimental subjects do.* Sandy was taking plenty of choline and B-5 when she first used arginine. See "choline" in the Safety Appendix for doses and precautions.

Since acetylcholine is necessary for arginine- and ornithine-induced GH release, drugs that block the effect of acetylcholine will block their GH-releasing effects. They will also block the GH-releasing effects of exercise and the prescription antihypertensive drug clonidine. (Bruni, 1978; Casanueva, 1984; Casanueva, 1983; Casanueva, 1980; Delitala, 1982; Leveston, 1980; Salvadorini, 1980) These drugs are called anticholinergics. They include atropine, scopolamine, hyoscyamine, and belladonna. Almost all antihistamines are also anticholinergics, which means that many nonprescription allergy and cold medicines will block the effects of these GH releasers. Fortunately for ulcer patients, cimetidine (an H_2 histamine receptor antagonist) does not suppress GH release, at least in rats. (Martin, 1980) In general, any drug that dries up your mouth or other mucous membranes and relaxes your muscles is fairly likely to have anticholinergic effects.

Potassium: Chronic intracellular potassium depletion blocks the GH-releasing effects of arginine and adversely affects blood sugar regulation. (Podolsky, 1972) This is presumably true for the GH-releasing effects of ornithine, too. A blood test for potassium will not necessarily tell you if your intracellular potassium is depleted because the bulk of your potassium is intracellular (inside of your cells), not in your blood. In this experiment, only 1 out of 5 intracellular-potassium-depleted patients had low blood potassium. A whole-body potassium[40] radiation counter was used to measure intracellular potassium, but this test is time-consuming, expensive, and available at only a few research hospitals. Potassium was restored to normal intracellular levels by a potassium supplement of 13.5 to 15 grams per day of potassium chloride (plus dietary potassium), which was given for at least 2 weeks.

The simplest way of avoiding intracellular potassium depletion is to make sure that you get roughly the Recommended Daily Allowance of potassium every day, either in your diet or as a supplement. The RDA of potassium is 1.9 to 5.6 grams per day. Fruits, vegetables, and their juices are rich in potassium; the amount can often be found on juice can nutritional information panels. Potassium is *not* a GH releaser, and having more than enough will not give you more GH. Extremely large amounts of potassium could slow or even stop your heart. Many popular diets are deficient in potassium, sometimes with lethal results, as was the case with some of the liquid protein diets. You probably have plenty of potassium if you eat lots of fruits, vegetables, and their juices. If not, we suggest that you take a potassium supplement of about 2 grams per day. This can be provided by about 4 grams per day of potassium chloride. Take it in divided doses with meals to avoid gastric irritation. You can even use it in place of common table salt (sodium chloride), but do not inadvertently use too much.

It is interesting to note that the popular recreational drug alcohol acts as a diuretic, and its use causes increased loss of potassium in the urine. Wine is relatively rich in potassium, so the potential potassium depletion problem is apt to be worse with hard liquor that contains no potassium at all.

The nutrient amino acids *phenylalanine* and *tyrosine* are *involved* in GH release, too. Some very popular commercial GH releaser products use these nutrients, believing them to be GH releasers. These two amino acids do not release GH at acceptable doses, but they are intimately involved with the natural GH release system. The details of this involvement are rather complex, but they are important to health professionals dealing with the obese, particularly if these clients are hypertensive or have cardiac arrhythmias, so we have put it into a technical note at the end of this chapter.

EFFECTIVE GROWTH HORMONE RELEASER USE

Growth hormone releasers must be used properly, or you will not get the benefits of your GH being restored to late-teenage or young-adult levels. Close attention to these details can make the difference between the success and failure of this technique. If you cannot follow instructions, don't even bother to try using GH releasers; most likely, they won't work for you.

Effects of Other Amino Acids and Proteins on GH Release

In order to get GH-releasing amino acids into your brain where they can release growth hormone, they have to pass a very picky membrane called the blood-brain barrier. They don't get in by passing through microscopic holes. These amino acid molecules are picked up outside the blood-brain barrier by specific transport molecules that act like little taxis which ferry the amino acids across the barrier and into your brain. There are a limited number of these taxis, however, and they can carry only a limited number of amino acid molecule passengers per hour.

This is why it is counterproductive to eat food containing protein, or to take certain other amino acid supplements less than 3 hours before taking, while taking, or less than 2 hours after taking the amino acid GH releasers. GH releasers that are not amino acids do not have this limitation.

Proteins consumed at the wrong time could block transport of the GH releaser amino acids into your brain by taking most of the transport taxis for themselves. Because of the body's limited ability to transport these amino acids across your blood-brain barrier, we think that ornithine might be more than twice as effective as arginine when taken in the relatively high doses that some competitive bodybuilders and athletes may wish to use.

Since ornithine costs twice as much as arginine, and since ornithine is twice as potent for releasing GH as arginine when taken in normal doses, it might seem that there is no reason for choosing one over the other. This is not true, however, in cases of very high dosage, because there is a limit on how much can be transported into the brain. At sufficiently high doses your blood-brain barrier transport system will be saturated, and the more potent ornithine is less likely to run into this limitation. Remember, however, that ornithine is not found in the diet, whereas arginine is.

Effects of Sucrose and Other Carbohydrates on GH Release and Function

The glycemic index of a food is a measure of how much that food elevates your blood sugar. (Jenkins, 1981) *Elevated blood sugar causes insulin release. All high-glycemic-index foods such as cane sugar, beet sugar, grape sugar, carrots, or mashed potatoes cause the release of lots of insulin, which can block the GH receptors, counteract the anti–fat storage effects of GH, and promote the storing of excess calories as body fat. Avoid high-glycemic-index foods for about 3 hours before using GH releasers and for about 2 hours afterward.* For more information on glycemic indexes, see Chapter 7, "Not All Calories Are Created Equal—Eat to Lose!" and the table of glycemic indexes in the "Supermarket Shopping Guide," Appendix 6.

You need to produce and release some insulin, but you do not want to have too much, or you will become very efficient in storing almost any sort of calories that you eat as fat, and you will find it very difficult to lose that fat. (Assimacopoulos-Jeannet, 1976; Bray, 1983; Cahill, Jr., 1979; Christy, 1979; El-Khodary, 1972; Larner, 1980; Lotter, 1977; MacKay, 1940; Murad, 1980; Ratzmann, 1978) This is why you should pay close attention to the glycemic indexes of the food that you eat. A high-glycemic-index food will raise your blood sugar a lot and hence cause the release of a lot of insulin, which will then promote the conversion of those calories to body fat as well as block the effects of your GH.

High levels of blood sugar release lots of insulin, which can rapidly use up too much of your blood sugar, causing reactive hypoglycemia. Reactive hypoglycemia is low blood sugar occurring as a reaction to insulin release caused by previous high blood sugar. Reactive hypoglycemia will make you crave more carbohydrates to get your blood sugar back up to normal. This is exactly what happens at a cattle or hog feedlot. The animals are given lots of high-glycemic-index carbohydrate-rich corn and grains, and this leads to the animals almost continuously stuffing themselves. The process is called feedlot fattening, and the animals put on a lot of fat very fast, with the help of all the insulin released by this type of diet. Take a good look at the junk food that you eat, and note how much of it has a high glycemic index. The phrase "pigging out" is very apt when applied to gorging on high-glycemic-index foods.

Note: The word "hypoglycemia" literally means "low blood sugar." In this book we use the term "hypoglycemia" to mean a blood sugar level significantly below the level that a particular person normally has, and low enough to cause noticeable discomfort in that particular individual. In our usage, a person who had missed a couple of meals, had a blood sugar drop of 30 percent, and consequently felt lightheaded, would be called hypoglycemic. Medical texts often reserve the use of the term "hypoglycemia" to mean a more severe drop of blood sugar to less than half of normal levels. The medical text usage is reasonable when dealing with pathological and life-threatening conditions, but a *dangerously* or *pathologically* low blood sugar level is not required to induce discomfort, hunger, and carbohydrate craving.

If you use the term "hypoglycemia" when talking to your physician, be sure to say that you are referring to a less severe blood sugar decline than the pathological 50 percent drop that he or she normally associates with the word. Note, too, that some people say that they are "hypoglycemic" simply because they feel tired or not quite right. This is not a proper use of the term. In many of these cases, their symptoms have nothing to do with their blood sugar levels. (Freinkel, 1979)

Effects of Hypoglycemia on GH Release

A large shot of insulin will cause GH release, and so will the insulin release caused by a large increase in blood sugar. (Christy, 1979; Holvey, 1972; Josefsberg, 1983; Kenny, 1972; Murad, 1980; Ratzmann, 1978) The insulin uses up your blood sugar, and when you become severely hypoglycemic (with blood sugar only about 50 percent of normal), you release GH, which blocks the sugar-using effects of the insulin and prevents your blood sugar from dropping further.

Massive (100-gram) doses of glucose can even cause sufficient insulin release so that the severe reactive hypoglycemia that usually occurs about 3 hours later causes GH release to terminate the effects of the remaining excess insulin. A lot of that blood sugar will be converted into stored fat with the help of the insulin before the GH is released. This is not a recommended GH release method; it will make you fatter, not leaner. Such severe reactive hypoglycemia is also a serious physiological stress and should not be provoked except by a physician performing a glucose tolerance test. We mention this because some idiot somewhere may start selling glucose as a cheap GH releaser, having seen but not really understood a paper on the subject, or perhaps being out to make a quick buck and not caring whether it really works as a fat loss aid.

Effects of Starvation on GH Release

Semistarvation diets such as the Pritikin Program are very popular, and this particular diet may owe some of its beneficial effects to enhanced GH release.

Combined severe protein and calorie malnutrition (PCM) cause two related pathological conditions called kwashiorkor and marasmus. If the dietary protein is very low, growth hormone levels rise to conserve body protein and slow down the eventually deadly loss of lean body mass, even though this impairs one's ability to convert dietary carbohydrate into stored fat. If the protein deficiency continues but the carbohydrate deficiency is corrected, the GH level does not drop as it would if there were enough protein in the diet, too. This is because body protein must still be conserved, even at the expense of sacrificing a potential increase of fat stores. (Pimstone, 1972)

The popular Pritikin diet may work, in part, by simulating this GH release mechanism. Pritikin recommended 600 to 1000 calories of food per day. This is a semistarvation diet. The food must be low in fat. The protein content of Pritikin's diet is 10 to 15 percent, which provides about 15 to 30 grams per day of protein. This is only about 1/5 to 1/3 the FDA's U.S. Recommended Daily Allowance of protein. The Pritikin Program requires a great deal of hard exercise to prevent serious lean body mass loss.

Does the Pritikin Program facilitate GH release? It is plausible, but we do not know yet. We would very much like people interested in the Pritikin Program to send us before-diet and during-diet serum GH data and data on serum levels of a related hormone, somatomedin. Please be sure that the blood samples are drawn at the same time of day and that the meal schedule is the same on both days. Our address is in Appendix 2, "How to Join Our Research Program."

Fortunately, one can use GH releasers rather than a semistarvation low-protein diet to enhance GH release.

Effects of Hypothyroidism on GH Release

Hypothyroidism can cause deficient GH release. Normal levels of thyroid hormone are required for normal synthesis of GH in your pituitary gland. (Samuels, 1976) Thyroid hormone is *not* a GH releaser. If you are hypothyroid, your physician can easily correct it. Do not take more thyroid than is necessary to provide you with normal thyroid hormone function. See Chapter 12 for more on hypothyroidism.

Effects of Alcohol on GH Release

The pure alcohol equivalent of roughly one bottle of wine can prevent the normal nighttime GH increase. (Leppaluoto, 1975) We do drink wine with gourmet meals and do not consider the dinnertime use of moderate amounts of alcohol to be a problem, but it probably would be better to forget about having a nightcap if you are using GH releasers. The experiment reported here did not involve the chronic use of large amounts of alcohol, so the mechanism of GH release suppression probably did not involve potassium depletion.

Effects of Sleep on GH Release

Good sound sleep is important for normal GH release. (Christy, 1979; Murad, 1980; Prinz, 1976; Quabbe, 1971) Tryptophan supplements can help you get good-quality sleep and release a big GH pulse. See the Safety Appendix for dose information. Tryptophan uses a different blood-brain barrier transport carrier than arginine and ornithine do, so they don't compete with each other and can be used together. Jet lag can wreak havoc with your sleep schedule, nocturnal GH release, and body fat. If you travel across time zones, see our chapter on jet lag in *The Life Extension Companion.*

Effects of Exercise on GH Release

When you were a teenager, a little exercise usually paid off with much more impressive results than in later years. Experiments funded by the National Institute on Aging have shown that the large exercise-induced GH release of one's teens becomes blunted during the twenties, and that there is little or no exercise-induced GH release after the age of about thirty. (Bazzarre, 1975; Hanson, 1973; Johnson, 1974; "Muscle," 1980) In fact, an NIA study found something quite surprising: if you compare two men in their forties who have the same height and bone structure, both will generally have the same lean body mass and muscle mass even though one is an extremely lean 100-mile-per-week fanatic longtime marathon runner and the other is badly overweight and completely sedentary. Of course, the fat man is a lot more likely to die from cardiovascular disease or cancer, but that is not our point. If you want exercise to rapidly burn fat and put on lots of muscles after thirty, GH releasers are very useful, perhaps even essential.

Vitamin B-6 augments exercise-induced GH release. (Moretti, 1982) Sandy was taking large doses of B-6 when she lost all that fat and built up her muscles with her six weeks of peak output exercise. See the Safety Appendix for dose information.

In our opinion, peak output exercise is likely to be a better releaser of GH than the same number of calories expended over a longer period of time in less intense aerobic exercise. Unless the exercise is intense enough to exhaust the muscle in half a dozen to a dozen repetitions, there is little physiological stimulus to increase muscle size, since peak, not long-term, muscle output is proportional to muscle size. The primary response to aerobic exercise is not to increase muscle size or to burn fat, but instead to increase stamina by increasing the number of mitochondria (little "power plants") in the existing muscles.

Even 5 minutes per day of peak output exercise after taking a GH releaser on an empty stomach (exercise 1½ hours later for capsules, 1 hour later for powders) can dramatically improve your results and the rate at which you achieve them. GH releasers alone will not give you bulging muscles, though GH releasers are very effective at preventing those bulging muscles from fading away rapidly when you stop exercising. We strongly encourage all healthy individuals to engage in peak output exercise. When the payoff is so great and the time required is so small, even confirmed exercise haters like ourselves may pump a little iron. See Chapter 14, "Peak Output Exercise: The Astronauts' Fast Exercise Method."

Effects of Injury on GH Release

Bodybuilders, particularly those over thirty years old, have a saying, "No pain, no gain." You don't hear this from the teenagers, though. Sandy seems to have figured it out. After your twenties, you release little or no GH as a response to exercise, but you continue to release some GH as a response to injury! The evolutionary advantage of injury-released GH is obvious: you will heal faster, with less chance of serious wound infection. The older bodybuilders can still get GH released by overstressing their muscles and slightly injuring them. We recommend strongly against this practice. Repeated minor injuries can gradually turn a fine muscle into an inflexible hunk of "muscle-bound" scar tissue.

Remember the daredevil Evel Knievel? That fearless wild motorcycle driver in the Captain America–like uniform would do some stunt that would send him to the hospital with a bunch of broken bones, be out the next day, be racing and daredeviling again within a week, and every few weeks go back to another hospital with a new batch of broken bones for another amazingly short stay. You don't hear about him anymore because he is no longer doing those bone-breaking stunts. We think that we know what happened. Evel Knievel didn't turn chicken, but he did grow older. We know that it started to take much more time to heal his broken bones than in the past. Age reduces injury-induced GH release, and we think that his healing time became too long for it to be practical for him to continue in his injury-prone profession. We hope that someone will tell him about GH releasers.

THE CASE OF THE WRECKED RACE CAR DRIVER

One of our experimental subjects is a world-class race car driver who has held several hundred world records. We have seen literally tons of his trophies! He is in his fifties and now an off-road racer, which is an extremely punishing sport. He crashed, seriously injuring his back. His personal physician assembled a team of specialists who said that he would be out of commission for six months. This prognosis was unacceptable to our race-car-driving friend; he would miss some important races. After he promised not to get back into his 550-horsepower race car until his doctors were completely satisfied with his X rays and general medical condition and had given him permission to do so, we told him how to accelerate wound healing by using GH releasers. His doctors said that our suggested nutrient supplements were harmless, but that they were a complete waste of time and would have no effects whatsoever.

Only six weeks—not six months—later, he was back in his unlim-ited-class off-road race car and was racing with the full but amazed consent of his physicians. They said that they had never seen such rapid healing in a person of that age. The GH releasers had restored the youthful growth hormone performance that he had had when he was a teenaged race car driver over thirty years ago.

P.S. Our race car driver's personal physician now uses many of our techniques on himself, his family, and his patients. In fact, he gives many of his patients copies of our *Life Extension: A Practical Scientific Approach.*

Effects of Obesity on GH Release

Obesity can reduce but does not usually eliminate the growth hormone release caused by most GH releasers. (Hanson, 1973; Murad, 1980; Ratzmann, 1978) One paper reported an experiment on 18 obese women who were an average of 181 percent of their "ideal" weights. GH release from the prescription amino acid drug L-Dopa was poor in 14 of these patients, but GH release from arginine was good in 16 of the 18 very obese women, increasing GH to an average peak of 12 times its initial levels. (D'Alessandro, 1974) This is about two thirds of the response that would be expected in persons of normal weight.

The antihypertensive prescription drug propranolol, a beta blocker, restores L-Dopa-induced GH release in the obese to normal. (Barbarino, 1978) With niacin, however, GH release did not occur in the very obese. (Irie, 1970) Most people who want to lose weight have a body fat percentage that is already under 35 percent, hence there will be relatively little reduction in GH releaser effectiveness, except perhaps in the case of niacin.

Hyperobese individuals have body fat percentages over 50 percent. Until a year ago, we did not think that GH releasers would be effective in the hyperobese because of the negative results of experiments on genetically hyperobese diabetic mice. Then we met two *nondiabetic* hyperobese men who had used 12 grams of ornithine per day in conjunction with a "slight reduction in calories, but I was never really hungry." (Growth hormone's anorectic [appetite-suppressing] effects may have helped, too. See Chapter 9, "Appetite Control Without Willpower: Nutrients That Curb Appetite!," for further information.)

Both of these men had a lifelong problem with hyperobesity. *One man lost 150 pounds in 8 months. The other man lost 100 pounds in 6 months. Both have been successful in keeping the fat off by continuing to use the GH releaser.* Both of these men had lost weight before on diets which left them so hungry that they were obsessed with constant thoughts of food. Naturally, they were unable to live indefinitely in such perpetual severe hunger and had regained all the lost weight.

These weight losses were faster than we consider desirable. We discourage people from losing more than 1 or 2 pounds per week. A conservative rate of weight loss will impose considerably less physiological stress on you, yet at this rate you can lose 50 to 100 pounds per year. Excessively rapid loss can be self-defeating; if you lose weight too fast, your hypothalamus may think that there is a famine and trigger a metabolic change that can make it exceedingly difficult to lose any further weight, even on a dangerous starvation diet.

Two hyperobese men are a very small sample. We do not know whether arginine and ornithine will work as effective GH releasers in all nondiabetic hyperobese individuals. At least in these two cases, ornithine worked far better than any diet, no matter how restrictive, either of the men had ever tried.

Experiments on hyperobese animals and humans show that prescription beta blockers (normally used to control high blood pressure) such as propranolol mitigate the reduction of GH releaser effectiveness normally caused by obesity. (Barbarino, 1978) Beta blockers should not normally be used in diabetics, but we do suggest their medically supervised use by the nondiabetic hyperobese. Since the hyperobese often suffer from hypertension, the use of beta blockers is very logical in this situation.

WARNING: All hyperobese persons must be under the close and continuing supervision of a physician, regardless of the fat loss techniques that they intend to apply.

WARNING: Diabetics should not *use GH releasers because the GH will block the effects of insulin and may worsen other diabetic pathologies. Diabetics should* not *use beta blockers such as propranolol.*

Effects of Depletion on GH Release

Depletion of brain noradrenaline can seriously impair the release of GH. This depletion can be caused by anergic (no energy) depression, abuse of stimulants (especially cocaine and amphetamines), certain prescription drugs such as reserpine, excessively heavy or extended use of adrenaline-like compounds such as phenylpropanolamine and most prescription diet pills, deficiency of any of several essential nutrients, and, to a lesser extent, jet lag, extreme stress, and prolonged overwork. Noradrenaline replenishment can be achieved by taking antidepressant dose supplements of the amino acid nutrients tyrosine or phenylalanine plus the necessary vitamin cofactors. *See the Safety Appendix before using these nutrients.* Further information on this subject can be found in our *Life Extension: A Practical Scientific Approach* and *The Life Extension Companion.*

Depletion of pituitary growth hormone will not be a problem with the doses of GH releasers that we suggest. Your pituitary contains a lot of GH; one report states that it is up to 10 percent GH by dry weight. (Murad, 1980) Another paper says that it is about 1 percent GH by whole weight, a comparable figure. (Tanner, 1972) A big hour-long GH peak of the sort that you will find in a very heavily exercising teenager (30 microunits of GH per milliliter of serum) depletes only 1 to 2 percent of the supply. (Frohman, 1972; Tanner, 1972) Remember that we want healthy late-teenage or young-adult GH peak levels, and persons that age don't run out of GH. Remember, too, that even elderly adults have about as much GH in their pituitaries as youngsters; it is just harder to trigger its release.

Effects of Down-Regulation on GH Release

When you take certain hormones, you may release less of your own hormone of the same type. This process is called down-regulation. It would be self-defeating if your use of GH releasers caused the release of GH but that additional GH then down-regulated your unstimulated GH release. This process has been investigated, and it has been found that additional injected human GH does not decrease normal human GH release. (Gerich, 1976) This finding should also apply to the additional GH released by GH releasers.

Effects of the Unknown on GH Release

We certainly do not know everything there is to know about using GH releasers. This is still an experimental technique, and there is yet much to learn. GH releasers do not seem to work in a few people whose clinical test results appear normal. We have had reports of three people who were in apparent good health, who were not borderline diabetics, who did not have any known pituitary abnormalities, who took pure arginine or ornithine, who said that they followed our instructions, and who did not get noticeable results. We do not know why. Fortunately, this does not seem to be a very common phenomenon.

In one set of laboratory tests, about 10 percent of apparently normal human subjects do not release significant GH when given arginine. When retested, some of these people subsequently show a normal release. Another paper reported the results of arginine as a GH releaser in over 500 people; the failure rate in normal subjects was 14 percent. (Josefsberg, 1983) We expect the failure rate for ornithine to be similar. The failure rate is probably a little lower with L-Dopa in nonobese subjects. Daytime doses of tryptophan have about a 40 percent failure rate in normal people. (Woolf, 1977) Circadian biological clocks are definitely involved in the normal serotonin-initiated sleeping release of GH and are set for nighttime, not daytime, GH release.

THE CASE OF THE DETERMINED FASHION DESIGNER

You may be a woman who wants to lose fat but does not want big muscles. GH releasers can help you, too. They are not just for the physical fitness fanatic.

Here is a case history of a woman fashion designer who was quite obese, but not hyperobese. It will illustrate the effects of our recommended doses of GH releasers taken at the proper times and under the proper conditions, including choline plus vitamin B-5 to ensure ample supplies of the acetylcholine that is needed for arginine and ornithine GH releasers to work, vitamin B-6 to promote GH release, and the use of GTF chromium and low-glycemic-index foods to control blood sugar and insulin.

If you ignore these factors, GH releasers may do little for you. The effective use of GH releasers is conditional on these other factors. You cannot just start swallowing capsules of GH releasers like diet pills and expect them to do the rest.

Anna Cartwright, a rock and show business clothing designer who owns "One Of A Kind Designs" in North Hollywood, California, is another of our experimental subjects. Anna has designed and/or made many of our leather clothes, as well as those for many rock groups. She is a relatively tough case, having been plagued by excess fat all her life; she simply has fat genes. Her father was a diabetic and very obese, and she apparently inherited his thrifty fat-conserving and storing genes, and perhaps his proclivity for poor blood sugar and insulin regulation. Though she is not diabetic, she frequently suffered from reactive hypoglycemia and carbohydrate craving. Unlike most people who want to get rid of some fat, she was obese enough for there to be some degree of increased medical risk from her condition.

Anna was a very determined woman. She was determined to whip herself into shape so that she could wear the fashions that she created. She designed special clothes to cloak her figure, but what she really wanted was to have a figure that her designs could emphasize rather than conceal. Imagine the frustration of being a fashion designer who couldn't wear most of her own designs! She wanted to be slim very badly and was willing to work hard and starve herself to do it.

She was persistent. She tried almost everything that she had heard of or read about. Years of repeatedly trying a wide variety of calorically restricted diets combined with lengthy exercise produced the usual results: unpleasant constant hunger and arduously earned weight losses that always ran into a weight plateau at a loss of 10 to 15 pounds . . . which she always promptly regained as soon as she stopped starving herself. The last diet weight loss/weight regain cycle left her 5 pounds heavier than when she started. Even being constantly hungry combined with running 4 miles per day, 6 to 7 days per week, left her with a fat problem. She had tried fighting her fat genes, and they eventually won every time. Anna did not want to be hungry for the rest of her life, which, because of her genes, is what a conventional diet and exercise approach would have required.

When she began our fat loss program on May 4 Anna weighed 182 pounds nude and had a body fat percentage (as determined using a Lange professional-model skin-fold caliper) of 31 percent. (Because of her pattern of fat distribution, we suspect that this may have been a significant understatement.) She is 5 feet 11 inches tall. According to the 1983 Metropolitan Life Height and Weight Tables, she was 6 pounds above the maximum medically acceptable weight for her height based on her large frame.

By August 22 she was down to 168 pounds, which is only 2 pounds more than the average weight for her height and frame size. She lost 14 pounds in 15½ weeks; she was careful to keep her weight loss rate down to about a pound per week so as not to provoke her thrifty genes into a pseudo-famine fat storage rampage that would cause a weight plateau. She plans to lose about another 10 pounds, so that she will be at the low end of the normal weight range. Her body fat percentage on August 22 was measured as 28.4 percent, an indicated loss of about 2.6 percent body fat.

What does this loss mean in terms of dress size measurements? *Along with the loss of 14 pounds, Anna lost 2½ inches from her hips and 2 inches from her waist, without* ever *going hungry!* She accomplished this in spite of drinking a lot of normally fattening beer and eating ice cream, things that she had given up on previous diets to no avail.

Anna was careful about the glycemic index of her foods, too, so that the insulin released by high-glycemic-index foods wouldn't block the effects of the GH released by the ornithine and tryptophan. This substitution of sweet low-glycemic-index foods for equally sweet high-glycemic-index foods also helped to solve her reactive hypoglycemia problem, and she is no longer bothered by carbohydrate cravings. She ate lots of fruit and vegetables and usually avoided high-fat items.

Anna's level of physical activity was moderate and did not involve peak output exercise. She walked a few miles per day and bounced about 45 minutes on her trampoline twice a week. She had done much harder exercise on previous diets but had never achieved these results, even with uncomfortable caloric restriction. *In contrast to the way she'd felt on the calorically restricted diets that made her weak, lethargic, and irritable, Anna felt that she had a markedly improved level of mental energy and physical strength and stamina.* She does the walking and trampoline bouncing for *fun,* because she is so full of energy that she feels the *need* for physical activity. She has a car and does not do any exercise unless she actually *feels* like doing it.

She said that she now feels much better than before she started the program.

Anna's fat loss program included a high-potency anti–free radical vitamin-mineral supplement 4 times per day (with meals and at bedtime) that contained 15 micrograms GTF (glucose tolerance factor) chromium and 40 milligrams of B-6. She also took 3 grams of choline with 1 gram of vitamin B-5 daily, about 5 grams of ornithine before bedtime, 1 tablespoon of brewer's grain fiber before meals, about 1.5 grams of phenylalanine in the morning as needed to control her appetite (see Chapter 9), and about 1.5 grams of tryptophan before bedtime as needed (average use of phenylalanine and tryptophan: 4 days per week). She never went hungry during the program, and because of her fat genes she is probably more resistant to fat loss than you are.

Note, too, that she only had to use eight (low-glycemic-index foods, GTF chromium, GH releasers, fiber, choline plus B-5, phenylalanine, tryptophan, and mirror, tape, and scale biofeedback) of the seventeen major metabolic modification techniques that we describe in this book. (See Chapter 13 for information on biofeedback.)

Anna's long-sought dream is finally becoming a reality. She has had to modify all of her clothes to fit her new figure. She is looking forward to doing it all over again as she loses another ten pounds or so. Anna, once medically obese but now average, has chosen the low end of the normal weight range for her height and frame as her goal. She is going to look like one of her fashion models. She has also had quite a bit of additional business lately: she has been busy altering clothing for some of our male rock star experimental subjects. She has had to take in a lot of waistbands and enlarge a lot of clothes at the chest, shoulders, arms, and neck. These techniques have worked on all of them: no hunger, less body fat, and more muscle.

The most important point is that Anna and her rock star friends now have a long-term solution to their fat problem, a solution that they can live with indefinitely since it does not involve caloric restriction, hunger, or obnoxious amounts of exercise.

P.S. When we checked this case history with Anna for accuracy, she mentioned that she now puts on a bikini and goes down to the swimming pool and gets whistled at! If this seems unlikely for a 168-pound woman, remember that Anna is tall and has a large frame, and that muscle is much more dense and compact than fat. One's appearance depends more on one's height, bone structure, and muscle-to-fat ratio than on one's absolute weight; keep these factors in mind when choosing a goal for your own personal program.

Expect Fat Loss, Not Necessarily Weight Loss

GH releasers alter your body's muscle-to-fat ratio, not necessarily your weight! Remember that fat loss is the only desirable form of weight loss, so you shouldn't worry if your scale may not show a weight loss. You may have put on 5 pounds of muscle and lost 5 pounds of fat. Since a man has a lot more of the natural anabolic steroid testosterone than a woman, and since this hormone works synergistically with GH to build muscles, men are more apt to experience this effect than women. In fact, men may even gain weight, especially if they are engaging in peak output exercise. The weight gain from elevated GH levels is generally muscle, not fat, however. (Bazzarre, 1975; Drop, 1982; Illig, 1970; Job, 1983; Kaplan, 1972; Prader, 1972; Tanner, 1971; Tanner, 1972; Tanner, Whitehouse, 1972; Zachmann, 1970)

Of course, GH at reasonable late-teenage to young-adult blood levels does not completely block the fat storage stimulus of insulin, so it is certainly possible for some people to eat enough food to cause fat deposition, especially if much of that food releases a lot of insulin due to its high glycemic index. Remember that the two hyperobese subjects who used ornithine as a GH releaser did reduce their caloric intake slightly, though not enough to make them hungry. The anorectic (appetite-suppressing) effects of GH may have helped them to eat a bit less without hunger. See Chapter 9 on appetite control.

How can you know that you have lost fat if your bathroom scale says that you haven't lost weight or have even gained weight? Your tape measure will show a change in your proportions, men's waistlines and women's hips shrinking, and biceps, calves, chest, and neck expanding, particularly if you are a man. Your skin-fold caliper will also allow you to actually measure your body fat percentage, and hence your fat loss.

Measure your success by your body fat, not your weight. Pay atten-tion to your tape measure and skin-fold caliper, and relegate your bathroom scale to being supplemental information, not your primary guide. See Chapter 16, "Measuring Your Own Progress," for further information.

GH Releaser and GH Frauds, Ignorance, and Errors

GH itself works only by injection. Oral preparations that contain GH are completely ineffective. Considering the current cost of GH, we are willing to bet that there isn't any GH in them, anyway.

Some bodybuilders are paying big money for something called "bovine growth hormone." That's a lot of bull! Cattle GH works well in cattle and rats, but it is completely ineffective in humans, even when taken by injection. Animal GH (except monkey or ape GH) does not work in humans. Now, after an absurdly long and expensive delay, the FDA permits the manufacture of inexpensive human GH from microbes that have been genetically engineered to contain the DNA blueprints for human GH. They were forced to finally act by an outbreak of a deadly brain viral infection in several people receiving the human cadaver GH.

Injected GH has substantial dangers. The National Institutes of Health recently had to discontinue distribution of its own human cadaver GH extract because of possible contamination by a virus that causes slow progressive brain damage and eventual death. (Brown, 1985; Koch, 1985; Gibbs, Jr., 1985) Much of the gray- and black-market human GH is extracted from cadavers behind the Iron Curtain. It isn't surprising that totalitarian states such as the Soviet Union are major extractors of hormones from dead people; if the Soviet state says that it wants your dying grandmother's pituitary, you don't have any choice. And when the Soviet state tells athletes that they must take potentially hazardous injections of this extracted GH, they don't have any choice, either.

Apart from the moral issue, there may be a substantial additional danger with these Soviet bloc human GH extracts. If the extract isn't sufficiently purified, it may be contaminated with neural proteins that could trigger a disastrous autoimmune reaction. Your immune system might be fooled into attacking your own brain as if it were a tumor or an infection. This type of attack, called an autoimmune encephalitis, results in progressive brain and spinal cord destruction, with effects similar to those seen in multiple sclerosis, another autoimmune brain and spinal cord disease. Soviet extracts are notorious for questionable quality control. Neither of us would risk using them even if we were hypopituitary dwarfs.

Most commercial GH releasers currently on the market are ineffective, because of either incorrect formulation, inadequate dose, or incorrect instructions. Some of the most expensive products are the most worthless. Unfortunately, that doesn't mean that some of the cheapest products work. The nutrient amino acid GH releasers are expensive when taken in effective doses. L-Dopa is very cheap per unit of GH release potency, but it should not be used without medical supervision.

Lysine is cheap, but does the lysine-arginine combination really work? The companies selling lysine containing alleged GH releaser mixtures have done nothing to confirm the rather meager data that supports its use. Unfortunately, this is par for the course. Nutrient supplement firms rarely put any money into biomedical research, unlike the major nongeneric pharmaceutical houses. By the time this book is published we will have firsthand information, since we will be performing the necessary experiments on ourselves. To find out, send a *stamped self-addressed envelope* to our address in Appendix 2; ask for the lysine GH data.

Serious muscle competitors such as bodybuilders and athletes are especially likely to be GH fraud victims. They are willing to pay a lot of money for something that they think will increase their GH levels more than the next competitor's.

Many of them are using Soviet bloc human GH of questionable quality. Others are using gray- or black-market "human GH" that supposedly comes from a reputable Scandinavian pharmaceutical house. We say "supposedly" because it is much easier to counterfeit one of their ampoule labels than a twenty-dollar bill, the Treasury men won't be after you for counterfeiting, the legal penalties are much lower, and you can sell that counterfeit ampoule full of water for over one hundred dollars.

THE CASE OF THE BODYBUILDER AND THE BIONIC BALDERDASH

We know of one bodybuilder who has paid several thousand dollars for an alleged "bionic GH releaser brain implant." Electrical stimulation of certain areas of the pituitary and hypothalamus with electrodes implanted in the brain will cause prolific GH release. The bodybuilder went repeatedly to what appeared to be a doctor's office. Some hair was shaved from the top of his head. He was then anesthetized. When he woke up, his head hurt and was wrapped in bandages. When the bandages came off, sure enough, there was a scar right on top of his head. He went back for a few more "brain surgery" sessions for "adjustments." Each time he was anesthetized, and when he woke up he was bandaged and had a fresh wound on top of his head. Each time, he paid the "doctors" more money.

It was a big fraud. One doesn't do pituitary or hypothalamic surgery in a doctor's office. It is a *major* operation that requires a modern fully equipped hospital and a big surgical team headed by a brain surgeon. You don't just wake up from the anesthetic and go home an hour later, either. Moreover, you do not generally operate on the pituitary or hypothalamus by going in through the top of the skull. You would have to cut through the entire thickness of the corpus callosum, which connects the two hemispheres of the brain, with this approach, and then work on the target glands through the deep narrow hole that you had cut. That is very difficult as well as needlessly causing a lot of brain damage. The pituitary and hypothalamus are very inaccessible. They lie along the midline of the brain just above the roof of your mouth and behind your eyes. Surgical approaches can go in and up through the roof of your mouth, or go in through your nose or the upper part of your face. That bodybuilder paid a small fortune for a few anesthetic hangovers and scalp scars.

Before you use GH releasers, you should first learn more about insulin and blood sugar, and how they are regulated by the foods that you eat. This information is in Chapter 7, "Not All Calories Are Created Equal—Eat to Lose!" and Chapter 8, "Sweets: How to Have a Sweet Tooth Without Putting On Fat."

Unlike most of the other methods described in this book, GH

releasers need to be part of an integrated program that involves improved control of your blood sugar and insulin. For example, Sandy was also taking niacin, a form of vitamin B-3 which altered her blood sugar regulation. You will learn about niacin in Chapter 8. Don't worry, though; you will probably be able to eat all the sweets you want once you understand what is going on inside of you when you eat them.

CAUTION: Before using any growth hormone releaser, even if it is a nutrient, study the Safety Appendix first! These nutrients are recognized by the U.S. Food and Drug Administration only as foods; they are not approved as GH releasers or as aids to fat loss or muscle building. These uses are experimental. Join us in being responsible guinea pigs and study the safety information first.

In conclusion, in this chapter we have shown you that:

1. A natural pituitary hormone, growth hormone (GH), plays an important role in the control of your body's muscle-to-fat ratio. It promotes the maintenance and building of muscle and the burning of fat for your body's energy needs. GH inhibits increases in your body fat stores. In many respects, growth hormone's effects are opposite to those of insulin, which promotes the storage of excess calories as body fat. GH is also important in maintaining normal function of your immune system and in the healing of injuries.

2. Natural secretion of GH by the pituitary gland declines markedly after early adulthood and continues to decline into old age. One common result is the accumulation of body fat, generally interpreted to be a survival feature: to provide famine insurance. Decreased GH output is probably also responsible for much of the loss of lean body mass that takes place as we age.

3. It is possible to increase pituitary GH secretion back up to normal late-teenage or young-adult levels by using specific nutrient supplements, such as the amino acids arginine and tryptophan and the vitamin niacin. To be effective, GH releasers must be used in an integrated program of the right supplements taken at the right time in the proper doses along with a coordinated eating schedule.

4. GH releasers may be used by healthy nondiabetic nonpregnant adults of any age to build muscles with a minimum of exercise, to maintain muscles after they are built up, to reduce body fat stores,

and to prevent the deposition of body fat. If desired, they can be used in conjunction with a conventional reduced-calorie diet to greatly decrease or eliminate the 25 percent loss of muscle mass that ordinarily takes place during weight loss, without the usual need for heavy exercise.

5. GH releasers promote fat loss, not necessarily weight loss. Pay attention to your figure and your measuring tape, rather than your scale.

TECHNICAL NOTES ON LYSINE, TYROSINE, PHENYLALANINE, CLONIDINE, PROPRANOLOL, AND L-DOPA

Lysine is an essential nutrient amino acid that is chemically related to arginine and ornithine. It is one of the most widely used ingredients in commercial products that are alleged to release growth hormone. We have seen three scientific papers that deal with lysine as a GH releaser.

The first paper tested lysine in 5 normal healthy young-adult human subjects. Some GH release was shown by 4 out of 5, but peak GH levels above 30 nanograms per milliliter of blood occurred in only 2 out of 5 subjects. That is over 10 times the pre-lysine GH levels measured in this experiment. These subjects had fasted overnight. The 30 grams of intravenous lysine caused a slight reduction of blood sugar, but not to a hazardous extent. This blood sugar decrease may be due to lysine's well-known ability to release insulin as well as GH. Indeed, lysine can induce severe hypoglycemia in some sensitive children because of the release of very large amounts of insulin. (Knopf, 1965)

By way of comparison, this paper also reported some GH release in 5 out of 5 subjects with arginine, and 4 out of 5 subjects had a GH peak exceeding 30 nanograms per milliliter with 30 grams of intravenous arginine. That is over 20 times the pre-arginine GH levels measured in that particular experiment. The pre-releaser GH level difference between the two experiments is a normal variation. (Knopf, 1965)

The second paper (Pecile, 1972) did not actually measure GH levels; it only examined an aspect of bone growth in rats as an indirect measure of GH. This growth can, however, be affected by many factors other than GH.

The third paper (Isidori, 1981) actually measured GH levels in humans after oral arginine and an arginine-plus-lysine combination. It claimed that the arginine and lysine together gave a far larger GH release than either one taken alone, even in the same total quantity.

There are some problems with this third paper, however. There was apparently something wrong with the authors' experimental technique. They measured an increase of GH after 1.2 grams of oral arginine. This GH peak was twice the unstimulated GH level, but it occurred after only 30 minutes, which is much too soon. When arginine is administered by intravenous injection, the GH peak occurs after about 60 minutes, and arginine is absorbed from the gut relatively slowly. When they doubled the oral dose to 2.4 grams of arginine, they observed *much* less GH than with 1.2 grams of arginine or with no arginine at all! Since this data is inconsistent with many other scientific papers on the GH-releasing effects of arginine, we must conclude that something was wrong with their experiment.

Insulin levels were tripled by the oral arginine-lysine combination, with the insulin peak occurring at 30 minutes. This short period of time after an oral dose of a slowly absorbed substance again suggests that something unusual was going on, possibly cephalic growth hormone release and insulin release responses. A cephalic insulin response means that the brain orders the pancreas to release insulin in anticipation of food, rather than because nutrients have reached the pancreas or brain. Could there have been a cephalic GH response in these subjects? GH can definitely be released by psychological factors. (Spitz, 1972)

The third problem is that the unstimulated GH levels of their 15 healthy young male subjects were about 5 to 10 times higher than the unstimulated GH levels in other studies. This can be explained, at least in part, by their subjects' ages; they were 15 to 20 years old, which is when GH release is at its postfetal maximum and can be stimulated relatively easily. Will comparable results be obtained with middle-aged people?

We think that their confusing results might possibly have been due to stress- and injury-induced GH release caused by the hypodermic needle punctures made to take blood samples. These interfering effects have caused some confusion in the scientific literature. (Spitz, 1972)

Why not just use arginine or ornithine and forget about lysine? First, the strong synergistic effect reported in this one paper would greatly reduce the required dose . . . if these results can be replicated in middle-aged humans. Moreover, lysine is much cheaper than arginine or ornithine. Because of this, many commercial preparations alleged to release GH contain a lot of lysine, even though the data on this subject is equivocal. We could find no confirmation of the 1981 experiments.

Is lysine plus arginine an amazingly good GH releaser? And even if it is, what will be the effects of tripling one's insulin level? Furthermore, lysine is known to compete with arginine and ornithine for transport across the blood-brain barrier, thereby reducing brain concentrations of two amino acids that are unequivocally GH releasers. We do not know whether there really is a synergistic effect of an arginine-lysine mixture, particularly in middle-aged adults rather than teenagers, but we do know how to find out. It is time for another experiment on our favorite guinea pigs, ourselves! The publishing schedule for this book doesn't leave us with enough time to do the experiments and report the results here. Since weight loss books are in greatest demand in the spring, we would have to delay our book for a full year just to include this new data. We think that this would be a mistake. GH releaser frauds, errors, and ignorance run rampant, and the public is shelling out hundreds of millions of dollars for what are usually poorly formulated products with incorrect instructions. In this context, a year's delay simply doesn't make sense.

To get the results of our own experiments on a low-cost lysine-plus-arginine mixture, just send a stamped self-addressed envelope *to our address in Appendix 2, "How to Join Our Research Program." Ask for the lysine GH data.*

Tyrosine is an essential nutrient amino acid. With the help of *vitamins B-6* and *C,* it can be converted to a brain neurotransmitter called dopamine, or to a related brain neurotransmitter called noradrenaline; this is the brain's version of adrenaline.

Phenylalanine is another nutrient amino acid that can be converted to these two neurotransmitters in a similar manner, except that more of it is likely to be turned into noradrenaline and less into dopamine. Both noradrenaline and dopamine can cause the release of GH. Injury can cause GH release, and noradrenaline is probably involved in injury-induced GH release. One experiment on 6 humans showed some GH release in 5 subjects, and a release peak above 30 nanograms of GH per milliliter of blood in 2 subjects; however, the doses used were at least 20 times higher than we could recommend. (Knopf, 1965)

Elevated brain dopamine levels can cause GH release, but a general brain increase in noradrenaline does not produce this effect. Noradrenaline stimulates two types of noradrenergic receptors, the alpha type and the beta type. Stimulating the alpha-type receptors can release GH, whereas stimulating the beta-type receptors blocks GH release, whereas blocking the alpha receptors blocks GH release and blocking the beta receptors releases GH. (Barbarino, 1978; Buckler, 1969; Imura, 1971; Lal, Tolis, 1975; Martin, 1980; Massara, 1970; Massara, 1972) Because of this compensating effect, there is no point in trying to increase brain noradrenaline above normal under most circumstances. We know of no evidence that either phenylalanine or tyrosine are GH releasers in doses that are medically acceptable for chronic use.

If, however, a person has hypertension (high blood pressure), a common antihypertensive prescription drug combination is an alpha receptor stimulant such as clonidine combined with a beta receptor blocker such as propranolol. *Both propranolol and clonidine cause GH release in humans.* (Barbarino, 1978; Gill-Ad, 1979; Imura, 1971; Lal, Tolis, 1975; Massara, 1970; Massara, 1972) This combination is a good GH releaser, and a logical combination for many of the overweight people who have high blood pressure.

For people who don't have hypertension, it is important to make sure that brain noradrenaline and dopamine are not subnormal, as is likely with many reduced-calorie diets, some vegetarian diets, most reduced-calorie vegetarian diets, severe overwork, stress, or anergic (lack of energy) type depression. Anergic depression and severe overwork and stress can promote obesity in some people. The lack of energy, aggressiveness, and ambition often experienced on a severely calorically restricted diet is frequently due to an inadequate supply of the phenylalanine and tyrosine that you need to make noradrenaline and dopamine. We believe that tyrosine or phenylalanine supplements with vitamins C and B-6 can be useful in many of these cases.

WARNING: Be sure to study the Safety Appendix before using tyrosine or phenylalanine. The doses of these nutrient supplements must be individualized. Even though they are nutrients that you probably get in your diet every day, their misuse could be deadly in certain medical conditions.

L-Dopa is an amino acid that is used as a prescription drug and is rarely found in foods. It was discovered because of the strange case of the cattle that couldn't be fattened. Cattle in certain feedlots, primarily in Georgia, just wouldn't fatten no matter how much corn and grain they ate. They put on weight all right—lots of solid muscle —*but there was too little fat* for the meat to be graded USDA Choice, let alone Prime. The cause was a rare amino acid called L-Dopa found in the Georgia-grown velvet beans that were the high-protein part of the cattle feedlot formula. The cattle digested the velvet bean protein, and some of the L-Dopa entered the cattle's brains, where it was converted to the neurotransmitter dopamine, which released so much growth hormone that the animals couldn't put on fat no matter how much they ate!

WARNING: Uncooked velvet beans contain proteins that are toxic to your kidneys, so don't try to go on the Georgia cattle feedlot miracle diet!

Tests sponsored by the National Institute on Aging showed that 500 milligrams per day orally of the prescription amino acid L-Dopa restored youthful GH release to healthy men in their sixties. No adverse side effects were reported in this study. (Meites, 1976; see also Barbarino, 1978; Boyd, 1970; D'Alessandro, 1974; Lal, Martin, 1975; Laron, 1972; Mims, 1973; Sonntag, 1982) L-Dopa use requires medical supervision and additional dietary antioxidants.

In our opinion, L-Dopa can play a useful role in medically supervised *fat (not necessarily weight) loss programs.* It is important to note that this suggested dose of pure L-Dopa produces brain levels that are much lower than those used in Parkinson's disease treatment. The side effects observed in Parkinson's disease treatment are predominantly caused by the much higher effective brain L-Dopa and dopamine levels involved, the peripheral decarboxylase inhibitor drugs that are a part of most L-Dopa-containing anti-Parkinson drugs, the preexisting brain damage that Parkinson's disease patients have, and, in our opinion, inadequate nutritional antioxidants to control L-Dopa and dopamine autoxidation.

CAUTION: L-DOPA is a prescription drug, and its use, even at these low doses, requires medical supervision. See the Safety Appendix before L-Dopa use, and see our Life Extension: A Practical Scientific Approach *for further information on the added requirement for nutritional antioxidants and for further safety-related information.*

6

Growth Hormone Releaser Dosage Schedules

The exact schedule for taking growth hormone releasers is very important. You can't get the full fat loss and muscle-building benefits if you don't take the GH releasers at the right time. A number of supposed growth-hormone-releasing products on the market contain use instructions that give incorrect times and conditions. These products are ineffective when taken as directed, even if they are properly formulated (which they usually are not).

RULES FOR GROWTH HORMONE RELEASER SCHEDULING

All of these rules apply to all amino acid GH releasers, such as arginine, ornithine, methionine, tryptophan, and L-Dopa. The comments pertaining to the consumption of high-glycemic-index foods apply to all GH releasers, not just to those that are amino acids. (The comments pertaining to high-glycemic-index foods also apply to any fat loss aid that can cause significant hyperglycemia, such as very large doses of niacin.)

1. Take the GH releasers on an empty stomach. "Empty" is a condition that depends on what you have eaten as well as the amount. For GH releaser scheduling, "empty" means empty of protein and other blood-brain barrier transport competing amino acids, and empty of high-glycemic-index foods. (See the next chapter for glycemic indexes.) "Empty" also depends upon how much food you have eaten. If you ate an average meal, 3 hours is adequate to empty

your stomach. If you ate a huge feast, it may take overnight to digest your meal. If you eat a low-glycemic-index low-protein food, your stomach is still "empty" as far as GH releaser scheduling is concerned.

2. If you intend to exercise, wait for about 1½ hours after taking your GH releasers. (Wait only about 45 minutes for L-Dopa.) If you take the GH releasers as powders rather than capsules, 1 hour is enough. If your GH releasers are in pills (not recommended), the longer time required for the pills to dissolve usually increases the delay to very roughly 2 hours, but the disintegration times of tablets can vary a great deal. Even a few minutes of peak output exercise at the right time is amazingly effective in increasing muscle mass and seems to be a big help in decreasing fat stores, too.

3. Your largest spontaneous GH release occurs naturally about 90 minutes after you fall asleep. Hence, taking your GH releasers just before bedtime is an excellent plan. Remember that tryptophan releases GH by a different mechanism from that of arginine and ornithine, which in turn is different from that of the prescription drug L-Dopa. Arginine and ornithine do not compete with tryptophan, methionine, or L-Dopa for transport across the blood-brain barrier, so tryptophan can be used with these other amino acid GH releasers. Since tryptophan is involved in the natural nighttime GH release, and since it will help put you to sleep, the logical time to take it is before going to bed. L-Dopa does compete with tryptophan to some extent, but we don't consider this to be a serious problem because of the relatively small quantities of amino acids that are involved.

4. Teenagers release GH pulses without any external stimulus. These pulses occur every 3 to 5 hours on the average. If you use more than one dose of GH releasers in a 24-hour period, we suggest that you space them at least 3 to 5 hours apart. We advise *against* trying to maintain the relatively high GH peak levels continuously; that might be fine if you were a rat, but that is not the way it is in healthy late-teen to early-twenties humans.

You can create any schedule that you like, provided that you follow the above principles.

Here are some *examples* of schedules that work.

The accompanying charts show you exactly when you can take your GH releaser nutrient supplements for best results. In designing these schedules, we have considered both foods that might interfere with either GH release or the effectiveness of released growth hormone. We have also considered the natural unassisted schedule that your body follows for the release of GH. If you deviate from these schedules in a way that violates any of the above four principles, you are not likely to obtain the fat-reducing, muscle-building benefits that you would otherwise get from GH releasers.

These are typical daily schedules. You can modify them to fit your own daily pattern provided that you follow the rules given at the start of this chapter. For example, if you eat breakfast at 5:00 A.M., 1 hour earlier than the schedule below, just move the GH dosage time to 1 hour earlier, at 8:00 A.M. and do your exercises 1 hour earlier, at 9:30 A.M. Peak output exercise only takes 5 minutes; hence it can even be done at work, in many cases.

ONCE-A-DAY GH RELEASER SUPPLEMENT SCHEDULE
Without Exercise

Take all your GH releasers at bedtime. This should be at least three hours after your last meal containing protein or high-glycemic-index foods.

ONCE-A-DAY GH RELEASER SUPPLEMENT SCHEDULE
With Exercise

TIME OF LAST MEAL	TIME TO TAKE GH RELEASERS	TIME TO EXERCISE
6:00 A.M.	9:00 A.M.	10:30 A.M.
	or	
12:00 noon	3:00 P.M.	4:30 P.M.
	or	
6:00 P.M.	9:00 P.M. or later	10:30 P.M. or later

Our own personal experience suggests that the best time to take GH releasers in a program with peak output exercise seems to be 1½ hours before bedtime, with the exercise immediately before going to bed. With this schedule, you have a GH peak from the releasers during your exercise, immediately followed by the natural sleep-induced GH release peak. (Remember that arginine or ornithine releases GH by a different route than that of tryptophan, which is involved in sleep-induced GH release, so there shouldn't be any interference.) This way, your exercise is followed by about 3 hours of elevated GH. The exercise also releases endorphins, your body's natural morphine-like sedatives, which will help put you to sleep.

TWICE-A-DAY GH RELEASER SUPPLEMENT SCHEDULE
With Exercise

TIME OF LAST MEAL	TIME TO TAKE GH RELEASERS	TIME TO EXERCISE
6:00 A.M.	9:00 A.M.	10:30 A.M.
	and/or	
12:00 noon	3:00 P.M.	4:30 P.M.
	and/or	
6:00 P.M.	9:00 P.M. or later	10:30 P.M. or later

You can take the last dose 1½ hours before bedtime and exercise at bedtime.

If you wish to take GH releasers, exercise, and snack between meals, too, your schedule will be a bit more complex.

If the snack does not contain a high-glycemic-index food or a lot of protein, you do not have to wait the extra 2 or preferably 3 hours to take your GH releasers. While ice cream does contain sugar, scientists have found that this sugar is not released quickly enough into the bloodstream to produce a big increase in insulin levels. Protein release is probably similarly moderated. Hence, ice cream is a low-glycemic-index food and is an acceptable snack after which you do not have to wait to take your GH releasers!

Most of our personal experience and that of our experimental subjects has been with one dose of the amino acid GH releasers per day, both with and without exercise. (We use niacin 4 times per day.) A few gung-ho bodybuilders and athletes normally use one dose of amino acid GH releasers before a daily workout, and another before a very short bedtime workout. If you do not exercise, we suggest that

TWICE-A-DAY GH RELEASER SUPPLEMENT SCHEDULE
With a Snack and Exercise

TIME OF LAST MEAL	TIME TO TAKE GH RELEASERS	TIME TO EXERCISE
6:00 A.M.	9:00 A.M.	10:30 A.M.
12:00 noon		
	and/or	
Midafternoon snack		
6:00 P.M.	9:00 P.M. or later	10:30 P.M. or later

You can take the last dose 1½ hours before bedtime and exercise at bedtime.

you take your daily amino acid GH releaser(s) in a single dose at bedtime. If you do exercise, we suggest taking your arginine or ornithine, methionine, and/or L-Dopa in a single dose before exercise, and your tryptophan at bedtime.

ONCE-A-DAY GH RELEASER SUPPLEMENT SCHEDULE
With Two Snacks and Exercise

TIME OF LAST MEAL	TIME TO TAKE GH RELEASERS	TIME TO EXERCISE
6:00 A.M.		
9:30 A.M. Midmorning snack		
12:00 noon		
3:00 P.M. Midafternoon snack		
6:00 P.M.	9:00 P.M. or later	10:30 P.M. or later

You can take the GH releaser dose 1½ hours before bedtime and exercise at bedtime.

You now know enough to figure out your own GH releaser dose schedule and optional exercise schedule. You will probably have a different schedule for weekends. You will find the schedule forms in Appendix 1, "Your Own Case History." Please fill them out now.

You may wonder why we have said nothing yet about the *amount* of GH releasers that you may take. You should not try to use the doses that were used in these short-term medically supervised tests. You will find our recommended dosage information in the Safety Appendix. The doses given there are the maximum total amounts that a person in good health can normally take per day on a regular basis. We put the dose data in the Safety Appendix to make certain that you read the safety information before using the GH releasers!

7

Not All Calories Are Created Equal—Eat to Lose! or Losing Fat While Snacking on Three Pints of Ice Cream per Day

Our last two chapters explained the relation between your body's muscle-to-fat ratio and your growth hormone level and your growth-hormone-to-insulin ratio. *To burn fat and help build muscle, you want to keep your GH up, like a healthy human in the late teens or early twenties, and keep your insulin as low as possible while still maintaining a normal blood sugar level.* Whether or not you use GH releasers, it is very important for you to control your blood sugar and insulin levels properly.

When you eat carbohydrates, they either are sugar already or are converted to sugar, so your blood sugar goes up. This in turn causes certain cells in your pancreas (the islets of Langerhans) to release insulin into your blood to metabolize that sugar. If you are getting more calories than you need, your insulin helps to convert those excess calories you ate into stored body fat. The insulin, moreover, blocks the fat loss and muscle-building effects of growth hormone. That is why carbohydrates have such a well-deserved reputation for making you fat.

Here is the great news: not all carbohydrates are created equal. Different carbohydrates have very different effects on elevating your

blood sugar; hence they cause different degrees of insulin release.
Equal numbers of calories of rice, pasta, and ice cream do not have
the same effect as the same number of calories of soft drinks, candy
bars, potatoes, and carrots. Scientists have found that different foods
cause sugar levels to increase in your bloodstream at different rates
and to different peak levels. These effects are not always what you
would expect. For example, a cup of carrots will raise your blood
sugar *much* more than a cup of ice cream!

*The glycemic index of a food is a simple yet very important concept
that is central to our fat loss program.* The glycemic index is a ratio.
Give a group of healthy normal human experimental subjects an
ounce of glucose (grape sugar). Measure the rise in their blood sugar
caused by the glucose. Give them an ounce of food Z. Measure the
rise in their blood sugar caused by food Z.

$$\text{glycemic index of food Z} = 100 \times \frac{\text{blood sugar rise from food Z}}{\text{blood sugar rise from glucose}}$$

Glucose (grape sugar) has a glycemic index of *100.*

Honey (a mixture of sugars) has a glycemic index of *87.*

Sucrose (beet and cane sugar, either white or brown) has a glycemic
index of *59.*

Fructose (fruit sugar) has a glycemic index of *20.*

Carrots have a glycemic index of *92. That means that an ounce of
carrots will raise your blood sugar considerably more than an ounce of
pure cane or beet sugar!*

Complex carbohydrates is a term frequently used for starches.
Many nutritionists believed that complex carbohydrates had a much
lower glycemic index than sucrose; hence they recommended potatoes instead of sugar as a carbohydrate source.

Scientists studying diabetes, where blood sugar control is a severe
problem, found something very surprising. Complex carbohydrates
do not necessarily have a low glycemic index, and sucrose-filled desserts do not necessarily have a high glycemic index. (Jenkins, 1981)
Instant mashed potatoes have a glycemic index of 80, which is worse
than sucrose. Sweet potatoes are considerably better with a glycemic
index of 48. Pasta, a staple of the Pritikin diet, is better yet at 42.
One of the lower glycemic indexes was 36 for ice cream, barely
higher than skimmed milk at 32! Although ice cream is full of su-

crose, it has a remarkably low glycemic index. We suspect that this is because the ice cream's microscopic fat-water emulsion structure slows the release of the sugar into your blood.

The glycemic index is your guide to delicious fat loss carbohydrate eating. If you eat high-glycemic-index foods they are more likely to keep your blood sugar relatively high, and this will make the amount of insulin in your blood relatively high. This high level of insulin in your blood will cause two effects that are very detrimental to our fat loss program.

1. A high level of insulin will increase your conversion of dietary carbohydrates, dietary fat, and dietary protein to body fat.

2. A high level of insulin will block the fat-mobilizing and muscle-building effects of your growth hormone, whether or not it is augmented with the use of GH releasers.

Whenever possible, substitute a low-glycemic-index food for a high-glycemic-index food. This is especially important before bedtime snacks, because of the natural release of GH during sleep, and before using GH-releasing nutritional supplements. Wouldn't you really prefer 300 calories of ice cream to 300 calories of carrots?

The glycemic index must be interpreted with care, however. Recently a group of scientists found that when specific carbohydrates are combined with other food constituents, as is usual in a meal, the single-food-at-a-time glycemic index is not a good predictor of the resulting blood glucose and insulin levels. (Coulston, 1984) For example, they found that plasma glucose concentrations following meals containing equal amounts of carbohydrate as rice, spaghetti, or lentils were similar and somewhat lower than meals containing potatoes. Yet the glycemic indexes of rice, spaghetti, lentils, and potatoes are 72, 50, 29, and 70, respectively. In a similar manner, calculating a glycemic index for a fruit or fruit juice from the proportions and glycemic indexes of its constituent sugars may not yield an accurate result. Some fruits and natural fruit juices that contain a lot of high-glycemic-index glucose and sucrose have low glycemic indexes when experimentally measured, perhaps because of the presence of fiber. (Jenkins, 1984)

Thus the glycemic index is best used to compare single-food items. It is particularly useful in evaluating snacks, which, unlike a meal, are likely to be comprised of a single food, such as ice cream or potato chips. We are looking forward to the day when the interactions between foods are well enough understood to permit a reasonably accurate calculation of the glycemic index of a meal from the characteristics, proportions, and glycemic indexes of its constituents. Such research will have great practical value to the blood-sugar-and-insulin-conscious meal planner.

In general, we would expect that combining foods might sometimes result in a lower glycemic index than expected, but we would be surprised if there were many combinations that elevated the glycemic index of the mixture unexpectedly. (Alcohol may be an exception to this, since it is known to speed the gut absorption of a wide variety of substances.) In other words, a high-glycemic-index food *may* be all right when taken with other foods, particularly if they have a high soluble-fiber content, but a low-glycemic-index food is acceptable either alone or in combination.

The importance of the glycemic index was vividly demonstrated by a bodybuilder (John P. Rosen) who is a weight trainer at the famed original Gold's Gym in Venice, California. He heard Durk on a "Merv Griffin Show" explaining how GH releasers work; why the glycemic index of foods is important, especially when using GH releasers; and that ice cream had a low glycemic index. The bodybuilder thought that Durk was crazy, that you couldn't burn fat and grow muscles while snacking on ice cream. He set out to prove Durk wrong.

The bodybuilder experimented with ornithine and vitamin B-6 over a period of 10 weeks. During this period he consumed very large quantities of ice cream; he generally added 2 to 3 pints of ice cream to his regular daily diet! He also frequently ate several candy bars every day. His food intake was 3750–4600 calories per day. He did not use any anabolic steroids during this period.

In 10 weeks he lost 3½ inches from his waist and added 1 inch to his chest while pigging out on ice cream!

Taking 3½ inches off the waist of an already lean bodybuilder would be a major accomplishment for any diet, but to put on muscle at the same time is unprecedented. Even though he gained a substantial amount of muscle, as demonstrated by his 1-inch chest-size increase, he lost 6½ pounds. None of this loss was electrolytes because he was consuming large amounts of carbohydrates. Since he gained muscle, this means that he lost more than 6½ pounds of fat from his initially very lean body. His loss of subcutaneous fat caused a great improvement in his muscular definition, which plays an even more important role in his improved appearance than his added muscle.

The bodybuilder said that the same amount of exercise combined with his usual high-protein, low-carbohydrate, low-fat, low-calorie diet had never done anything like that for him before, nor for any other bodybuilder that he had ever heard about. Such diets had enabled him to lose fat, though much more slowly, but they had also cost him muscle. He had never before been on a program where he actually gained a substantial amount of muscle while losing a lot of fat! And he had done it while pigging out every day on a huge amount of *low-glycemic-index* ice cream!

See Appendix 6, "Supermarket Shopping Guide," for a table of glycemic indexes. Take it with you when you shop for food. Pay attention to it, and you probably won't have to buy another diet book next year.

8

Sweets: How to Have a Sweet Tooth Without Putting On Fat

The enjoyment of sweets is a nearly universal pleasure among people in technologically advanced countries. In this chapter we look at the effects of different sweets on your body fat storage mechanisms. We will describe how your body regulates your blood sugar and insulin levels, and how errors in that regulation can help make you fat. These errors can cause high insulin levels and therefore enhance the storage of dietary calories as body fat. These errors can also lead to the carbohydrate craving of reactive hypoglycemia. We will then explain how you can improve your blood sugar and insulin control to help solve these problems. Since diabetics have especially severe blood sugar and insulin control problems, we suggest that diabetics and borderline diabetics give this chapter special attention.

EFFECTS OF VARIOUS SWEETENERS ON BLOOD SUGAR AND INSULIN REGULATION

There are many different sugars in foods. Sucrose (cane or beet sugar) is most commonly added to food to sweeten it. In this chapter we examine the different properties of several other sugars and compare them to sucrose. We'll tell you about a natural sugar you probably eat every day that is better for your fat loss program than sucrose.

Reactive hypoglycemia (uncomfortably low blood sugar) is a common side effect of eating too much sucrose, the ordinary table sugar that is contained in candy, desserts, some soft drinks, some fruits and vegetables, and many other everyday foods. Many people have become "strung out" on sugar and eat large amounts of it, becoming overweight as a result.

When you eat sugar, the hormone insulin is released into your bloodstream. The insulin is released because it enables your body to use the sugar either for energy or to make stored fat. The effects of the increased insulin release can continue for a relatively long time, while the sugar is metabolized more rapidly and leaves your bloodstream. The large quantities of insulin that are released in response to a high-sucrose meal can subsequently cause an overreaction, driving your blood sugar level down too low. When blood sugar levels are too low, you will crave sugar and other carbohydrates that your body can convert to blood sugar. A person with a sugar craving may then eat another high-sucrose meal, which causes the release of another big dose of insulin, driving the levels of blood sugar down below normal again, and thereby starting the whole vicious cycle over again. This cycle is called reactive hypoglycemia.

The problem is not confined to sucrose; it exists with any high-glycemic-index snack or meal. The risk of reactive hypoglycemia can be minimized by eating foods with a low glycemic index (foods that do not increase blood sugar levels too much). That doesn't mean that you have to give up sweets. Fructose (fruit sugar) has a relatively low glycemic index and is one of the sugars that sweetens most "unsweetened" fruit juices. Ice cream has a remarkably low glycemic index, even when made with sucrose. Fructose-sweetened ice cream is even better. It does not significantly increase blood sugar; that means that fructose-sweetened ice cream has a glycemic index that is close to zero.

We would like to see a whole line of fructose-sweetened foods, including snack foods like candy bars, cookies, and ice cream. Fructose, which is natural fruit sugar, would be a natural for a line of jams and jellies. Fructose tastes just as good as sucrose and has the virtue of not being as likely to trigger the carbohydrate craving caused by the wide cyclical blood sugar swings of reactive hypoglycemia. Pure fructose can be found in the dietetic section of some supermarkets. It is more expensive than sucrose (it may cost five times as much), but it can be used in cooking foods. Cooking with fructose may require some recipe modifications because of its somewhat different cooking properties. It is also 3 to 70 percent sweeter than sucrose (Brunzell, 1978), so, frequently, less of it can be used, leading to a reduction in calories as well as cost. The different sugars all have about the same number of calories per pound. See Appendix 6, "Supermarket Shopping Guide," for some fructose recipes and information about cooking with fructose.

The differences between the amounts of insulin released in response to sucrose, fructose, and glucose are very marked. In one study of the insulin responses in human subjects to 50-gram (about 2-ounce) fructose and glucose doses, the fructose insulin response was only 1/3 to 1/2 that of the glucose insulin response. (Crapo, 1984) Another study compared 100-gram oral doses of glucose, sucrose, and fructose. The fructose elevated insulin levels to 2 times their fasting values, but the glucose and sucrose both elevated insulin to 4 times fasting values. The sucrose insulin peak was shorter in duration than the glucose peak, though. (Bohannon, 1980) And in another study, insulin responses of 10 normal subjects to fructose- or sucrose-sweetened cake were examined. Insulin levels in response to sucrose cake rose to *twice* the levels of that of fructose cake. (Crapo, 1982) Studies have proved that fructose is less likely to cause reactive hypoglycemia than glucose or sucrose because it stimulates lower insulin levels. It is interesting to note that the sucrose caused a more severe reactive hypoglycemia than the glucose. (Bohannon, 1978; Bohannon, 1980)

Sucrose is not necessarily bad for you; you can simply eat more fructose or other low-glycemic-index carbohydrates before experiencing an insulin and blood sugar regulation problem. The consumption of small to moderate amounts of sucrose mixed with other foods is not likely to create these problems in normal individuals. If you eat a lot of sweets, particularly on an empty stomach, you should consider switching to fructose. Note, too, that sucrose is certainly not the worst carbohydrate, either; 100 grams of carrots or mashed potatoes eaten alone will give you worse blood sugar and insulin regulation problems than 100 grams of sucrose. Those food faddists who consider sucrose to be the invention of the devil should now direct more of their complaints at the many carbohydrate-rich foods that have a glycemic index higher than that of pure sucrose.

You do not want high levels of insulin circulating in your bloodstream. High levels of insulin will generally rapidly use up your blood sugar; this reactive hypoglycemia makes you crave more sugar and other carbohydrates. Insulin stimulates fat synthesis from any ingested calories that are not immediately burned. Insulin also blocks growth hormone. Fructose is considerably less likely to cause these problems than sucrose.

Besides sucrose and fructose, there are several other naturally occurring sugars, which differ in their glycemic indexes and other properties:

Corn sugar: See glucose.

Corn syrup contains mostly glucose with some fructose and a few percent of other sugars. There are three forms of corn syrup frequently used as sweeteners: dextrose (glucose), high-fructose corn syrup, and ordinary corn syrup (a mixture of sugars). Ordinary corn syrup has a glycemic index that is even higher than sucrose because of its high glucose content. Some high-fructose corn syrups have a much more moderate glycemic index, as you will see below.

Dextrose is another name for glucose, so it has a glycemic index of 100, way above the 59 glycemic index of sucrose. You will sometimes find dextrose listed as an ingredient in foods. See glucose below.

Fructose is a sugar that commonly occurs in natural foods such as fruits and vegetables. It is not commonly added as a pure sugar to foods as a sweetening agent. *Fructose has a low glycemic index. On the scale of 0 to 100, fructose is 20.* That means that it causes only a small rise in blood sugar levels and hence only a small insulin release. (See glucose for a quantitative comparison of insulin release with sucrose and glucose.) It is slowly absorbed from your digestive tract. It is much less likely than sucrose or glucose to cause a subsequent insulin-induced excessive drop in blood sugar. There is much less chance of reactive hypoglycemia. Fructose doesn't cause subsequent carbohydrate and sugar craving. In fact, it is capable of relieving carbohydrate hunger, fatigue, and anxiety without their cyclical reactive hypoglycemic return. (Rodin, 1983; Rodin, 1984) Another possible advantage is that substitution of fructose for sucrose may lower the incidence of dental caries. (Makinen, 1974)

Fructose has been a major sugar in our food supply for millions of years, and we are equipped by evolution to metabolize fructose very well. In fact, the usual American diet contains 15 to 50 percent of its carbohydrate calories as naturally occurring fructose in its free form or combined in disaccharides or polysaccharides. (A polysaccharide is a big carbohydrate molecule made from many small sugar molecules attached together. Starch is a polysaccharide. Sucrose is a disaccharide; it is a molecule of glucose attached to a molecule of fructose.) In honey, the concentration of fructose is 40.5 percent. Many physicians recommend that their diabetic patients substitute fructose for other sugars in their diet, because of its much lower glycemic index. But before you decide to switch to fructose for your own personal fat loss program, be sure to read the Safety Appendix.

Glucose is a naturally occurring sugar, like sucrose and fructose. It is found in grapes and grape juice and in many other fruits and vegetables. *Glucose has a very high glycemic index. On the scale of 0 to 100 on the glycemic index, glucose is 100; it increases blood sugar levels rapidly and markedly.* Glucose is the standard sugar on the glycemic index, and all the other sugars are compared to it. (Jenkins, 1981) Glucose is rapidly absorbed from your digestive tract. Glucose is the sugar used by your body and brain cells as their primary source of energy. Interestingly, while your body requires insulin to use glucose, your brain cells do not. Even if you substitute fructose for all the sucrose and glucose in your diet, your body can make glucose from other dietary carbohydrates, such as starches. If fructose is the only significant carbohydrate in your diet (which we do not generally recommend), your liver can slowly make glucose from fructose. Since this process is much slower than the rapid absorption of glucose from your gut, it does not provoke a big release of insulin. Your liver can even make glucose from protein; this occurs on a low-carbohydrate diet.

When you are using growth hormone releasers, you do not want to ingest a lot of quickly absorbed glucose. In many people, the increased blood sugar itself will reduce GH release. Moreover, the relatively large insulin release that results from the relatively large blood sugar increase can block the effects of growth hormone, increase your conversion of that blood sugar to stored body fat, and promote reactive hypoglycemia, which will make you crave more sugar. If you took very large amounts of GH releasers, you might even release enough GH to block most of the effects of your high levels of insulin and cause severe hyperglycemia, far too much blood sugar, like an insulin-resistant diabetic.

HFCS, or high-fructose corn syrup, is a mixture of fructose, glucose, and small amounts of other sugars. One of the problems with fructose is that it is expensive. It may cost up to 5 times as much as sucrose. High-fructose corn syrup costs less, sometimes even less than sucrose. Unfortunately, the word "high" means different things to different people. HFCS may contain as little as 42 percent fructose and as much as 53 percent glucose and 5 percent other sugars. This HFCS may have a glycemic index higher than sucrose. At its best, HFCS contains about 90 to 95 percent fructose, along with a small amount of glucose (3 to 7 percent) and other carbohydrates (2 to 3 percent). Upon testing by a group of scientists supported in part by the American Diabetes Association, high (90 percent)–fructose corn syrup still caused a significantly higher increase in blood glucose concentration than did pure crystalline fructose. (Akgun, 1981) Nevertheless, while it was not recommended for diabetics, 90 percent high-fructose corn syrup is certainly preferable to sucrose in our fat loss program.

Look at food labels to find out what sweetener is added. Even if it just says "sugar," it may not be sucrose. According to the Washington-based Sugar Association (representing cane and beet—ie., sucrose—producers) only a handful of smaller soft drink companies are still using cane or beet sugar. (Colford, 1985) The rest are using high-fructose corn syrup, which may simply be labeled "sugar." The Sugar Association has a publicity campaign to make consumers aware that "sugar" on a label is not necessarily sucrose, apparently thinking that they can persuade the consumer that anything other than sucrose is an inferior or artificial substitute. We think that this campaign will backfire when consumers learn of the benefits of fructose from our book. We favor voluntary labeling that actually states the percentage of each sugar.

Honey is a mixture of sugars, with 40.5 percent being fructose. Unfortunately, honey has a very high glycemic index, 87, much higher than sucrose at 59, and only slightly less than that of glucose,

100. Honey ice cream probably has a much lower glycemic index than honey itself.

Inositol: See xylitol.

Mannitol: See xylitol.

Maple syrup is approximately 62 percent sucrose, 35 percent water, 1 percent glucose and fructose, and 1 percent malic acid. Although we have not seen a published report of maple syrup's glycemic index, we would expect it to be about as high per unit of sweetening power as sucrose. Despite its probable high glycemic index, it certainly does taste good!

Sorbitol: See xylitol.

Sucrose is the most commonly used natural sugar. Its major source is sugar beets and sugar cane, but it also occurs in smaller amounts in fruits and vegetables, along with other sugars. It has an agreeable sweetness and flavor profile that has made it a big favorite. *Unfortunately, sucrose also has a relatively high glycemic index of 59.* It is absorbed rapidly from your digestive tract. This means that it will cause a rapid large blood sugar rise, which results in a large release of insulin, which will promote the conversion of much of that sugar to stored body fat, rapidly using up the sugar. (See glucose for a quantitative comparison of insulin release with glucose and fructose.) In many people this large insulin release can cause reactive hypoglycemia. (One delightful exception to that rule that we've noted is ice cream, where the blood sugar rise is surprisingly small.) Hypoglycemia can cause carbohydrate craving, fatigue, and sometimes anxiety and depression.

Xylitol, inositol, mannitol, and *sorbitol* are four closely related natural sugars. They do not cause insulin to be released, nor is it required for their use. They passively and slowly diffuse into your bloodstream; they are not rapidly carried from your gut to your bloodstream by special active transporter molecules, as is the case with sucrose and glucose. Little is converted to glucose, resulting in a much lower increase in blood sugar (glucose) levels than the equivalent amount of glucose. In quantities over about 50 grams per day, these sugars can cause diarrhea and other problems. In people with a certain rare genetic defect, large amounts of these compounds may cause aldol-type cataracts, too, but these can be prevented in experimental animals by supplements of the nutrient bioflavonoid rutin.

Synthetic sweeteners do not increase blood sugar levels at all; they have a glycemic index of zero.

Aspartame (trade name NutraSweet) is a chemical combination of two amino acids, aspartic acid and phenylalanine. It has a clean, sweet taste (like sucrose and fructose) but does not increase blood sugar levels. It is now being used in soft drinks and a wide variety of other foods. In double-blind taste tests, at least 30 percent of the women and 50 percent of the men perceived an aftertaste; however, in the same experiments, at least 60 percent of the women and 50 percent of the men perceived an aftertaste with sucrose, too! The reported aftertastes were somewhat different for aspartame and sucrose. "The aspartame aftertaste was described as having a lingering sweetness, a bitter-sweetness, and a slightly powdery sensation, while the sucrose aftertaste was described as sweet, drying, with only a slight bitterness." (Samundsen, 1985) Both of us detect this slightly different aftertaste, but to us it is nowhere near as intrusive and obnoxious as the far more bitter aftertaste of saccharin.

Dr. Richard J. Wurtman of MIT has pointed out that you can get increases in brain levels of phenylalanine if low-protein foods such as soft drinks containing aspartame are consumed on an empty stomach. He is concerned about possible behavioral changes as a result. Phenylalanine levels in the brain also increase in response to carbohydrate foods or ingestion of phenylalanine as a single amino acid. Except for people with specific metabolic problems in handling phenylalanine (see the Safety Appendix), we do not see a significant health hazard in the normal use of aspartame. Aspartame is recognized as safe by the FDA, the expert food and medical regulatory bodies of more than forty-eight nations, the European Economic Community, and the Joint Expert Committee on food additives of the World Health Organization of the United Nations.

Remember to compare aspartame's risks to those of sucrose, not to those of some nonexistent perfect sweetener in the sky. That perfect sweetener may never arrive, and even if it does, a lot of obese people will die from the increased cancer and cardiovascular risks while they are waiting for it and eating sucrose. And even if it were invented one day, it would take a long time to clear the FDA's approval process. It took sixteen years from the discovery of aspartame in 1965 to its U.S. approval in 1981! The sucrose lobby had more than a little to do with it. If sucrose had been invented recently as an artificial sweetener, we doubt that it would ever be approved . . . especially if there were a fructose lobby.

A number of studies on animals and humans have shown that phenylalanine can suppress appetite. (See Chapter 9, "Appetite Control Without Willpower: Nutrients That Curb Appetite!") It is possible that the increase in brain phenylalanine levels associated with heavy aspartame use on an empty stomach could suppress appetite. If so, that could be a very desirable result for most people, considering that people usually consume aspartame-sweetened foods and drinks to lose weight.

In one study of obese individuals in a metabolic ward, scientists secretly substituted aspartame-sweetened foods for those same foods sweetened by sucrose. This substitution resulted in an immediate reduction of spontaneous unrestricted-eating food energy intake (calories) of 25 percent. (Porikos, 1977) There is no reason to think this couldn't work if it was done openly, rather than secretly, by people who really wanted to lose weight. (In the case of an eating disease, such as bulimia, though, it may not work.) This aspartame substitution may have worked because the experimental subjects got the same satisfaction on fewer calories (see Chapter 13, "Changing Your Behavior: How to Act Slim") and/or it may have had something to do with the appetite-depressing effect of the phenylalanine in the aspartame. In any case, it is a big improvement over giving up sweets or going hungry.

Cyclamate, another synthetic sweetener, has had a similar rocky road. In fact, cyclamate was banned as a result of poorly designed sugar-lobby-sponsored tests in which combinations of saccharin, cyclamate, and cholesterol were studied in animals for the ability to cause or promote cancer, again at absurdly high doses.

In a recent legal case, a defunct company sued the U.S. Government because its business, based upon a cyclamate-sweetened low-calorie low-glycemic-index canned fruit line, was destroyed by the cyclamate ban. The company correctly argued that cyclamate had not been shown to promote cancer because it had been tested along with saccharin, not as a single agent. At the time these studies came out, we objected vehemently to them for this and other reasons. As a result of this case, the company won a settlement of nearly $6 million. We hope many more companies will successfully sue the federal government for being deprived of their business because of improper conclusions drawn by regulatory bureaucrats. We would like to see a class action suit against the FDA (the banning agency) by diabetics, the obese, and their heirs for damages caused by improperly depriving them of this safer-than-sucrose sweetener. Perhaps the government bureaucrats would think twice before making blanket bans if part of their agency's annual budget could be taken away by the courts as damage awards when they are held legally accountable for their wrongful and damaging actions.

Cyclamates continue to be used in many countries. We do not consider their use to be a significant health hazard. Cyclamates have been found safe by the Joint Expert Committee on Food Additives of the World Health Organization, the Scientific Committee for Food of the European Economic Communities, and the medical and food regulatory authorities in forty countries. Thanks to the sugar lobby, whose members consider it a greater potential commercial threat than the less-desirable-tasting saccharin, you cannot get cyclamate in the U.S.A. In Canada, which is not a major sugar producer, cyclamates are legal and saccharin is banned. Cyclamate is a lot better than saccharin to our palates, but it still doesn't taste quite right to us.

Saccharin has been used in many countries for a long time. It is a synthetic sweetener that has been very controversial because of some badly designed research supported by the sugar lobby that initially incorrectly identified it as a carcinogen. The results of subsequent properly designed scientific studies have indicated that saccharin is a very weak promoter of cancer in incredibly large doses in specially selected highly susceptible strains of laboratory animals. Saccharin cannot cause cancer itself but may promote the formation of cancer in the presence of carcinogens. The small quantities ingested by humans consuming dietetic foods or drinks are sometimes very unrealistically compared to the immense quantities required to promote cancer in animals especially bred to be very cancer-prone. It should be noted that if these special rats are given the sucrose in one can of soda pop each day, they will have an increased incidence of cancer. This does not mean that sucrose causes cancer. It means that sucrose makes these rats fat, and when they get fat, they get more cancer. Per unit of sweetness, saccharin is a lot safer than sucrose for these rats.

We do not consider saccharin to be a significant hazard and do not avoid it for that reason. We don't use it because both of us have a genetic trait that causes us to perceive saccharin as having an unpleasant, intensely bitter aftertaste. If you wish, you can do a small biochemical-genealogical study at your next family reunion by identifying which members of your family do and which don't detect this bitter aftertaste.

Even though these artificial sweeteners do not contain any sugar, they can still cause the release of insulin under certain circumstances in certain animals and people! How is this possible? Pavlov's dogs provide an answer. Pavlov, an experimental psychologist, found that if he rang a bell and then fed his hungry dogs, the dogs learned to associate the bell with the food. At first the bell meant nothing to them, and they did not salivate until they were given food. Eventually, though, the dogs would salivate the moment the bell rang, even if there was no food present. They had been conditioned to respond to the bell as they had originally responded to the food. This also applies to insulin release in people and animals. The taste of something sweet, such as saccharin, can cause what is known as a cephalic insulin response; the brain expects sugar and orders the release of insulin to get ready for it.

The cephalic insulin response varies a great deal from individual to individual, whether one is a rat or a man. A small percentage of animals and people respond strongly both to a sweet taste and to the sight and smell of food. They are called hyperresponders. Human hyperresponders released insulin while salivating over a steak that they had smelled and seen but not tasted. Does the sight of food often suddenly make you hungry? You may be a hyperresponder. There is a simple questionaire for identifying hyperresponders in Rodin, 1984. Experiments have shown that rats with a high cephalic insulin response are more likely to become obese when fed a cafeteria diet (a wide variety of different palatable foods) of the sort that humans usually eat. (Berthoud, 1985)

What can you do about it? Let us return to Pavlov's dogs. If the dogs were fed regularly after the bell rang, their conditioned response of salivating when the bell rang was reinforced. When Pavlov stopped feeding them after ringing the bell, the conditioned response gradually became weaker and finally disappeared. This is called the extinction of the conditioned response. We suspect that high-cephalic-insulin responders might be able to reduce their sweet-induced insulin release if they were consistent in using only artificial sweeteners, or at least used fructose rather than sucrose. If, however, a high-cephalic-insulin responder indiscriminately mixes high-glycemic-index sweets with low- or zero-glycemic-index sweets, the undesired cephalic insulin response will continue to be reinforced. Indeed, a high-cephalic-insulin-release responder might even suffer from reactive hypoglycemia after eating an artificial sweetener, since the released insulin would not have any additional sugar to use up. Niacin or a vitamin B-1 plus vitamin C plus cysteine mixture (see later in this chapter) could be helpful in at least some of these cases. *These blood-sugar-elevating and insulin-counteracting nutrients may be particularly useful to a hyperresponder who will be exposed to food but who does not wish to eat or to suffer from the insulin-induced hunger.*

EFFECTS OF OTHER NUTRIENTS ON BLOOD SUGAR AND INSULIN REGULATION

Chromium. Many people who have carbohydrate cravings, the symptoms of hypoglycemia, or poor blood sugar and insulin regulation may be helped by a nutrient called GTF (glucose tolerance factor) chromium or its precursor, the essential mineral trivalent chromium.

According to research performed by the U.S. Department of Agriculture, *most* Americans are probably chromium-deficient, so it is not surprising that blood sugar and insulin regulation problems are common in this country. GTF is a chromium-containing complex that is required for your insulin to activate the insulin receptors on your cells. Without GTF, it would be impossible for insulin to enable your cells to take in sugar as fuel for energy. The cells (and you) would die. In the past, most sources of chromium were thought to have poor bioavailability (ability of one's body to absorb and use a substance). More recent experiments have shown that inorganic trivalent chromium chloride is effective in raising human GTF levels. Some people seem to have an impaired ability to convert inorganic chromium to GTF as they become older. (Glinsmann, Mertz, 1966; Gurson, 1971; Hopkins, Price, 1968; Hopkins, Ransome-Kuti, 1968) For these people, GTF yeast is a good source of preformed GTF; it is available in health food stores.

If your insulin is not working properly because of inadequate GTF, you will find it difficult to use your blood sugar. (Mertz, 1969; Evans, 1973) This will make you feel as if you have hypoglycemia, where you do not have enough blood sugar, because in both cases there is not enough sugar getting into your cells. You may actually have hyperglycemia, excessive blood sugar, because your insulin cannot do its job of helping that sugar to enter your cells. You may also have hyperinsulinemia, too much insulin released in response to all that sugar in your blood and not enough sugar entering your cells. Fortunately, chromium supplements have been shown to lower insulin release in humans. (Doisy, 1976)

This impaired insulin function is why people who are chromium-deficient have an impaired glucose tolerance and may even resemble a mild case of adult-onset insulin-resistant diabetes. Indeed, some adult-onset diabetics have gained improved control of their blood sugar and a few have even had a reduction in their insulin requirements when using a chromium or GTF supplement. Scientific experiments have shown that genetically diabetic mice given yeast GTF chromium showed significant reductions in blood glucose (indicating improved insulin function), cholesterol, and triglycerides. (Tuman, 1974) Similar improvements in glucose tolerance and serum lipids have been demonstrated in adult humans (including eight mild adult-onset diabetics) with about 3 to 10 micrograms per day GTF chromium. (Doisy, 1976; Offenbacher, 1980) Similar results in normal humans have been obtained with 200 micrograms per day trivalent chromium. (Riales, 1981; Polansky, 1982)

Some people have hyperglycemia because their insulin is not working as well as it should. They may have large quantities of insulin in their blood, but they have damaged or blocked insulin receptors. These people may have insulin-resistant diabetes, and yet about half of them do not realize it. Diabetes is a very serious disease requiring prompt and continuing medical attention; nobody should attempt to self-treat it. *We think that everyone should have a physical exam that checks for diabetes before starting our fat loss program.*

WARNING: If you are a diabetic, do not reduce your insulin dose just because you are taking a GTF chromium supplement. Have your physician check your blood sugar and glucose tolerance; he or she will advise you if such an insulin dose reduction is desirable.

As we said earlier, many Americans are deficient in the nutrient chromium, and the problem tends to become worse as one becomes older. (Tipton, 1963; Tipton, 1965) This is especially true for women, who appear to lose a significant part of their total chromium stores with each pregnancy. This plays a role in the symptoms of reactive hypoglycemia and other blood sugar regulation problems that often appear after repeated pregnancies.

Glucose consumption increases your chromium requirements. This is presumably also true for sucrose, since it is broken down in your body into glucose and fructose. Chromium is released into the blood of normal subjects after a dose of glucose, but this release does not occur in those who have a poor glucose tolerance curve. (Glinsmann, Feldman, 1966; Levine, 1968; Gurson, 1978; Liu, 1978; Liu, 1982; Mertz, 1969) After you consume glucose (and presumably sucrose, too) more chromium is lost in your urine. (Mertz, 1969; Doisy, 1976; Liu, 1978; Gurson, 1978) We suspect that fructose would cause less chromium to be used up than an equal weight of sucrose or glucose would, because of its much lower insulin release.

Exercise increases your chromium requirements. (Anderson, 1982) When you exercise, you burn more blood sugar, so it is not surprising that you use more chromium in conjunction with the insulin required to utilize that sugar.

Refined sugar (sucrose) does not contain any nutrients other than sugar. Brown sugar (and molasses) also contains biologically significant amounts of chromium; however, the glycemic index is just as high. We recommend that you use fructose instead, with a chromium supplement. For a general review of chromium in nutrition, see Pi-Sunyer, 1984. See the Safety Appendix for the recommended chromium doses.

Niacin: You can alter your desire to consume sweets by altering your blood sugar regulation. Changing what you feel like eating sure beats self-deprivation and willpower. Niacin (also called nicotinic acid), a form of vitamin B-3, can be used for the treatment of hypoglycemia. (Shansky, 1981) The proper dose of niacin allows blood sugar levels to rise a bit and stabilize, but not rise enough to stimulate the release of insulin or be abnormally high. The rise in blood sugar is particularly important to your brain, which normally uses nothing but glucose for its energy source. Carbohydrate craving, anxiety, fatigue, "the shakes," and other symptoms of hypoglycemia can often be quickly terminated by niacin.

Many years ago Durk was a sugar junkie with a heavy habit. He consumed about 3/4 pound of sucrose per day in the form of sugar-sweetened Kool-Aid alone! He even added 70 percent more sugar than suggested on the package label. His total sucrose consumption was probably about a pound a day. That's a real sugar junkie. When we began to take large doses of niacin (a total of 3 grams per day in 4 divided doses) as part of our life extension experiments, things changed dramatically.

Durk did not drink the supersweet Kool-Aid for a week after he started taking the niacin. He had no urge to do so. The effect was almost immediate, occurring within a half hour after the first dose. Then one afternoon he noticed the pitcher in the refrigerator and took a little sip to see if it had spoiled. It tasted sickeningly sweet and, instead of being refreshing, now tasted horrid, even though it had not gone bad. Durk's flavor perceptions of sweetness had dramatically changed. He immediately spit it out, washed out his mouth with water, and has never felt like drinking it again. It should be noted that we did not know that niacin had an effect on blood sugar regulation until years later, and had not expected anything of this sort to happen.

With continuing use of niacin, Durk has never gone back to heavy use of sugar and, in fact, uses only moderate amounts of it except when confronted with a delightful array of gourmet desserts. Then we both pig out. In fact, Durk now drinks unsweetened fruit juices and almost always complains that they are too sweet! He dilutes them with lots of ice made from activated charcoal-filtered water to improve their flavor by cutting what to him is now excessive sweetness. Adequate doses of niacin may have a prompt and truly dramatic effect on your perception of and preference for sweetness. Note that Durk's enjoyment of sweetness has *not* been reduced; what has been reduced is the *amount* of sugar needed for that enjoyment, not the pleasure received from eating it. You will have to find out for yourself whether niacin will have such a dramatic effect on your sugar craving and reactive hypoglycemia. Everyone may not be as sensitive to these effects as Durk is.

A 5-year trial of 3 grams of niacin per day in over 1000 men for lowering serum cholesterol and triglycerides in cardiovascular patients provides some interesting data. The percentage of patients noticing a reduction in appetite and unexpected weight loss in the niacin group was about 3 times larger than in the control group of over 2000 men. This difference was statistically very significant. There was no difference between the placebo and the niacin group in the percentage of subjects having sugar in their urine, which would indicate excessive blood sugar levels. The fasting blood plasma glucose of the niacin group was slightly higher, and the plasma glucose 1 hour after a large dose of glucose was about 10 milligrams per deciliter higher. As expected, niacin slowed the removal of sugar from the blood. All these differences were small, but statistically significant. (Coronary, 1975)

Caution: Niacinamide, another form of vitamin B-3, does not *slow blood sugar removal and does* not *reduce excess serum lipids.*

Caution: See the Safety Appendix before using niacin and for proper doses for both medically supervised and unsupervised use. Diabetics and ulcer patients should not take niacin supplements unless advised to do so by their physician.

B-1–C–cysteine mixture: Excess insulin can be destroyed by the nutrient amino acid cysteine. This effect was first discovered by scientists working with tissue cultures, cells from mammals grown in bottles of nutrients. Insulin is added to these tissue cultures because the cells need it in order to use the glucose in the culture medium. Scientists discovered that if they added the nutrient amino acid cysteine to their cultures, they had to add far more insulin. (Hayashi, 1978; Rizzino, 1979) The cysteine reduces and breaks sulfur-sulfur chemical bonds (disulfide bonds) that hold the insulin molecule together. Insulin is very sensitive to this effect. The cysteine made the insulin fall apart, destroying its biological activity. The levels required for significant insulin deactivation can be obtained by taking a cysteine supplement orally.

The reducing action of cysteine can be strengthened by using a mixture of vitamin B-1, vitamin C, and cysteine. (Sprince, 1974) This thiol (a chemically reactive S-H group) reduction of disulfide bonds destroys insulin, but it does not destroy growth hormone. (Cerasi, 1972)

We have found that this nutrient mixture can substantially reduce the symptoms of reactive hypoglycemia starting within about 20 minutes after it is taken orally. Do not take it with high-glycemic-index foods; it might induce hyperglycemia. You can take it about 3 hours *after* high-glycemic-index food consumption if you frequently suffer from reactive hypoglycemia.

WARNING: Do NOT use cysteine alone. Diabetics should not use this mixture! See the Safety Appendix for precautions and dose.

EFFECTS OF EATING PATTERNS

Another method for improving your blood sugar and insulin regulation and therefore controlling your sugar and carbohydrate craving is to eat only small portions of sugars with a high glycemic index (such as sucrose). You get a much smaller insulin release when you eat multiple small snacks of sugar than when you eat the same total amount of sugar at one time. Try to keep portions small at each feeding. We are not suggesting self-deprivation, just spreading the same total sugar consumption out over a longer period of time. Of course, the proper use of niacin may help you to be just as satisfied with less sugar. Moreover, your insulin release is even smaller when your sugar snack is made from a low-glycemic-index sugar such as fructose.

We both love sweet foods and would never give them up, so we both use chromium, B-1–C–cysteine, and niacin nutritional supplements to alter our blood–sugar and insulin regulation. When possible, we eat foods sweetened with low-glycemic-index fructose or, as a second choice, high-fructose corn syrup. We hope that food manufacturers will get the message and switch to fructose and 95 percent high-fructose corn syrup so that more people can get off the sucrose roller coaster of hyperglycemia followed by a big fat storage promoting insulin release, subsequent reactive hypoglycemia, sugar craving, and eating more sucrose, which starts it all over again. (Don't forget that there are a lot of complex-carbohydrate foods with glycemic indexes even higher than that of sucrose. See the table of glycemic indexes in Appendix 6, "Supermarket Shopping Guide.")

We don't expect the sugar lobby to sit around and just let people switch to fructose, though, since the sugar lobby that helped make so much trouble for saccharin, cyclamates, and aspartame wants you to use only their product, which is sucrose, not fructose. They have reason to be concerned. As we mentioned before, the large soft drink companies are now using the less expensive high-fructose corn syrup instead of sucrose. Although high-fructose corn syrup can be more expensive on a dry weight basis, fructose is considerably sweeter than sucrose under these conditions, so less needs to be used (adding fewer calories, too). Fructose is sweeter than sucrose in an acid medium and at cold temperatures, conditions met by most soft drinks only as long as they are cold. You may have noticed that a warm soft drink that has lost its acidic carbonation doesn't taste as sweet as it once did.

The Washington-based Sugar Association feels that it is inappropriate to label fructose and HFCS as "sugar." We are glad they feel this way. We hope manufacturers will let people know what sugars their products contain so that consumer choice can promote the greater use of 95-percent-fructose HFCS and pure fructose.

There are two very different ways that the sucrose industry can deal with fructose competition. One way is to launch a propaganda campaign for sucrose and against fructose, and attempt to get food laws and regulations passed that will interfere with the desires of the consumers for more fructose. The public relations personnel at the Sugar Association have already started along this route because that is all they know how to do. The other way to deal with this problem is to innovate, to improve their product with scientific research and development.

We suggest that instead of attacking the use of fructose and HFCS, the Sugar Association spend a little of its political and propaganda war chest on some science instead: genetic engineering. It would be technically simple to delete a gene required to make glucose in sugar cane and sugar beets. Sucrose is a disaccharide; it is a molecule of glucose joined to a molecule of fructose, hence it should be relatively easy to produce designer genes for sugar cane and beets that produce only fructose. Since this can be done by the straightforward classical technique of mutation-induced gene deletion or inactivation and since it does not require the use of recombinant DNA, there are no onerous and irrational regulations to delay the introduction of these new improved crops.

There is no reason for increasing fructose sales to threaten cane and beet sugar producers other than their own shortsightedness in not improving their traditional product. With pure fructose selling for about five times as much as pure sucrose, a major sucrose producer with the foresight to put its money into science instead of lobbying could make a lot of money instead of fighting a losing battle against the inevitable.

9

Appetite Control Without Willpower: Nutrients That Curb Appetite!

There are two very different ways you can reduce your caloric intake. One involves your using sheer willpower to eat less food, even though you actually feel like eating more. You constantly have to fight feelings of hunger and have to give up your favorite fattening foods. *The other way—our way—is to use nutrients and/or foods that have been shown to modify your appetite biochemically so that you feel full and satisfied with fewer calories.* You don't feel hungry, because you eat until you are full. You don't give up your favorite fattening foods. You will probably eat less of the latter, but it will not be because of willpower but because you have modified your appetite and really *feel* like eating less. Hard thinking certainly beats self-deprivation!

In this chapter we will describe how to use nutritional supplements and special snacks that specifically reduce carbohydrate craving and spoil your appetite, how to use other nutrients to make you feel just as full and satisfied with less food by triggering the same brain mechanism that makes you feel full after a big meal, and how to use nutritional supplements to help alter the times that you want to eat. We will also explain how to combat true food addiction with nutrient supplements and optional prescription drugs that are not diet pills. We will explain why eating less, whether due to self-deprivation or to appetite control, can reduce your intake of essential nutrients that help protect you from cancer, cardiovascular disease, and infectious disease, and how you can prevent this increased risk.

We will even tell you how one of the nutritional supplements discussed in this chapter has an additional benefit: it can give your sagging tummy an overnight lift by improving your abdominal muscle tone without any exercise at all!

Carbohydrate craving may be controlled with the essential nutrient amino acid tryptophan. Your brain makes serotonin from tryptophan (with the help of vitamins C and B-6). Judith Wurtman and Richard J. Wurtman, scientists at MIT, have found that craving for carbohydrates is controlled, in both animals and humans, by the quantity of serotonin in the brain. (Wurtman, 1981) Serotonin is an inhibitory neurotransmitter, a substance that brain cells use to communicate with each other which tends to inhibit brain cell firing. Serotonin is the brain substance that puts you to sleep at night. Serotonin also controls impulsive aggressive urges. The Wurtmans found that if you increase the amount of serotonin in your brain, you can reduce your subsequent desire to eat carbohydrates. It does not affect your hunger for protein.

Carbohydrates increase the entry of tryptophan into your brain. (Fernstrom, 1971; Fernstrom, 1978) Dr. Judith Wurtman reports that 200 calories of carbohydrates are an adequate snack for this purpose. (Wurtman, 1983) Your brain rapidly makes serotonin from the tryptophan, and your increased brain serotonin acts as a signal to your brain to inhibit further carbohydrate eating. (Wurtman, Moses, 1983) It also has another effect that you have probably experienced on many occasions: it tends to make you a bit sleepy. The common drowsiness that takes place after lunch *(never* give a lecture just after lunch!) is due to the carbohydrate-induced increase of brain serotonin. Two-hundred-calorie low-glycemic-index carbohydrate snacks can be eaten an hour or so prior to peak craving periods to suppress *subsequent* carbohydrate eating. This can be a major help to people whose principal binge eating is of carbohydrates. See *The Carbohydrate Craver's Diet,* published by Houghton Mifflin and Ballantine Books (which, unlike most diet books, was written by a nutrition scientist, Dr. Judith J. Wurtman of MIT).

The tryptophan and hence the serotonin in your brain can also be increased by taking a tryptophan supplement either on an empty stomach or—even more effective—along with a low-glycemic-index carbohydrate such as fructose.

The tryptophan can enter your brain more readily when your stomach contains no other protein or competing amino acids. The tryptophan has to compete to some extent with certain other amino acids (but not arginine or ornithine) to enter your brain by transport across your picky blood-brain barrier. By taking the tryptophan alone (or, better yet, with some fructose) about an hour before you anticipate substantial carbohydrate consumption, you avoid that competition and reduce your desire for carbohydrates during that meal. The use of tryptophan alone as a supplement was effective in suppressing carbohydrate snacking in 5 out of 11 subjects in one of the Wurtmans' studies. You will have to find out by self-experimentation whether it works for you. In the same 11 subjects, fenfluramine, one of the better prescription appetite control drugs, reduced carbohydrate consumption in 8 persons. (Wurtman, 1981)

Here is one of our formulas for controlling carbohydrate craving:

> fructose
> GTF (glucose tolerance factor) or trivalent chromium chloride
> niacin
> tryptophan
> vitamin B-6
> vitamin C

(The use of niacin to alter blood sugar regulation was described in the last chapter.)

See the Safety Appendix for suggested doses.

A common type of sugar/carbohydrate craving occurs in the premenstrual syndrome, also called PMS. PMS also frequently involves depression and irritability. (Smith, 1969) In a recent study, premenstrual syndrome was correlated with biochemical evidence indicating low levels of serotonin. (Taylor, 1982) Because of this biochemical change, one would expect an increased appetite for carbohydrates. We expect the following formula to be helpful in cases of premenstrual syndrome with carbohydrate cravings:

> fructose
> GTF (glucose tolerance factor) or trivalent chromium chloride
> inositol
> niacin
> niacinamide ascorbate (a vitamin B-3–vitamin C complex)

tryptophan
vitamin B-6
vitamin C

(Irritability and anxiety are common in PMS. We have dealt with this in three ways. First, the fructose, tryptophan, B-6, and C increase brain serotonin levels, reducing irritability and anxiety. Second, the nutrients inositol and niacinamide mildly activate the same brain receptors as Valium, thus decreasing anxiety. We feel that the complex niacinamide ascorbate gets more niacinamide across the blood-brain barrier than ordinary niacinamide. Third, the niacin helps keep blood sugar up, and the chromium also helps to improve blood sugar regulation.)

See the Safety Appendix for dosage information.

You've probably all heard your mother complain that you were spoiling your appetite by eating snacks before your meal. She was furious that you wouldn't be eating as much of her carefully prepared cooking. *Now that you are overweight, though, spoiling your appetite with the right type of snacking is a sensible strategy to help you attain your desired weight.* But you must choose your appetite-spoiling snack and the time that you eat it with care, or you might actually end up eating *more* calories. This could occur either because you ate a high-calorie snack and didn't reduce subsequent eating by at least that much, or because you ate a snack with a high glycemic index and the big insulin release and subsequent reactive hypoglycemia made you eat more, and store more of those calories as fat, too.

Your spoiler snack must *have a low glycemic index and be low in conventional fats. Fruit, unsweetened fruit juices, or fructose are good choices. The spoiler can be high in protein and/or high in a low-glycemic-index carbohydrate.* It can optionally contain a special type of fat called MCT, medium-chain triglycerides. MCTs will be discussed in Chapter 11, "Fat Metabolism: How You Can Change It."

A low-glycemic-index fructose snack before meals causes reduced subsequent food consumption compared to a high-glycemic-index glucose snack. In one study of 30 human volunteers, two different 192-calorie before-dinner drinks were prepared. Ten subjects got a drink containing 192 calories of glucose (about 2 ounces), while 10 others got a drink with the same number of calories, but containing fructose rather than glucose. Ten others got plain water. Two hours after the experimental drink, the subjects were presented with a sumptuous buffet and told to eat all they wanted. The people who had had the high-glycemic-index glucose drink ate 250 calories *more* per person on the average than the controls who got the water. The group receiving fructose ate 226 calories *less* per person on the average of the buffet than those who got only a glass of water. The fructose group actually ate a total of 476 calories less than the glucose group! This is why insulin is sometimes called the "hunger hormone." (Rodin, 1983; Rodin, 1984) It is a vivid demonstration of the difference between a high-glycemic-index snack and a low-glycemic-index snack.

There was another surprise, however. Since the fructose group ate 192 calories of fructose and subsequently ate 226 calories less of the buffet than the group that drank plain water, they experienced a net reduction of 34 calories. While this reduction in total calories is small, it is statistically significant. (Rodin, personal communication, 1985) *Eating the fructose snack actually decreased total caloric consumption (snack plus subsequent meal) by about 17 percent of the calories contained in the snack. You really can eat to lose!*

A high-protein snack taken well before a meal may be a useful way to reduce eating in that meal without resorting to willpower and experiencing hunger. In rats, protein-rich meals keep the rats satiated longer than meals of equal calories of either carbohydrates or fat. (Booth, unpublished observations, 1970) In humans, it has been found that diets containing only 13 percent protein result in constant hunger, whereas different diets proportionally low in carbohydrates or fat but high in protein were as satiating as normal food. In one study of human subjects, a protein-poor or protein-rich lunch was eaten. Two and a half to three hours later, a supplementary meal of average protein content was provided. Total caloric intake for the two meals was lower when the lunch had a high protein content. (Booth, 1970)

Here is our formula for an appetite-spoiling snack that includes some of the nutrients and foods we discuss in this chapter. We suggest you consume the snack formula about 1 to 2 hours before lunch and dinner, then eat your regular meal until you feel full and satisfied. It can also be used to make small snacks when you feel like eating between meals.

>   caffeine (optional)
>   fiber
>   fructose
>   fruit juice (unsweetened)
>   GTF (glucose tolerance factor) or trivalent chromium chloride
>   hydrolyzed protein (optional)
>   MCT (medium-chain triglycerides), which must include an antioxidant
>   protection system (optional)
>   niacin
>   tryptophan
>   vitamin B-6
>   vitamin C

See the Safety Appendix for recommended quantities.

See the Suppliers' Appendix for sources of similar products.

Normally we would not suggest simultaneously taking both a protein supplement and an amino acid supplement that has to enter your brain to be effective. With most individual amino acid supplements, the competition from the amino acids in the protein would markedly reduce brain transport of the expensive pure amino acid. Tryptophan, however, seems to have its own special transport system, along with a more general one that it shares with phenylalanine and tyrosine. The hydrolyzed protein will undoubtedly reduce your tryptophan uptake to some extent, but we think that it is still worthwhile in this particular application. The problem created by amino acid blood-brain barrier transport competition seems to vary from one individual to another. You will have to find out whether you get better results with or without the protein by experimenting on yourself.

Caffeine is an optional ingredient in our appetite-reducing snack. It is an effective anorectic (reduces appetite) and thermogenic agent (makes you burn calories for heat). Too much caffeine can cause "jitters," anxiety, and a subsequent letdown. You will note that caffeine is a common ingredient in nonprescription appetite reducers. As with other stimulants, you will tend to become tolerant to caffeine's central-nervous-system-stimulating effects, including its appetite-inhibiting effect.

What is it that makes you feel full and satisfied after a big meal? It is the release of certain natural substances in your brain such as chole-cystokinin, *also called CCK.* CCK is a nonsteroid polypeptide (many amino acids connected together to form a rather large molecule) hormone whose molecule contains 33 amino acids. It is released by your intestines when food enters them, and in the hypothalamus gland in your brain. Experimental studies indicate that it acts as a satiety signal (Smith, 1976; Gibbs, 1973; Gibbs, 1976); that is, it tells you that you are full and should stop eating. Rats that are given injections of CCK directly into the proper area of their brains act as though they feel full and satisfied, even if they are slowly dying of starvation. The CCK brain-injected rats will starve themselves to death next to a pile of their favorite food. Rats that have had surgical damage done to the part of the hypothalamus that has the CCK receptors behave in exactly the opposite manner. These rats are pathologically hungry; they will stuff themselves with food until they kill themselves.

WARNING: There are a number of alleged CCK products being sold at health food stores, department stores, and by mail order. They are NOT effective. See the next chapter, on diet pills, for further information.

Even though you cannot buy an effective CCK preparation, you can purchase effective CCK releasers. This is similar to the case of growth hormone; you can take nutrients that release the hormone, rather than taking the hormone itself as a drug.

Tryptophan and L-phenylalanine are good CCK releasers. (Meyer, 1972)

An essential nutrient amino acid, L-phenylalanine, *has been found to be a potent appetite inhibitor. It works by causing the release of CCK in your brain and also by naturally increasing your brain's nor-adrenaline.* Noradrenaline is your brain's version of adrenaline and is a stimulant chemically related to amphetamine. The anorectic (appetite-suppressing) effectiveness of L-phenylalanine has been demonstrated in both animals such as rats (Gibbs, 1973) and rhesus monkeys (Gibbs, 1976) and humans. (Morley, 1982; Smith, 1981) D-phenylalanine does not work for this purpose because it is only a very weak releaser of CCK.

The L-phenylalanine should be taken on an empty stomach because phenylalanine has to compete with other amino acids to get into your brain through your transport-limiting blood-brain barrier. If you have food containing protein in your stomach, less phenylalanine will get into your brain.

You can take the L-phenylalanine either just when you rise in the morning or just before retiring for bed, depending on your rate of conversion of phenylalanine to noradrenaline. Some people are fast converters of phenylalanine to noradrenaline; if they take it at bedtime, they wake up too early and can't get back to sleep. Fast converters should take it as soon as they wake up. If a slow converter takes the phenylalanine in the morning, it may still be coming on strong at bedtime, causing insomnia. Slow converters should take it at bedtime so that it starts to take effect in the morning and is wearing off at bedtime. If you find you develop insomnia when taking the L-phenylalanine in the morning, try taking it just before going to bed. Insomnia may also be a sign of an excessively high dose.

We have found that tryptophan supplements (which are converted to the inhibitory neurotransmitter serotonin) are very useful for preventing irritability and excessive aggressiveness, which can be enhanced in some people, especially some males, by L-phenylalanine.

Vitamins C and B-6 are necessary cofactors for converting phenylalanine to noradrenaline (and also for converting tryptophan to serotonin); if you have marginal supplies of these nutrients, the anorectic and stimulating effects of phenylalanine will be reduced. Moreover, if you have been taking little or none of these vitamins and have found a satisfactory dose of phenylalanine, and then start taking a high potency C- and B-6–containing supplement, you will find that the same amount of phenylalanine is now an overdose because of your newly improved conversion efficiency.

D-phenylalanine, DL-phenylalanine, and L-phenylalanine are unlike stimulants such as amphetamine and phenylpropanolamine, which cause you to use up your noradrenaline faster than you can make it, thereby causing its depletion and an eventual development of tolerance, crash, depression, and subsequent abnormally great rebound hunger. Phenylalanine is made into noradrenaline, which is then released; there is no depletion. In fact, L-phenylalanine at 100 to 500 milligrams per day for two weeks has been successfully used in a scientific experiment on human amphetamine abusers to replete their amphetamine-depleted noradrenaline and terminate their depressive crash. A molecule of the synthetic D-phenylalanine is the mirror image of a molecule of the natural L-phenylalanine. DL-phenylalanine is an equal mixture of D-phenylalanine and L-phenylalanine; this mixture is recognized as a food by the FDA, as is the natural essential nutrient L-phenylalanine. When we refer to "phenylalanine," we mean all three.

Because phenylalanine is a noradrenaline precursor and repleter instead of a depleter, you will not have the usual problems with the rapid and extensive development of tolerance. Some of our experimental subjects have been successfully using L-phenylalanine every day as an anorectic for 1½ years without loss of effectiveness or having to increase their dose.

WARNING: Before you take phenylalanine supplements, there is dosage data and several important warnings in our Safety Appendix which you should read and heed. Dosage must be individualized. Even though phenylalanine is a nutrient, there are certain medical conditions and drugs with which phenylalanine could be extremely dangerous. Do not take phenylalanine supplements while using ephedrine or phenylpropanolamine.

It is well known that depression can result in overeating and overweight in some people. Both the essential nutrient amino acid phenylalanine and the nutrient amino acid tyrosine are proven antidepressants. (Gelenberg, 1980; Borison, 1978) In one study of human subjects, 100 to 500 milligrams of L-phenylalanine a day for two weeks resulted in 80 percent success in relieving depression. Tyrosine is effective at similar doses. These are helpful in cases of anergic depression, where you are tired, drag yourself around, and can't get anything done.

The other major type of depression, where you are depressed but angry, is often responsive to the nutrient amino acid tryptophan. In one case we saw, a friend had developed an agitated, angry depression and had beaten his girlfriend and was attacking himself severely. He was afraid that he might kill himself. He might have done so if the police had not intervened. One dose of 3 grams of tryptophan and he felt far better within an hour. See our *Life Extension: A*

Practical Scientific Approach and *The Life Extension Companion* for further data on the use of these nutrients in depression.

WARNING: Depression can be caused by a variety of serious illnesses such as hypothyroidism. If you are depressed, you must not assume that phenylalanine and/or tryptophan is an appropriate therapy; have your physician perform a complete physical exam. An incorrect self-diagnosis could be very hazardous to your health. Do not use phenylalanine or tyrosine in cases of agitated or irritable depression, since this may make the agitation and anger worse. Before using phenylalanine, tyrosine, or tryptophan for depression or any other purpose, see the Safety Appendix. You will also find data there on how to make the individual dose adjustments that will be required. Do not take phenylalanine or tyrosine supplements while using ephedrine or phenylpropanolamine.

Some people seem to become addicted to food. Like classical heroin addiction, this addiction includes withdrawal symptoms such as anxiety and restlessness. Food addicts don't eat because they feel hungry in the normal sense; indeed, their stomachs may be uncomfortably full, yet their cravings drive them to stuff more food down their throats. The food addict continues to eat in order to stave off the sickness that comes with withdrawal. This type of food addiction is biochemical, not psychiatric, in nature. Fortunately, there are simple technological fixes for the biochemical "appetite" that drives this type of food addict. (True psychiatric eating disorders still must be dealt with by traditional methods.)

It is well known now that endorphins, the brain's versions of opiates like heroin, are involved in the food satiation system. (McCarthy, 1981) Animals and humans given naloxone, which blocks endorphin receptors (so the endorphins have no effect), reduce their eating because the kick from it is blocked. Eating may act like a little internal hypodermic syringe of heroin for some people who have a hard time resisting the urge to repeatedly inject themselves. Naloxone (a very safe prescription drug) blocks the effects of opiates and endorphins. Naloxone cannot be taken orally, but it can be taken by injection or insufflation (snorting the powder up one's nose).

The endorphin satiation receptors are different from the CCK satiation receptors and are not affected by the CCK releaser L-phenylalanine.

Stress is another factor that has been observed to cause some people to eat more. In rats, stressing them induced eating. (Morley, 1980) When they were then given naloxone, the rats behaved exactly as if they were being withdrawn from opiates: they got the "shakes," showing that the natural opiate system had been chronically activated by the stress.

A new opiate antagonist called naltrexone can be taken orally and is being used by ex–heroin addicts to help them stay off opiates. New methods of administration for these opiate antagonist drugs are being developed. One, a slowly diffusing patch, will be available soon for use by heroin addicts who are trying to remain dope-free. Before attempting to use naloxone or naltrexone, however, be sure to see our Safety Appendix. These are prescription drugs and, although very safe, must be used under a physician's supervision.

Anyone whose eating seems addictive should consider asking their physician if they can try an opiate antagonist. If your eating problem does not involve addiction in your endorphin system, you will feel no effects, except, according to one paper (Cohen, 1985), a reduction in appetite. If your eating is indeed truly addictive in the sense of involving your endorphin system, the use of an opiate antagonist will cause some degree of opiate addiction withdrawal symptoms. These will last no more than two weeks, after which you will be free of this addictive eating so long as you take the antagonist. Even short-term (a couple of months) use of an opiate antagonist may be very useful in helping you break old ingrained habits and make a long-term change in your eating behavior.

Another possible way to handle food addiction is to block the aversive sensations of withdrawal by taking the anti–high blood pressure drug clonidine. Clonidine has been found effective in reducing or eliminating withdrawal symptoms in heroin *(JAMA,* 1980), alcohol (Wilkins, 1983), and cigarette (Glassman, 1984) addiction. It is a logical drug for food-addicted overweight people who also have high blood pressure. An added benefit is that it increases growth hormone output, particularly in the obese. This is a powerful prescription drug and should be used only under the supervision of a physician.

Taking D-phenylalanine or DL-phenylalanine with vitamin C is one way to maintain high levels of brain endorphins (and the euphoria that often goes with them). (Ehrenpreis, 1979) These nutrients reduce the rate at which certain enzymes break down the endorphins in your brain. They may be helpful weight loss aids to people who are addicted to eating and eat to keep their brain endorphin levels high by providing a low-calorie method of accomplishing the same result. Remember that L-phenylalanine does not produce this effect.

It may seem odd that we suggest dealing with food addiction by either blocking the endorphin receptors or assisting them. *Even though the effects are the opposite, they both disconnect the endorphin reward system from eating.* Both approaches, moreover, have been successfully used in human heroin addicts to help them stay off opiates. In a similar vein, clonidine's blocking of withdrawal symptoms disconnects relief from these unpleasant feelings from the act of eating. *We would like to see these methods used as adjuncts in medically supervised behavior change programs for food addicts.* Unfortunately, most good medically supervised weight loss clinics are almost exclusively oriented toward behavior therapy, with the possible use of traditional diet pills as an adjunct. We know of no clinics that take advantage of these techniques, in spite of their having been in the scientific and human clinical literature for years.

Fiber is yet another food that can be used to modify your appetite. Fiber, even though it cannot be digested, is an important nutrient that may lower your risk of colon cancer, a major killer. (Reddy, 1983) Fiber reduces the amount of time food spends in your digestive tract by increasing its bulk and so helping to push it through. In Western societies, people typically have much longer digestive tract transit times (about three days) than do people in more primitive societies that eat a lot of fiber (about one day). (Scala, 1975) Because there are a lot of mutagens (mutation-causing substances) and carcinogens (cancer-causing substances) naturally present in food and others are created in your digestive tract, it is advisable to get old food out of the digestive tract promptly. The longer it stays inside, the more mutagenic and carcinogenic it is likely to become. Fiber is a very good solution for this problem. Because food is exposed to the gastrointestinal tract for a shorter time when there is plenty of fiber, some of the food's calories may not be absorbed. See below for an easy way to measure your own digestive tract transit time. *This issue of gut transit time is of great importance to dieters.* If it is three days on a typical 2500-calorie-per-day low-fiber Western diet, what is it going to be on a 1000-calorie-a-day diet? It will, of course, be much longer than the already too risky three days and might even be over a week. Fortunately, fiber and choline plus vitamin B-5 supplements can deal with this problem very effectively.

We have seen some evidence that fiber itself will actually help cause a loss of weight. Obese male college students were used in an 8-week study that involved voluntary unenforced caloric restriction. A wide variety of foods were eaten, including 12 slices of bread per day. The subjects could eat as much food as they wanted, but were also told that they would have to reduce their caloric intake in order to lose weight. The 7 subjects who received regular white bread lost an average of 13.9 pounds. The 6 subjects who received special high-fiber bread lost an average of 19.4 pounds. The subjects did not know whether they received the regular bread or the high-fiber bread. The white bread contained 1 gram of fiber per day, while the high-fiber bread provided 25.5 grams per day. Because of the high-fiber content that partially replaced flour, the special bread had 30 percent fewer calories per slice. The weight loss in the two groups was entirely due to reduced caloric intake, but it was easier for the high-fiber group to cut their calories, so they ate less than the other group. (Mickelsen, 1979)

Fiber can certainly help to make you feel full with less food—at least for a while. Chinese food is generally high in vegetable fiber; it fills you up but leaves you hungry a few hours later. Scientific experiments with humans on 800-calorie-per-day diets showed that a high fiber content resulted in greater satiety and feelings of fullness with less hunger compared to a low-fiber diet. (Anderson, 1980) *You can use fiber to make yourself feel full and to shift your hunger to a different time. Fiber can also be used to slow the absorption of nutrients from your gut.*

These properties are valuable in your fat loss program because they can help you ameliorate the big insulin peak that is usually released if you absorb a lot of typical low-fiber high-glycemic-index American food in a short time, and they can help you adapt your hunger to a more desirable schedule. If you feel hungry before going to bed, fiber can help make your stomach feel full, while a small fructose-containing snack will help deal with the biochemical aspects of your hunger, if necessary. Tomorrow morning, you might eat a bigger breakfast than if you had had a big high-calorie meal before bedtime, but a big breakfast won't wreak havoc on your very important nighttime GH release peak. If that big meal before bedtime has a high glycemic index, it will probably induce you to eat more in the morning than if you had eaten nothing at all at bedtime.

Caution: Fiber absorbs vitamins and minerals, too; the degree that it does this depends upon the particular type of fiber. It is most prudent, if you plan to ingest a lot of fiber, to take a high-potency multi-vitamin-mineral supplement at the right time *to prevent deficiencies.* See the Safety Appendix for our suggested supplement.

Take your fiber supplement anywhere from 1 to 2 hours before a meal, to make your stomach feel full and to decrease digestive tract transit time. Take your multi-vitamin-mineral supplement immediately after *the meal to limit its exposure to the fiber that might otherwise absorb some of it.* If you want to reduce the glycemic index of the meal, you will have to take the fiber with it, and use a vitamin-mineral supplement to make up for the losses.

A suitable fiber supplement would be the fiber found in "dried brewers' grains." This is what is left (along with some protein) after the grain has been used in brewing beer, the yeast having eaten most of the digestible sugars and starches. Rice and oat bran are good fibers, too. Citrus pulp and pectin are also good. The latter are by-products of the frozen orange juice industry; unfortunately, most people do not like a thick fiber-filled orange juice.

The soluble fibers that make a viscous solution, such as pectin and oat bran, are the most effective in slowing the absorption of carbohydrates, and thereby reducing their glycemic indices. Indeed, they are so effective that they have been used in diabetic diets for this purpose. These fibers also are the most effective in reducing serum LDL cholesterol. (Kirby, 1981; Anderson, Chen, 1979; Anderson, Chen, 1980; Anderson in Spiller, 1980; Jenkins, 1975; Anderson, Ward, 1979; Kiehm, 1976; Vetter, 1984)

We suggest that you use a mixture of different fibers, since they have somewhat different protective properties. *The human studies* that demonstrated a reduction in colon cancer involved the consumption of fiber from many different foods.

Caution: See the Safety Appendix before you purchase a fiber supplement. Some of them may not be wholesome.

To summarize the benefits of fiber:

1. It fills your stomach, delaying hunger, allowing you more flexibility in meal scheduling.

2. It slows absorption of nutrients, including sugars, and hence can lower the effective glycemic index of carbohydrates ingested with it.

3. It can reduce serum LDL cholesterol, a cardiovascular risk factor.

4. It helps promote weight loss by making caloric restriction easier.

5. It cleans out your digestive tract.

6. It may reduce your risk of colon cancer and possibly other gut cancers. The National Cancer Institute recommends 25 to 35 grams of fiber per day.

WARNING: It is also possible to speed food out of the colon with enemas. The latter are frequently recommended in so-called health books. The problem with this technique is that a lot of vital electrolytes, such as potassium, are lost with the other contents of the digestive tract. *Losing a sufficient quantity of potassium by frequent enemas could potentially lead to lethal cardiac fibrillation, where the heart quivers but does not pump blood.* You die within a few minutes unless a paramedic gets to you with a defibrillator. Fiber does not have this risk.

Choline, a nutrient found in fish and available as an inexpensive supplement, can be a helpful adjunct to an appetite modification program. Choline is made into acetylcholine by both your body and your brain, with the help of vitamin B-5. Acetylcholine increases the muscle tone of your digestive tract and reduces gut transit time by speeding peristalsis (the wavelike contractions that move food through your gut).

You can measure your digestive tract transit time by a simple procedure. Take about 25,000 I.U. (International Units) of beta-carotene (an orange-colored nutrient found in carrots and available as a nutritional supplement in health food stores) with your fattiest meal of the day (the beta-carotene dissolves in fat). Then keep track of how long it takes for your feces to emerge orange-colored. The measurement is not a true measure of your digestive tract transit time if you have diarrhea during that time. (Beta-carotene is a very desirable supplement for regular use in your general health maintenance and enhancement program. It can significantly reduce the incidence of gut and skin cancer and is amazingly effective at preventing smoking-induced lung cancer. [Shekelle, 1981] See our *Life Extension: A Practical Scientific Approach* and *The Life Extension Companion.)*

Choline may have another use in your fat loss program. There is some evidence that choline or cholinergics (similar substances that stimulate the same cell receptors) may act peripherally (in your body) as modulators of appetite. (Garattini, 1981; Seiden, 1977) This view is based on animal experiments in which cholinergic agonists (substances that act like acetylcholine or which increase its effects) increase low rates and decrease high rates of bar pressing to earn a food reward. In human terms, this suggests that more acetylcholine may make you more likely to spread your eating out over time and reduce your desire to gorge on a huge amount of food all at once. This is desirable in your fat loss program.

Choline has another big benefit for people with flabby stomachs. Many people with flabby stomachs do not have as much fat over their abdominal muscles as they think. Their problem is, at least in part, poor abdominal muscle tone. Vigorous exercise of these abdominal muscles will slowly improve their muscle tone. *Supplements of choline chloride with vitamin B-5 can quickly raise your muscle tone with no exercise at all.* In fact, the common choline overdose symptoms—muscle tension headache or tight muscles, especially in the neck and shoulders—are due to too much muscle tone. See the Safety Appendix for suggested dose.

Growth hormone is reported to have anorectic (appetite-suppressing) effects. (Cahill, 1979) This is an added bonus to the use of growth-hormone-releasing nutrients that we described in Chapter 5.

One way of attempting to control excess carbohydrate eating that does NOT seem to work in the long run is to go on a low-carbohydrate diet. The ketosis induced by a strict low-carbohydrate diet can temporarily reduce your carbohydrate craving, but the craving will come back with a vengeance as soon as you deviate from the diet. After laboratory animals have been on a low-carbohydrate diet for a few weeks and then allowed once again to eat as much carbohydrate as they desire, they responded by binging, eating more than they otherwise would. (Wurtman, Moses, 1983) Sound familiar?

In the last chapter we have already described how you can use the B vitamin niacin to reduce sugar and carbohydrate craving by altering your blood sugar regulation. We also described how chromium supplements and low-glycemic-index snacks and foods decrease the release of insulin, which has been called a hunger hormone, further improving your blood sugar regulation and reducing carbohydrate craving even further. In addition, we described the use of a mixture of vitamin B-1, vitamin C, and the nutrient amino acid cysteine to inactivate excess insulin during hypoglycemic episodes.

Wouldn't you rather control your caloric intake and composition by altering your appetite and feeling full than by forcing yourself to eat less and being hungry? You now have the tools to do just that.

Caution: Reduced food consumption is likely to reduce your intake of nutrients such as beta-carotene, selenium, zinc, and vitamins A, C, and E that help to protect you from cancer, cardiovascular disease, and infectious disease. See the Safety Appendix for our suggested high-potency multivitamin-mineral supplement formula. If you would like to learn more about the protective effects of nutrients, see our *Life Extension: A Practical Scientific Approach* and *The Life Extension Companion* for further data.

10

Diet Pills:
What You Need to Know

It is easy to see why diet pills are so popular. Taking a pill for weight control is very simple and almost effortless; it can be done without hard work or hard thinking. For many years the most widely used diet pill was amphetamine, with potentially serious side effects, including addiction and psychosis. Modern prescription diet pills are safer and about as effective, yet they are not without risks. We describe many methods in this book that you can use to lose fat safely and effectively without taking these pills. But even though you don't *need* to use them anymore, we recognize that many people will continue to use diet pills, so we include this chapter to describe the limits to their effectiveness and their potential risks.

This chapter contains information about the most popular appetite control remedies, including caffeine and phenylpropanolamine (nonprescription), prescription diet pills, other prescription drugs being used experimentally for appetite control (even though approved by the FDA only for other purposes), and natural hormones that have been used experimentally as aids to weight loss.

NONPRESCRIPTION DIET DRUGS

Caffeine is a thermogenic agent—that is, it increases the amount of fuel used by your body to create body heat (calories). (Himms-Hagen, 1981) Caffeine has been measured, at doses equivalent to about 2–6 cups of coffee to produce a slight (10 percent) increase in basal metabolic rate in people. See Chapter 12, "Thermogenesis: The Cool

Way to Lose Fat" for more information on caffeine as a thermogenic aid.

Caffeine is also an *anorectic* (appetite depressant). Note that many nonprescription anorectic products contain caffeine, usually in combination with phenylpropanolamine. Caffeine, in therapeutic doses, can increase circulating levels of natural chemical messengers called catecholamines (such as adrenaline, noradrenaline), which are themselves anorectics. The per-capita intake of caffeine in the United States is above 200 mg daily. (1000 mg = 1000 milligrams = 1 gram) A cup of coffee supplies about 85 mg of caffeine, a cup of tea provides about 50 mg of caffeine and 1 mg of theophylline, a cup of cocoa contains 250 mg of theobromine and 5 mg of caffeine, and a 12-ounce cola drink contains about 50 mg of caffeine, half of which is added by the manufacturer.

Many herbal diet aids contain very large amounts of caffeine; far more plants than just coffee and tea contain caffeine. Common caffeine-containing herbs and plants that are frequently used in these preparations include: kola (nuts from *Cola nitida* or from other *Cola* and *Sterculiaceae* species, also called Sudan coffee, Bissy nuts, gooroo nuts, guru nuts); guarana (seeds from *Paullinia cupana* var. *sorbilis,* which usually contains 2.7 to 5.8 percent caffeine, plus other psychoactive drugs) (Henman, 1982); yoco (bark from *Paullinia yoco);* and mate (from *Ilex paraguariensis).* The amount of caffeine in a particular herb can vary widely from batch to batch, so each batch should be quantitatively analyzed and the herb quantities adjusted to give a standard caffeine dose which should be stated on the package. Unfortunately this is rarely if ever done. To make matters even worse, very few herbals that contain caffeine are labeled as such, and very few herb users know what is in their herbs.

Theophylline is chemically very similar to caffeine, and its effects are also similar. Theophylline is used therapeutically as a treatment for bronchial asthma. Overdoses of it produce a more profound and potentially dangerous stimulation of the central nervous system (brain and spinal cord) than does caffeine. Ordinary tea contains physiologically active amounts of this drug. (Rall, 1980)

Theophylline is an anorectic in mice made obese by damage to their hypothalamus (theophylline causes a 13 percent reduction in voluntary food intake) and in genetically obese rats (9 percent reduction), but it did not affect appetite in lean mice, or normal mice and rats made obese with a diet having far higher fat and higher protein content than is normal for these rodents. Tolerance to theophylline's anorectic effects seemed to develop after 2 or 3 weeks of continuous use. Despite the fact that it did not affect their appetites, theophylline nevertheless caused dramatic fat loss in both normal mice (which had only 41 percent of the body fat of the control group!) and rats (which had only 50 percent of the body fat of the control group!) that had become obese on the high-fat diet. The obese animals continued to eat the high-fat diet without reduction in appetite while they lost a great deal of body fat compared to the control group, which ate the same obesity-inducing high-fat diet. This fat loss occurred because theophylline is a potent thermogenic drug. Tolerance to thermogenic effects was not reported. (Dulloo, 1984) (See Chapter 12 on thermogenesis for more information on theophylline.) See the Safety Appendix before taking theophylline.

Theobromine, although chemically related to caffeine, has almost no central nervous system stimulating activity. It probably has no value as an anorectic.

Ephedrine is very similar to the natural hormones adrenaline and noradrenaline, and also like the nonprescription anorectic phenylpropanolamine. Some herbal diet preparations contain ephedrine, though they are rarely labeled as such. Ephedrine is an anorectic, and it is a powerful thermogenic agent as well. (See Chapter 12 on thermogenesis for more information on ephedrine and ephedrine-containing herbs.)

Warning: Do not use an ephedrine-containing product while taking phenylalanine or tyrosine supplements. Before using an ephedrine-containing herb, be sure to see the Safety Appendix!

Phenylpropanolamine is a sympathomimetic (adrenaline-like) drug that is about as potent as adrenaline in its pharmacological properties but produces less central nervous system stimulation. It is chemically related to amphetamine. It is a popular anorectic that is available without prescription. It has been found to decrease feeding in rats without increasing locomotion (body movement). Human studies have shown that the drug can be used to lose weight effectively. (Silverstone, in Silverstone, 1982) It also has thermogenic properties. After a few weeks, however, tolerance develops.

Tolerance occurs with phenylpropanolamine because the brain is depleted of noradrenaline by it. Phenylpropanolamine blocks the reuptake of noradrenaline (recycling of used noradrenaline), which temporarily leads to extra noradrenaline stimulation in the synapses (gaps between nerve cells), but which eventually depletes the supply. You will note that the instructions on packages of phenylpropanolamine anorectics specify only temporary use. This is the reason.

Warning: Do not use a phenylpropanolamine-containing product while taking phenylalanine or tyrosine supplements.

PRESCRIPTION DIET DRUGS

An increasing variety of prescription drugs for the control of body weight are in widespread use. The rationale behind weight control drugs is that, properly used, they can either reduce energy intake (food) or increase energy output (heat and work). A kilogram (2.2 pounds) of fat represents 7000 calories. Thus if a person could increase the gap between energy intake and energy output to only 500 calories a day, the fat weight loss per week would be a half kilogram (1.1 pounds) if all the losses were fat. (Remember that fat loss rather than weight loss should be your goal. Without vigorous exercise or growth hormone releasers, about 25 percent of your weight loss would be expected to be lean body mass). A half kilogram of weight lost a week doesn't sound like a lot, but in a year this would represent a loss of 57 pounds. The modern prescription drugs we discuss have been designed to help make it easier for overweight people to lose weight. Most of these powerful drugs are appetite suppressants. They should be used only under a doctor's supervision. Do *not* exceed your doctor's prescribed dosage or duration of use.

Like any other drugs, the prescription drug weight-reducing aids represent a compromise between efficacy (causing a loss of weight) and unwanted side effects (such as insomnia). No drug of any kind is perfectly safe, and that is true for this class of drugs as well. The anorectic drugs we discuss below are for temporary use. Most of the weight loss takes place during the first three months or less. Unfortunately the weight loss also tends to be temporary. Rapid regain usually takes place after the anorectic drug is discontinued.

The most commonly used anorectic prescription drugs include amphetamines, phenmetrazine, phentermine, diethylpropion, mazindol, and fenfluramine. (See the review by Silverstone in Silverstone, 1982.) These and the other drug names given below are the generic names; the name on your pill bottle may be a trademarked brand name. Your doctor or pharmacist will be glad to tell you the generic name of your medication. You can also find out what you have in your pill bottle by looking it up in the *Physicians' Desk Reference* (published by the Medical Economics Company, with a new edition every year), which you can find at any public library and most large book stores. This reference book will also give you very detailed information about side effects and drug interactions. We strongly urge any user of prescription drugs to buy a copy of this book and look up all their medications.

Amphetamine (and the closely related dexamphetamine and methamphetamine) works by increasing brain release of noradrenaline (the brain's version of adrenaline) and blocking its reuptake (preventing recycling of used noradrenaline). In the short term, its effects include appetite suppression, as well as increased alertness, elevation of mood, and lowered fatigue. After a short time, however, the brain is depleted of noradrenaline, and amphetamine no longer produces these effects. Depression and rebound eating may result when the drug is discontinued. Common side effects of amphetamine use include insomnia, restlessness, irritability, tremor, excess perspiration, dry mouth, epigastric discomfort, constipation, and palpitations. Chronic amphetamine abuse can lead to psychological (including amphetamine psychosis) as well as medical problems. It is very habit-forming for many people. We recommend against using it, even temporarily. Although few doctors still prescribe amphetamine as an anorectic, it is so readily available in the drug black market that it is unfortunately easier to get than the much better modern prescription anorectics, which are generally of less interest to the illicit drug user!

Ciclazindol is a prescription drug weight loss aid which may not yet be available in the United States, although it is used abroad. It is an antidepressant chemically related to mazindol but not to amphetamine. This substance causes weight loss in people. One proposed mechanism for this effect is an activation of thermogenesis (burning excess calories for heat) in brown adipose (fat) tissue. (Rothwell, 1981) See Chapter 12, "Thermogenesis: The Cool Way to Lose Fat" in this book. Ciclazindol was effective in blocking noradrenaline uptake (recycling of used noradrenaline) in brown adipose tissue by more than 90 percent, which was greater than fenfluramine, imipramine, and dexamphetamine. It blocked uptake in brown adipose tissue more than it blocked uptake in brain tissue, which is very desirable in a weight loss drug. Blocking noradrenaline uptake in the brain produces amphetamine-like stimulant effects. Ciclazindol was effective at doses at which it did not cause CNS (brain and spinal cord) stimulation. Side effects include tiredness, headaches, and dizziness. See "Mazindol" for adverse interactions with nutrients and other drugs, contraindications, and side effects.

Diethylpropion is related to amphetamine. It has effects similar to amphetamine, but the heart and blood-pressure effects are less severe. In people the stimulant effects of diethylpropion on the brain and spinal cord are only 10–20 percent those of amphetamine. Adverse drug effects have been reported. They are usually mild and include restlessness, insomnia, constipation, and dry mouth. Unlike when amphetamine is used, psychosis following use of diethylpropion is rare.

Fenfluramine has central sedative rather than stimulant effects, unlike amphetamine and amphetamine-like drugs. Fenfluramine has a selective effect on eating behavior, causing a decrease in carbohydrate consumption. (Wurtman, 1981) It is thought that fenfluramine enhances serotonergic neurotransmission—that is, increases the effectiveness of serotonin. Serotonin is known to control carbohydrate cravings. The drug has no amphetamine-like central stimulant effects. Fenfluramine also has side effects which commonly include dry mouth, drowsiness, lethargy, light-headedness, and diarrhea. In some people, it may produce nausea, irritability, depression, and depersonalization. It may cause insomnia with nightmares. The drug should be reduced gradually rather than all of a sudden, to avoid the possibility of depression in some sensitive persons.

Mazindol is not a chemical relative of amphetamine, which makes it unusual among the anorectic drugs. But its properties are similar. It does not have much of a stimulant effect. However, it may potentiate the effects of catecholamines (adrenaline or noradrenaline) and should therefore never be used with sympathomimetic (adrenaline-like) drugs, catecholamine precursors (substances made into catecholamines, such as phenylalanine and tyrosine), or certain antihypertensive compounds. It is contraindicated (must not be used) in hyperthyroidism, anxiety states, and peptic ulcers. Annoying side effects are fairly common and include insomnia, nervousness, dizziness, dry mouth, nausea, and constipation.

Phenmetrazine, also related to amphetamine, has similar anorectic effects to amphetamine, though it has less of a stimulating effect on the central nervous system and heart. Its side effects are similar to amphetamine. This drug should not be used in anxiety states and thyrotoxicosis (hyperthyroidism). Adverse effects include restlessness, irritability, insomnia, tremor, tachycardia, dry mouth, and epigastric discomfort. Psychotic states indistinguishable from amphetamine psychosis have been reported.

Phentermine, also related to amphetamine, is a weak sympathomimetic (adrenaline-like) drug with less stimulant effect than amphetamine. It is about as strong an anorectic as dexamphetamine. Adverse drug effects can occur but are unlikely to require discontinuing the drug. These include insomnia, nervousness, nausea, dry mouth, and constipation.

The evidence suggests that these drugs are capable, at least in the short run, of promoting a significant weight loss. An analysis performed for the Food and Drug Administration found the average weight loss reported in 160 double-blind placebo-controlled studies was about 1/2 pound per week. (Munro in Silverstone, 1982) Even though most of these were short-term studies, nearly half of the experimental subjects dropped out, presumably due to unpleasant side effects. The drugs mentioned previously are roughly equal in their ability to produce a weight loss.

After a relatively short period of use, these drugs no longer depress appetite. It may be possible to overcome the tolerance that develops for the anorectic effects of amphetamine and the amphetamine-like drugs by taking phenylalanine or tyrosine supplements well after you stop using the amphetamine-like drug. Phenylalanine or tyrosine can be used by the brain to synthesize a new supply of noradrenaline, which is depleted by long-term use of amphetamine like drugs.

Warning: The combination of phenylalanine or tyrosine supplementation and anorectic drug use is potentially dangerous (high blood pressure 'and cardiac arrhythmia being two potential problems) and should be done only *under a doctor's close supervision.*

The use of phenylalanine or tyrosine starting several days after discontinuing the amphetamine-like anorectic drug is much less potentially hazardous for most people and may be able to prevent post-drug depression and rebound eating by replenishing your depleted noradrenaline stores. Before using phenylalanine or tyrosine supplements for any purpose, read our Safety Appendix. Increases in blood pressure may occur in a few sensitive individuals, especially when using phenylalanine during stressful situations. We suggest that even healthy people take their blood pressure twice a day for at least a week when they start using phenylalanine or tyrosine supplements, to make sure that they are not unusually sensitive to these effects.

DRUGS USED FOR WEIGHT LOSS BUT NOT FDA-APPROVED FOR THIS PURPOSE

Anabolic steroids are chemical relatives of the male steroid sex hormone testosterone. They promote muscle gain and fat loss, possibly by their synergistic effect with growth hormone. Growth hormone works without anabolic steroids, but anabolic steroids may not work as anabolics without growth hormone. Abuse of anabolic steroids can cause a great deal of damage, especially to your liver, kidneys, and cardiovascular system. The orally active anabolics are readily available on the black market, but they are also most likely to cause liver damage. We strongly recommend *against* their use for fat loss. If you feel the slightest urge to use them, rush on out to your nearest book store and buy a copy of *Death in the Locker Room* (Icarus Press, 1984), coauthored (with Goldman) by the same Dr. Klatz who wrote the "Physician's Foreword" and part of the "Changing Your Behavior" chapter (13) in this book. Reading this book should eliminate any temptation that you may have felt about using anabolic steroids.

We can think of only one reasonable use of anabolic steroids in fat loss: If a man has abnormally low levels of testosterone as determined by a clinical laboratory test, it is usually quite appropriate for his physician to raise those levels up to the normal range with biweekly or monthly injections of testosterone cypionate.

Antiestrogens are compounds that block one's estrogen receptors. Estrogens are female steroid sex hormones. Antiestrogens are widely used to block the effects of natural estrogens in women who have estrogen-sensitive cancers. In effect they temporarily mimic menopause. Men have estrogen receptors too, and some of them seem to be related to the differences in fat deposition patterns between males and females. Some male athletes and bodybuilders have been using a new nonsteroid antiestrogen to fight fat accumulation in their thighs and hips, areas of particularly great fat deposition in women.

Two types of antiestrogens are available. The older ones are derivatives of the male hormone testosterone, and are similar to and include the anabolic steroids. The new antiestrogen tamoxifen citrate is not a steroid hormone and is not chemically related to testosterone and the other anabolic steroids. Although we have had glowing reports on its effects from an Olympic athlete friend of ours, we certainly cannot recommend it for general use due to lack of knowledge of its long-term effects in men, and due to its known side effects. (See the *Physicians' Desk Reference.)* Nevertheless it is likely to be safer than the anabolic steroids, and we think that there may be a real future in developing this class of drugs for use as prescription fat loss aids, at least for men. Women considering this class of drugs should be aware that the drugs will cause atrophy of their breasts and genitals and cancel the protective effects that their estrogens have against cardiovascular disease, thereby giving them a cardiovascular risk factor similar to men's.

Bromocriptine given alone in one study without dietary restriction did not cause weight loss. (Harrower, 1977) However, fat loss can occur without weight loss with these growth hormone releasers. Appetite suppression did occur.

Cholecystokinin (CCK), a polypeptide hormone released in the brain and intestines in response to food is believed to be a satiation signal. It makes you feel full and satisfied, so you stop eating. Injected CCK has been shown to decrease food intake in rats (Gibbs, 1973), rhesus monkeys (Gibbs, 1976), and in humans. (Morley, 1982; Smith, 1981)

Caution: Products that are alleged to contain CCK are being sold in health food stores, department stores, and by mail. We are very doubtful that these nutrient-supplement manufacturers have actually either synthesized or extracted and purified a 33-amino-acid polypeptide. These are very technically complex and expensive processes. The vendors are probably just buying it from some other supplier. Moreover few if any manufacturers of nutrient-supplement products have the analytical capability to test the alleged CCK that someone is selling to them to see if it is really CCK. But even if they have obtained real CCK, there is no evidence that the oral CCK products work. When taken orally, CCK is digested like a piece of steak in your stomach. Oral administration is not the same as the production of CCK by your gut tissue and its direct release to the vagus nerve, which takes it to the hypothalamus in your brain. Don't buy these products.

A CCK anorectic is a good idea, in principle, but today's versions just won't do the job. It will probably have to be a nasal spray, as is the case with the prescription polypeptide pituitary hormone vasopressin. At this time there is no evidence that a CCK nasal spray would work; its molecule is four times as large as that of vasopressin and might not be able to get into the brain tissue. Moreover the proper dose and safety precautions have not yet been determined. Someday CCK may be a useful satisfaction-producing anorectic; what you can get now is a rip-off. Remember, though, that L-phenylalanine and L-tryptophan are good CCK *releasers.* See Chapter 8 on "Sweets."

Dehydroepiandrosterone (DHEA) is a steroid hormone now being *allegedly* sold in some health food stores as a weight loss aid. Unfortunately, the product being labelled as DHEA is actually a steroid plant hormone extract of a Mexican yam, which contains a chemical precursor to DHEA. Although this compound can be converted to DHEA in the test tube, there is no evidence that it is converted to DHEA in the human body. In addition the yam, like other root storage vegetables, is likely to contain a wide variety of toxins to control bacteria, fungi, insects, worms, and higher animals that would otherwise eat them. The potential risks of this extract have not been scientifically evaluated. There is no reason to expect it to have any benefits in terms of fat loss. It is a rip-off and possibly a dangerous one.

Real DHEA has created a lot of excitement lately as a potential future weight control aid. DHEA is a steroid hormone manufactured in the adrenal glands. Obese individuals excrete less of DHEA than do the nonobese. The amount of DHEA secreted falls markedly in humans between the ages of 20 and 30. In one study of a genetically obese strain of mice, DHEA given orally in sesame oil controlled weight gain and prevented obesity. (Yen, 1977) The food consumption of DHEA-treated mice was normal or slightly above normal, so appetite control was not the mechanism of DHEA's action. DHEA significantly decreased fat synthesis (lipogenesis) in the liver. We cannot yet recommend real DHEA as a fat loss aid, however, since the dosage required to produce the proper youthful serum level is not known and may require individualization (individual dose adjustment). In our opinion it is not ready for prime time.

Human chorionic gonadotrophin (HCG) is a nonsteroid hormone. It was used by the Simeons weight control centers. The evidence concerning its possible benefits is not convincing. These benefits are claimed to include appetite reduction, weight loss, and improved well-being. Double-blind studies have failed to find an advantage of HCG over placebo. (Bray, 1976) Don't waste your money. One study that did report positive results got extremely high weight losses in the placebo group too; we suspect that psychological and behavioral factors at this clinic were more important than the pharmacological effects of the drug.

L-Dopa is an anorectic. It reduces appetite and, according to some studies, may cause weight loss in both animals and people. (Leibowitz, 1978; Thomson, 1970; Vardi, 1976) Yet in one study, doses of up to 4.8 grams daily of L-Dopa failed to produce weight loss during a 6-month double-blind study of obese humans. (Munro, 1982) Remember that weight loss, not fat loss, was measured in this experiment.

Even more important is the fact that L-Dopa does not release growth hormone in the obese unless a beta-adrenergic blocker such as propranolol is used. (See the technical note at the end of Chapter 5.) Growth hormone is reported to have anorectic effects (Cahill, 1979), so if the anorectic effects of L-Dopa depend on GH release, it should not work on the obese unless propranolol or a similar drug is used with it. The cattle that were fed L-Dopa-containing velvet beans put on plenty of weight, but it was nearly all muscle and other lean body mass instead of the richly fat-marbled tissue that was needed to meet the requirements of USDA Prime and Choice grades. While heavy, these cattle were not obese.

In another study of obese humans, L-Dopa prevented the fall in oxygen consumption (a measure of metabolic rate, oxygen being needed to turn your food to water and carbon dioxide) that occurs with low-calorie feeding. (Landsberg, 1981) This finding is particularly exciting because it means that L-Dopa can circumvent some of your body's energy-conserving mechanisms that are activated by famine or pseudofamine.

L-Dopa is a prescription drug (even though it is an amino acid closely related to the nutrient amino acid tyrosine) and should be used under a physician's supervision, and only with supplemental nutrient antioxidants. See the Safety Appendix for further data.

Lisuride and *lergotrile,* two ergot derivatives related to bromocriptine, caused a 50 percent inhibition of food intake at doses that did not increase locomotor activity (body movement) or induce stereotyped behavior (of the sort that amphetamine causes) in animal studies. (Carruba, 1980) The dose of lisuride that caused a 50 percent reduction in food intake by animals was 1/45th of that required to obtain a similar effect with amphetamine.

Naloxone is an antagonist of certain of the effects of opiates, whether they are taken exogenously (like heroin) or are secreted endogenously (like the body's naturally made opiate-like endorphins and enkephalins). Opiates may play an important role in eating as a satiation signal. (McCarthy, 1981) Endorphin release is associated with overeating in certain genetically obese mice and rats. (Margules, 1978) In rats, rabbits, and cats deprived of food to get them very hungry, naloxone administration reduced the amounts of food eaten. In humans too naloxone reduced food intake by 28 percent without altering the individual perception of hunger. (Cohen, 1985) Therefore naloxone may be an effective weight loss aid. Other opiate antagonists are being developed that may be more practical. Naltrexone, for example, may be administered orally, unlike naloxone. We do not yet know what side effects might result from the long-term use of naloxone or other opiate antagonists as weight loss aids. We do know that heroin addicts have been able to use these substances to control their addiction. The use of naloxone or naltrexone for weight control is strictly experimental but should be considered by those whose eating patterns suggest addictive behavior.

Thyroid hormone plays an important role in thermogenesis, the burning of food calories for heat. Overweight persons with hypothyroidism may find that their condition improves with thyroid therapy. One of the problems the obese may have is a general unresponsiveness to TSH, thyroid-stimulating hormone (also known as thyrotropin), even if they are not hypothyroid. (Schmitt, 1977)

Relatively large doses of thyroid hormone have been used by some weight-reducing clinics. An excess of thyroid hormone can cause cardiac arrhythmia and heart failure. Moreover the weight loss resulting from excessive doses of thyroid hormone is said to be principally the result of protein catabolism (breakdown)—that is, the loss of lean body mass rather than of fat. (Munro, 1982)

You want a normal level of thyroid-hormone activity in your tissues, not abnormally high levels. Do not take any more thyroid hormone than is necessary for normal basal metabolism. If you have a deficiency in serum thyroid hormone levels or if you are relatively resistant to the effects of a given amount of thyroid hormone, your physician can usually easily correct it. More than this is definitely not better!

As research into fat loss continues, diet pills can be expected to becoming increasingly safer and more effective. But for the present, we must deal with the available drugs and their limitations. If you wish to try any of these, be sure to follow your doctor's directions. Use only the dosage your doctor specifies. If any adverse reactions occur, report them promptly to your doctor. He or she may suggest that you switch to a different drug. Do NOT use your friend's diet pills; such usage without professional guidance could be hazardous. Above all do not expect miracles. These drugs are only *aids* to weight control, and most are effective for a limited time only.

11

Fat Metabolism: How You Can Change It

If you want to get rid of fat, go right to the source, the biochemistry that governs your fat metabolism. Fat is metabolized by a number of different chemical pathways in your body. It is possible to change your pattern of fat metabolism so that less fat is synthesized from carbohydrates, more fat is utilized for energy needs (i.e., burned up), and less fat is stored. This can be done by taking certain nutrient supplements which alter fat metabolism. There are special fats that you can burn for quick energy, but which cannot be stored in your body. These special fats even promote the use of stored body fat; eating these special fats actually helps you to burn up your body fat stores!

We have already discussed the central importance that your growth hormone level and growth hormone to insulin ratio plays in determining your body's ratio of muscle to fat, and we have told you how to readjust both of these hormones. These alterations to your fat metabolism are so important that we have devoted separate chapters to them. You can do even more to alter your fat metabolism to suit a very well-fed twentieth-century high technology society, rather than leave your biochemistry, and your proclivity to store fat, back in the famine-filled Ice Age.

SPECIAL FATS

Not all fats are created equal, either. Some fats are metabolized quite differently from most of the fats that you eat every day. Because of these differences these unusual fats, the *medium-chain triglycerides (MCT)*, will become much more common in dietetic foods. Conventional fats and oils are *long-chain triglycerides*, also called *LCT*. MCT are not artificial like saccharin; they are found in coconut and other palm kernel oils (about 15 percent MCT can be extracted), and in butter. The process of separating it from the other 85 percent, which is LCT, is currently rather expensive. MCT has about 10 percent fewer calories per gram than LCT, but that is only one of MCT's advantages. (Kaunitz, 1958)

Fat in your diet, whether MCT or ordinary LCT, depresses your lipogenesis (synthesis of fats from carbohydrates or protein). The less fat you eat, the more fat you make from carbohydrates. When you eat fats, whether MCT or LCT, your body makes more of the enzymes involved in fat burning. LCT consumption does not induce enough of these additional enzymes to prevent some of the LCT from being stored as body fat. LCT, the ordinary fats and oils, can be added directly to your fat stores. *Neither the fatty acids of MCT nor MCT itself is deposited to any appreciable extent in your fat stores!* (Senior, 1968; Harkins, 1968) The MCT is quickly absorbed from your gut and carried by your blood to the rest of your body. Your mitochondria, especially those in your liver, very rapidly burn MCT for energy.

Experiments show that rats have to eat significantly more calories of an MCT-containing diet than of a similar LCT-containing diet to maintain constant body weight. With a 20 percent fat-by-weight diet, the rats that received MCT had to eat 12 to 20 percent more calories than the rats that received LCT (lard) instead. With a 33 percent fat diet, the MCT-eating rats had to eat 22 percent more calories than the LCT eaters. Cholesterol levels in the MCT-fed adult rats were lower by 35 to 57 percent. (Kaunitz, 1958)

Since MCT suppresses the synthesis of conventional storable LCT fats from carbohydrates, increases the production of enzymes involved in burning both MCT and LCT fats, is very rapidly burned, and cannot be stored as body fat, one might suspect that eating MCT would burn up some stored LCT body fat, causing a net reduction in body fat stores. Therefore MCT may be quite useful in foods as aids to fat loss. (Lavau, 1978)

Experiments confirm this. Rats were fed with three different diets:

low fat (8 percent of the dietary calories were corn oil LCT, 72 percent were carbohydrates, and 20 percent were protein); high-fat MCT (55 percent of the dietary calories were MCT, 5 percent were corn oil LCT, 20 percent were carbohydrates, and 20 percent were protein); and high-fat LCT (60 percent of the dietary calories were LCT in the form of corn oil, 20 percent were carbohydrates, and 20 percent were protein). The rats were allowed to eat as much as they desired. The MCT-fed rats had the same caloric intake as the LCT-fed rats. The rats fed low-fat food ate about 10 percent more calories. *After 8 weeks on the high-fat MCT diet, the rats had a decrease of 10 percent in their weight and 40 percent in their principal fat stores, when compared to the rats on the low-fat diet!* As expected, the rats on the high-fat LCT diet gained more weight and more body fat than those on the low-fat diet. (Lavau)

The expected enzyme changes were observed too. The capacity of fat storage tissue in both MCT- and LCT-fed rats to take up and use blood sugar (to make stored fat) under conditions of both normal and high insulin levels was decreased to about 1/3 that of the low fat diet rats. *This is why a low-fat diet is not necessarily the best way to lose fat.* Of course, the LCT-fed rats had so much readily storable fat in their high-LCT, high-fat diets that they gained body fat anyway. Since the rats eating the high MCT, high-fat diet could not store the fat that they ate, they lost fat, just as expected. This is truly a case of eating to lose!

MCT is a quick high energy source and is excellent for endurance athletics. Pure medium-chain triglycerides are currently being used by people with certain diseases that reduce their ability to absorb fats because MCTs are extremely easy to absorb. They are also FDA-approved and widely employed in intravenous solutions used for the long-term feeding of coma patients and others who cannot be fed orally. We hope that MCT manufacturers are also considering the possibility of developing new foods for more widespread use for fat loss purposes.

Warning: MCT absorption is normally so rapid that it might create a medical hazard; one's blood could be overloaded with MCT fats by absorbing them even faster than one can burn them. In order to be safe for use as a fat loss aid, MCT-containing foods must be carefully designed to slow down this excessively rapid absorption.

Moreover, a fat-containing product must contain a good antioxidant system to prevent the fat from becoming dangerously autoxidized (rancid). Just because a fat doesn't smell rancid yet does not mean that it is safe; vegetable oils and fats have to be about 35 times more autoxidized than is acceptably safe before they smell rancid. Be very cautious of MCT-containing products from vendors whose technical capabilities are an unknown. After the publication of this book, we expect to see droves of poorly designed, inadequately tested, and possibly hazardous MCT-containing products appearing on the market. Let the buyer beware! Before adding MCT to your diet, see the Safety Appendix.

FAKE FATS

Just as there are synthetic no-calorie sweeteners, there is now a no-calorie fake fat. It is a synthetic fat substitute that tastes like fat and has a mouth feel like fat, but you can't absorb it. It is called *sucrose polyester* and may also soon be appearing in processed foods where fats and oils are added. For example, it can effectively replace shortening in baked goods. It might even be possible to make aspartame-sweetened sucrose polyester whipped cream and ice cream that has only a few calories per pint.

Sucrose polyester has already been used in small clinical trials with overweight people and has been successful in causing weight loss without harmful side effects. In one study (conducted by Charles Glueck of the University of Cincinnati), the people lost nearly half a pound per day. Most people could not tell whether sucrose polyester or real fat was in their food. The material also reduces blood cholesterol levels. Even though it is made from sucrose, it cannot be digested, it is not sweet, and it releases no insulin.

The availability of this new food depends on FDA approval, which typically takes many years. The material was developed more than thirteen years ago by Procter & Gamble Company and is patented by them. While the FDA's concern with safety is laudable, it is often misplaced. In the past thirteen years, millions of people have died from the cardiovascular-disease and cancer-promotion consequences of real fats. The way the FDA philosophically views safety, these millions of deaths involving the alternative, real fat are not considered in the approval process. We believe that the *relative* safety of the competing foods or drugs should be considered and that the search for absolute safety is an unscientific chimera on which only a Washington bureaucrat could waste lives. Compare the relative risks of sucrose polyester to real fat in obese cardiovascular patients, and then get on with saving lives.

Polydextrose is an available high-tech synthetic product which helps reduce the caloric content of foods. It is a patented food ingredient developed by Pfizer Research. The FDA has finally approved polydextrose. It is a partially metabolizable, water-soluble polymer prepared from D-glucose with small amounts of sorbitol and citric acid. Most of this substance passes through your body unabsorbed. It can be used as a substitute for many of the functional food properties of sugar, such as its bulk and body effects. (However, polydextrose is not sweet.) In some applications it can be substituted for fat. Polydextrose has 25 percent of the calories of sugar and 11 percent of the calories of fat. If consumed in high quantities (50 to 130 grams a day), polydextrose can cause diarrhea. It is most likely to be found in baked goods and diet foods, though it is used in some other prepared foods as well. Read your food ingredient labels to find out when they contain polydextrose.

NUTRIENT SUPPLEMENTS FOR ALTERING FAT METABOLISM

Your mitochondria are the power plants of your cells. They burn essentially all fats that you use for energy and much of your carbohydrates, too. *Carnitine* is a natural amino acid-like substance that is required for transport of fatty acids across your mitochondrial membranes. Carnitine is needed in order to utilize fatty acids for energy. (Fat-processing enzymes called lipases split a triglyceride (fat) molecule into one molecule of glycerine and three molecules of fatty acids.) Carnitine is synthesized within our bodies, primarily in the liver and kidneys, from lysine and methionine. Except for some of us who are vegetarians, we also get carnitine in our diets. Carnitine is found in meat and some dairy products. Generally the redder the meat, the more carnitine it contains. Sheep, lamb, and beef are the three best natural sources.

It is generally accepted that carnitine also has a major function in thermogenesis (Borum, 1983), the process of burning calories to create heat (see the next chapter for details), a major method your body uses to get rid of excess calories.

Some studies indicate that carnitine can reduce serum lipids such as triglycerides, which, as we mentioned earlier, are fats in your bloodstream. In one study, triglycerides were reduced with DL-carnitine chloride supplements of 900 mg/day orally (Maebashi, 1978). On this point a study prepared for the Bureau of Foods of the Food and Drug Administration said, "Studies to date have been conducted on a limited number of subjects, but the absence of side effects of daily doses of 1.0 to 2.0 grams L-carnitine and the possibility of beneficial effects on serum lipoprotein profiles suggest further investigational drug trials." (Borum and Fisher, 1983) There are indications of toxic effects in some studies with the D- or DL-carnitine (including cardiac arrhythmia and muscle weakness), however, that are not found with equivalent doses of L-carnitine. DL-carnitine is an equal mixture of the mirror image D-carnitine and L-carnitine molecules. *Therefore do not use D- or DL-carnitine.*

A few preliminary studies indicate that L-carnitine may be of benefit to athletes. It may be able to help reduce body fat in athletes who are both taking an L-carnitine supplement and doing vigorous exercise as well. However, more research is needed. Since in endurance exercise fatty acids are the major source of body energy, it seems plausible that L-carnitine supplementation could be of value. L-carnitine supplements might increase the rate of fat utilization, thus facilitating a decrease in body fat. Studies of long-term use of carnitine for these purposes have not yet been done. Use of L-carnitine must be currently considered experimental.

Caffeine can inhibit the storage of fat in ordinary body fat, also called white fat. It can also stimulate the burning of fat in a special type of fat with lots of mitochondria called brown fat, the purpose of which is to burn fat, not store it. (Bukowiecki, 1973) We will have a lot to say about this special heat-producing fat in the next chapter.

Niacin (nicotinic acid, a type of vitamin B-3) can be used to alter your fat metabolism. Niacin inhibits fat synthesis in the liver and is effective in reducing serum cholesterol, triglycerides (fats), and LDL and VLDL, the low- and very low-density lipoproteins (fat-cholesterol-protein complexes) which have been associated with increased risks of cardiovascular disease and, perhaps, cancer. (Carlson, 1962; Charman, 1973; Coronary, 1975; Larner, 1980; Miettinen, 1969)

Your liver plays a major role in both your fat and carbohydrate metabolism. Your liver can convert blood sugar to free fatty acids and triglycerides, sending them to the rest of your body to be either stored or burned. Triglycerides are ordinary fats; they are comprised of 3 molecules of fatty acid chemically combined with 1 molecule of glycerin. Your liver can also convert its stored carbohydrate (glycogen), as well as fat and protein, to blood sugar, a process called gluconeogenesis. (Pike, 1975)

Niacin causes a dramatic drop in circulating free fatty acids while it elevates blood-sugar levels. It does this by reducing blood-sugar uptake by your liver; this blood sugar would normally be converted into free fatty acids and triglycerides (fats) and released into your bloodstream. (Miettinen, 1969) Niacin also shifts your muscle metabolism from burning free fatty acids to burning both blood sugar and the triglycerides (fat) stored within the muscle, while at the same time causing blood sugar (glucose) to be manufactured by and released from your liver. Experiments have been performed on humans that show that this shift of muscle energy supply does not impair performance in either peak output exercise or in heavy prolonged aerobic exercise. (Lassers, 1972) Experiments on rats which had been given niacin have shown that the amount of fat in the heart muscle is reduced, as occurs in heavy exercise. (Carlson, 1966; Froberg, 1969)

For example, in one study 14 patients with hypercholesterolemia (excess serum cholesterol) were treated with niacin as follows: 1 gram on the first day, 2 grams on the second day, and then 1 gram 3 times a day. After 2 weeks on the program, serum cholesterol was reduced on the average by 25 percent, and serum triglycerides were reduced on the average by 30 percent. (Miettinen, 1969)

Niacin's ability to alter fat metabolism was vividly demonstrated in this experiment; serum triglycerides are ordinary fats being carried around by your bloodstream. What happens to these transported fats? If you don't burn the fats promptly, they can be carried to your fat-storage cells and stashed away for a famine that will never come. High serum triglyceride levels and obesity are closely related. The proponents of the semistarvation Pritikin diet claim only an average 25 percent cholesterol reduction, and to attain that requires a great deal of heavy exercise as well. We would rather eat well and take our niacin.

In another larger study, 3 grams a day of niacin produced similar results which were maintained for 8 years while the subjects continued to take niacin. (Charman, 1973) These fat metabolism modifications have since been confirmed in the massive long-term Coronary Drug Project. (Coronary, 1975)

The reductions in VLDL can be very dramatic. Durk and Sandy were first measured for lipoproteins in 1978 (when lipoprotein typing was a new technology). They were measured at Dr. Lundgren's laboratory at Donner Research Laboratories (University of California at Berkeley). Dr. Lundgren is the scientist who developed lipoprotein testing, a technique now used in nearly every comprehensive physical exam. Sandy's VLDL peak was undetectable, both by electrophoresis and the ultracentrifuge, and lower than 94 percent of women in her age group. Durk's was also extremely low (lower than 92 percent of men in his age group), especially considering that both had eaten a *huge* fatty gourmet feast only about eight hours before. The results were so amazing that our specimens were run three times apiece to make sure that there was no mistake. Both of us had been using niacin supplements for about 8 years at that time. See our *Life Extension: A Practical Scientific Approach* and *The Life Extension Companion;* also see Gilman, Goodman, Gilman, 1980.

Caution: Before you begin taking niacin, however, you should read the cautions in the Safety Appendix. Diabetics and ulcer patients should not use niacin supplements unless directed to do so by their physician.

Vitamin E: Cellulite, lumpy fibrous body fat deposits, is very difficult to deal with using conventional caloric restriction diets. This is because cellulite is not just fat; it is fat in a matrix of fibrous cross-linked tissue. The tanning of leather, the aging of a gelatin dessert that loses its elasticity, becomes lumpy, and weeps fluid, and the loss of elasticity in your automobile's windshield wiper blades after long exposure to sunlight and ozone, are all examples of cross-linking. (Tanzer, 1973; Verzar, 1963) Cross-linking is the chemical binding of large molecular chains to each other. The result is rather like pouring some epoxy cement (which hardens by cross-linking) over a pile of rubber bands; when the cement cures (cross-links), you end up with a hard lump that isn't springy anymore.

Free radicals are a major cause of undesired cross-linking in biological systems; this cross-linking is the principal cause of the loss of skin elasticity with age, and it plays a major role in the aging process itself, as is described in the cross-linking theory of aging. (Bjorksten, 1968; Deyl, 1971; Kirk, 1962) Fats are especially subject to free radical attack, so it isn't surprising that fatty tissue can become cross-linked with age or by exposure to other sources of free radicals such as smoking or excess drinking. The use of free-radical-scavenging nutrient supplements should be able to slow the cellulite-forming process. If it is slowed enough, your body's natural repair mechanisms will be able to remove the fibrotic tissue faster than it is formed. Over a period of a year to a few years, the damaged tissue is replaced with new tissue that has not been pathologically cross-linked.

The fibrotic fatty tissues of fibrocystic breast disease, are in our opinion a possible model for the fibrotic fat deposits in cellulite. Vitamin E is a very important free-radical-scavenging nutrient; indeed protection from free radical attack on fats (called *lipid peroxidation)* is the only known biological function of this essential nutrient. Vitamin E may be effective in the treatment of fibrocystic breast disease in humans, according to a recent study. The study was double-blind and placebo-controlled, involving 26 women receiving 600 units of Vitamin E per day, with 8 other women receiving the placebo as a control. There was both subjective and objectively measurable regression of the fibrotic fat deposits in 22 of the 26 women receiving the vitamin E over a period of 8 weeks, whereas the control subjects receiving the placebo did not improve. (Sundaram, 1981)

The improvement described in this paper took place much more rapidly than we would have expected. The limited anecdotal data that we have suggests that one will usually not see any improvement in cellulite for a year and that further improvement occurs slowly over a period of years. There is a wide variety of reported responses, ranging from no effect to about 80 percent eventual cellulite reduction. Remember that these are *not* the results of double-blind placebo-controlled studies. On the other hand, we have heard of no cases of spontaneous cellulite remission (reduction in lumpiness) in obese persons who have not lost body fat, though this doesn't mean that it cannot occur. It should also be noted that spontaneous remission (usually only temporary) does frequently occur in fibrocystic breast disease. At present, we consider the use of 1000 units of vitamin E per day (best taken with a balanced free-radical-scavenging nutrient mixture such as we describe in the Safety Appendix) to be an unproven and experimental (but safe) therapy for cellulite.

Radiation-induced lung fibrosis is another free-radical-caused fibrotic disease. (Becklake, 1979) It is well known that X-ray radiation does its damage by creating hydroxyl free radicals in tissue and that antioxidants such as vitamin E, beta-carotene, and selenium can reduce that damage.

Retrolental fibroplasia is another fibrotic pathology caused by free radicals. In this case, it is due to exposure of premature infants to more oxygen (autoxidation of fats creates the free radicals) than their free-radical-scavenging systems can cope with. Vitamin E has been used to treat and prevent this damage. (Hittner, 1984) Vitamin E has also been used successfully to treat several types of primary fibrositis. (Steinberg, 1950)

We suggest that cellulite sufferers try 1000 units per day of DL-alpha tocopherol acetate (a form of vitamin E) plus a powerful free-radical-scavenging nutrient supplement formula such as the high-potency multivitamin-mineral formula in the Safety Appendix; it contains over a dozen free-radical-scavenging nutrients. We have no scientific studies on the treatment of cellulite itself with free radical scavengers, but we have heard several anecdotal reports on the disappearance of cellulite over a period of a year or more from people who were taking large doses of free-radical-scavenging nutrients for other purposes, with no expectation of any effect on their cellulite. There is no guarantee that it will work, but we think that it is worth a try.

There are literally hundreds of pages on free radicals, cross-linking, and protective nutrients, and hundreds of scientific literature references on these subjects in our *Life Extension: A Practical Scientific Approach* and *The Life Extension Companion.*

You may have fought your fat metabolism for years with conventional diets. Remember that your fat metabolism has evolved to keep you "safely" fat, *especially* in times of famine. The harder you fight it, the harder it fights you. So quit fighting it. Alter your fat metabolism to suit the twentieth-century cornucopia of modern high-yield agriculture.

12

Thermogenesis: The Cool Way to Lose Fat

Thermogenesis means the generation of heat. This heat is produced by burning fats, carbohydrates, and protein in your body. Heat is measured in calories. When you count calories, you are counting the heat producing potential of your food. If you can persuade your body to burn more calories than you eat, you will lose weight. We have explained in chapters 5 and 7 how you can make sure that your weight loss is all fat, not partly muscle.

Work and heat are both forms of energy. Your muscles have to do a lot of work to burn off a few calories; you would have to walk around carrying a 200-pound load for about 45 minutes to burn off the calories in a typical candy bar! Moreover, over 75 percent of those calories that you burned to do that work appear as heat (exercise-induced thermogenesis) rather than mechanical work, since your body is less than 25 percent efficient at converting the chemical energy calories in food into mechanical work calories. The bottom line, for example, is that well over 80 percent of the calories eaten by an NFL football player in heavy training heat his body and the air around him.

If most of the calories expended during exercise are given off as heat, could heat loss itself be used to help you lose fat? The answer is yes. *Thermogenesis, the process of burning calories to produce heat, can actually be used to help you lose fat without the exercise.* Some people can eat *twice as much* without becoming fat as other people with the same level of physical activity. (Rose, 1970) Individual differences in thermogenesis play a major role.

Some interesting experiments have been performed to compare

body fat loss in hamsters fed as much as they wanted of various diets and either allowed to exercise voluntarily or exposed to cooler temperatures without exercise. Voluntary exercise—running 7 to 10 km (4.2 to 6 miles) per day in a cage exercise wheel—caused a 17 percent decrease in body fat in the hamsters fed a high-fat diet but it had no fat loss effect in the hamsters fed a normal lab chow diet. Nevertheless the hamsters that had access to the high-fat diet became obese whether or not they exercised. The fat hamsters on the unlimited quantity high-fat diet were then chronically exposed to a 5° C environment, instead of their usual 23° C (73° F). They lost 80 percent of their body fat! Cold exposure caused loss of lean body mass unless the hamsters were on a high-fat diet too. Although both exercise and cold increased food consumption, the cold-exposed group still had much less body fat than the exercise group. (Bartness, 1984)

Since most Americans eat a high-fat diet, thermogenesis is an interesting approach to body fat loss. Isn't 5° C (41° F) too cold to be practical for people? Remember that hamsters come equipped with built-in fur coats. If you wear a head-to-toe fur coat, you might have to be in a really cold environment, but normally clothed humans exhibit cold-induced thermogenesis at 72° F, a very reasonable temperature which does not cause shivering. In women with a normal range of body fat percentages, a change from 28° C (82° F) to 22° C (72° F) caused an increased thermogenesis of about 7 percent. (Dauncey, 1981) If you eat about 2900 calories per day, that 7 percent is about 200 calories per day. This may not sound like much, but 200 calories per day adds up to about 25 pounds of fat over a year.

There are different types of thermogenesis, depending on the type of stimulus which activates it. (McMinn, 1981) Nevertheless a calorie burned is a calorie burned, regardless of the way it's burned.

Cold-induced thermogenesis—there are two types, nonshivering thermogenesis and shivering thermogenesis. The former can be a useful part of our program, but the latter is too uncomfortable for us to recommend.

Diet-induced thermogenesis—eating certain types of nutrients or an excess of calories can increase the number of calories that you burn. The wrong type of diet can suppress thermogenesis. (Rothwell, 1983; Stock, 1983)

Drug-induced thermogenesis—certain drugs such as caffeine, theophylline, ephedrine, phenylpropranolamine, and nicotine can trigger thermogenesis. Certain other drugs can inhibit thermogenesis. (Rothwell, 1981)

Exercise-induced thermogenesis—when you work up a sweat, this is what is happening. Exercise-induced thermogenesis takes place in muscle, not brown fat. Shivering thermogenesis is a type of exercise-induced thermogenesis, whereas much nonexercise and nonshivering thermogenesis takes place in brown fat. Recent evidence shows that nonshivering non-exercise-induced thermogenesis can also take place in human skeletal muscle. The wrong type of exercise can impair brown fat thermogenesis. The right type of exercise can not only increase your brown fat thermogenesis, it can increase your maximum brown fat thermogenic capacity.

Brown fat, also called brown adipose tissue, contains special fat cells whose purpose is to *burn* fat instead of *storing* it. Brown fat is especially adapted for thermogenesis. It is brown because it is crammed full of blood vessels and mitochondria (which are brown), your cells' power plants that burn fats and sugar to produce heat and other forms of energy. We will describe a variety of ways for triggering thermogenesis in your brown fat and even of increasing your supply of brown fat while decreasing your white fat. White fat is your body fat storage tissue. A little bit of brown fat can burn a great deal of stored white fat; when stimulated, brown fat can burn its own weight in regular white fat about every 12 hours. (Morgan, 1981)

A small amount of brown fat may explain a lot about why some people can eat all they want and remain lean while others restrict their eating and still get fat. Evidence supports the idea that brown fat is the site for much of your body's thermogenesis, the production of heat by burning fuel (calories). This important function is carried out by a few tiny deposits of brown fat found on the back of your neck, near your spine, and on the upper part of your back from your neck to your shoulder blades, around your kidneys, around your heart and aorta, scattered through your abdomen, and in your armpits and groin region. (Morgan, 1981; Stock, 1981) *Your brown fat may be only about 1 percent of your total body tissue, yet produce roughly as much heat—that means burn as many calories per hour—as the rest of your body.* (Elliot, 1980, quoting Bray)

When normal rats are fed a diet of laboratory chow, they eat just enough for their energy needs. But when they are fed a wide variety of highly delicious foods such as bologna, chocolate, popcorn, marshmallows, cookies, and so on, they overeat and gain weight. (Sound familiar?) This is called a cafeteria diet. But the rats don't gain nearly as much weight as would be expected from the number of excess calories they ate. *In fact, rats ate 80 percent more calories and gained only 27 percent more weight in cafeteria feedings. Scientists discovered the process called diet-induced thermogenesis, whereby overeating animals would burn up a lot of those excess calories to produce heat.* Animals with a genetic defect that makes them obese, on the other hand, do not do this to nearly as great an extent. Instead they conserve more of their body's energy and get fat.

There is an evolutionary advantage to diet-induced thermogenesis. If an animal has a diet that is low in essential nutrients such as vitamins or protein, it may have to eat a lot of food to get enough of the essential nutrients. Diet-induced thermogenesis helps prevent extreme obesity from developing in animals who must eat a lot of a low-quality diet. (Stock, 1981) An animal that is too fat may be well prepared for a famine, but it will have a hard time escaping from a quick lean hungry predator.

Diet-induced thermogenesis is stimulated by eating excess calories. (Landsberg, 1981) Both diet-induced and cold-induced nonshivering thermogenesis appear to be controlled by the same mechanisms. (Himms-Hagen, 1981) Some scientists studying obesity now believe that there may be a defect in thermogenesis in some obese persons (Jung, 1979), which may help explain why they gain weight. (They may have more difficulty using up excess calories in the production of extra heat.)

Brown fat is believed to be a major site of diet-induced thermogenesis and cold-induced nonshivering thermogenesis. The sympathetic nervous system's adrenaline and noradrenaline are the specific biochemical stimulants to brown fat thermogenesis. These same biochemicals also stimulate thermogenesis in human skeletal muscle. It is interesting to note that many obese animals are not only insensitive to sympathetic nervous system stimulation of diet-induced thermogenesis but also do not keep themselves as warm as the other animals in the cold, which further conserves energy. They do not have normal cold-induced nonshivering thermogenesis. (Himms-Hagen, 1981)

It is possible to increase or decrease thermogenesis with a wide variety of foods, drugs, and behavior.

EFFECTS OF FOODS

Sucrose and carbohydrate feeding promote thermogenesis, at least in normal individuals. (Landsberg, 1981; Bukowiecki, 1983) For the sake of a high GH/insulin ratio, you should obviously avoid high-glycemic-index carbohydrates such as glucose and sucrose. *Fortunately low-glycemic-index fructose is an effective thermogenic agent. In a human experiment fructose, as compared to glucose, caused only 25 percent as much insulin release but produced a 50 percent greater increase in thermogenic energy expenditure.* (Simonson, 1985)

Other nutritional factors affect thermogenesis. *Thermogenesis is suppressed by a low-calorie pure protein diet, very low-carbohydrate diets, very high-fat diets (in some species), and in the long run, diets that are iodine deficient.* Obviously many popular diets suppress thermogenesis, including low-salt diets, which may induce an iodine deficiency.

Dietary iodine is required for your thyroid to synthesize thyroid hormone, and normal amounts of thyroid hormone are required for normal basal metabolism and thermogenesis. With the continuing trend toward low-salt and low-calorie diets, iodine deficiency may once again become common according to the U.S. Department of Agriculture. The development of goiter (enlarged thyroid gland due to iodine deficiency) used to be common until the addition of supplemental iodine to salt. We may begin to see this disease once again as people use less salt; iodized salt is a major source of iodine for many people.

Most people who wish to decrease their consumption of salt, or who are on a calorically restricted diet (which is likely to contain less iodized salt) should take an iodine supplement containing the Recommended Daily Allowance of iodine, 150 micrograms per day in the form of potassium iodide. Iodine supplementation may even be advisable for most people, due to the smaller amounts of salt now being added to processed foods. Do not take extra large iodine doses; you will not get any additional benefits, and you may be harmed by them.

Caution: Women in families with high incidence of thyroid disorders should take iodine supplements only if directed to do so by their physician. (Bagchi, 1985)

L-carnitine is needed to move fatty acids into your mitochondria for burning. The ability of your mitochondria to rapidly take in large amounts of fatty fuel may be improved by increasing your carnitine intake. Some athletes seem to improve when given carnitine, though we know of no double-blind placebo-controlled studies regarding this point. Since red meat is the major dietary source of carnitine, carnitine supplementation may be particularly helpful for those who do not eat red meat. Carnitine, or its dietary precursors lysine and methionine, may be useful adjuncts to thermogenesis. *Warning: Do not take D-carnitine or DL-carnitine.* (Borum, 1983; Borum, Fisher, 1983) See Chapter 11 for more on L-carnitine.

Niacin may be useful as an adjunct to other thermogenic techniques. The peripheral vasodilation produced by niacin (the niacin flush) causes lots of hot blood to be routed through capillaries in your skin, so your skin feels hot and is considerably warmer than normal. This means that your body will lose heat faster than normal. We have no reason to think that niacin specifically stimulates brown fat thermogenesis as ephedrine does, but it certainly increases your heat loss for the duration of the flush, particularly if you are wearing cool or few clothes. An oral dose of 200 mg of niacin will elevate face and neck temperatures by 2 to 3° F for about an hour. Niacin causes vasodilation in your skin but not in your muscles. (Bean, 1940) Niacin does seem to promote the burning of fats stored within muscles (Lassers, 1972), so it may be a useful adjunct to the nonshivering, non-exercise-induced muscle thermogenesis which can be stimulated by thermogenic drugs.

In our opinion, niacin might be useful in counteracting some of the peripheral vasoconstriction that is caused by adrenaline-like compounds such as phenylpropanolamine and ephedrine. This might allow the brown-fat-generated heat that is triggered by these drugs to escape with less of a body temperature rise. Rise in body temperature inhibits production of more brown fat. An injection of adrenaline greatly reduces the hot skin flush caused by niacin, but the skin temperature is still a bit above normal. (Bean, 1940) Normally the adrenaline alone would cause the skin to become significantly cooler due to vasoconstriction. Niacin can also be used to counteract the rise in serum lipids caused by adrenaline-like drugs.

EFFECTS OF DRUGS

Drugs that increase thermogenesis include caffeine, theophylline, nicotine, phenylpropanolamine, ephedrine (Stock, 1981; Bukowiecki, 1983; Dulloo, 1984; Astrup, 1985), beta-adrenergic receptor agonists (examples are fenoterol, isoproterenol), alpha-adrenergic receptor antagonists, and possibly ciclazindol (Rothwell, 1981), and L-Dopa. (Landsberg, 1981) Drugs that block or diminish thermogenesis include alpha-adrenergic receptor agonists (an example is clonidine), and beta-adrenergic receptor antagonists (an example is propranolol). The drugs that we discuss here are not approved by the FDA as thermogenic agents, though most are approved for other purposes.

Caffeine is a very popular recreational drug that increases thermogenesis in brown fat and inhibits fat storage in the ordinary white fat. (Bukowiecki, 1983) It is interesting to note that people often have a cup of coffee after a meal, when diet-induced thermogenesis would be expected to take place. Frequently people smoke a cigarette (containing nicotine, another thermogenic drug) along with the coffee. This may be an adaptive behavioral control mechanism to help prevent weight gain. Recently the combination of caffeine and phenylpropanolamine was found to synergistically increase brown fat thermogenesis in rats. *(Synergy* means that the effects when both are used together are greater than the sum of the effects of the two drugs when each are used individually.) (Wellman, 1985)

Tolerance to the behavioral and anorectic effects of caffeine develops after a few weeks of use. Tolerance to its thermogenic effects may occur more slowly. See the chemically closely related theophylline below. See our Safety Appendix for warnings about using caffeine.

Theophylline, found in small amounts in tea, is a potent thermogenic drug in a variety of animal models of obesity. Theophylline did not cause fat loss in genetically obese mice or in normal lean mice; in fact these two groups of experimental animals ended up with slightly more body fat than the control animals. (An increase from a body fat percentage of 6.91 percent to 7.15 percent in the normal mice.) Theophylline caused genetically obese rats to have only 65 percent of the body fat of the untreated genetically obese control rats. Genetically normal mice made obese by hypothalamic damage (Perkins, 1981) had only 73 percent of the body fat of their controls. (Dulloo, 1984)

One recent study reported particularly good results with theophylline. Genetically normal rats and mice can be made obese by giving them a diet with far more fat and more protein than is normal for rodents. The diet-induced obesity is probably a good model of the most common kind of human obesity. *The theophylline-treated mice that had been made obese with a high-fat diet had only 41 percent of the body fat of the untreated control group on the same diet! The theophylline-treated rats that had been made obese by the high-fat diet had only 50 percent of the body fat of the untreated control group on the same diet!* During this experiment, both the theophylline-treated and the untreated control groups of rats and mice continued to eat the diet that had made them fat in the first place. The control groups of rats and mice ate the same high-fat diet but did not receive the theophylline. The theophylline strongly affected body fat but did not cause a loss of lean body mass. (Dulloo, 1984)

In fact, the theophylline-treated mice eating the high-fat obesity-inducing diet had lower *body fat percentages than the untreated lean mice eating a normal non-obesity-inducing relatively low-fat lab chow diet.* (There was no lab-chow-fed group of lean normal rats for a similar comparison.) (Dulloo, 1984) Why does theophylline work so much better in the high-fat diet animals? A high-fat diet can cause an increase in noradrenaline levels. Theophylline (and caffeine) act as stimulants in both the brain and in brown fat cells by increasing the effects of a given amount of noradrenaline.

You do not have to eat a high-fat diet to increase your noradrenaline levels, however. You can also increase your noradrenaline stimulation with ephedrine or phenylpropanolamine. Caffeine and phenyl-propanolamine synergistically increase brown fat thermogenesis because the phenylpropanolamine increases your noradrenaline and caffeine increases the effects of a given amount of noradrenaline. (Wellman, 1985) Theophylline works like caffeine. The combination of ephedrine and theophylline has not been tested for thermogenic synergy, but on the basis of their individual results and mechanism of operation (Dulloo, 1984), we expect powerful synergy and even better results. Due to the slightly increased body fat in the theophylline-treated normal mice which had been fed a normal diet, we do not recommend the use of theophylline as a fat loss aid without the use of ephedrine unless one is on a high-fat diet. Even if one is on a high-fat diet (definitely *not* recommended), the thermogenic effects should be much stronger with the added ephedrine.

Although the development tolerance to the anorectic effects of theophylline was noted in these experiments after 2 to 3 weeks, tolerance to its thermogenic effects during the 7-week-long experiments was not reported. (Dulloo, 1984)

Theophylline is chemically very similar to caffeine, and its effects are also similar, except that overdoses of it produce a more profound and potentially dangerous stimulation of the central nervous system (brain and spinal cord) than does caffeine. *Do not use more than the recommended dose of theophylline. See the Safety Appendix before using theophylline.*

Ephedrine is a very powerful thermogenic drug. It is found in the herbs used in some diet aids as anorectics. As is the case with similar drugs, tolerance develops to the anorectic effects within a few weeks. Ephedrine is very similar to the natural hormones adrenaline and noradrenaline, and also like the nonprescription anorectic phenyl-propanolamine. Ephedrine works by increasing noradrenaline stimulation.

Genetically normal rats and mice become obese when given a diet far higher in fat and higher in protein than they normally consume, like many humans on a high fat diet. *The diet-induced obese rats receiving ephedrine had only 32 percent of the body fat of the control rats fed the same diet but not given ephedrine! The diet-induced obese mice had only 44 percent of the body fat of their controls! Ephedrine caused loss of body fat, not lean body mass.*

In genetically normal mice made obese by hypothalamic damage, those treated with ephedrine had only 58 percent of the body fat of their similarly damaged control mice. Ephedrine-treated genetically obese rats had only 50 percent of the body fat of their controls, and ephedrine-treated genetically obese mice had 82 percent of the body fat of their controls. Ephedrine-treated normal lean mice on a normal diet had 86 percent of the body fat of their controls.

On the basis of experience with its very successful and extensive long-term use by asthmatics, we would expect that ephedrine might cause somewhat less of a problem with the development of tolerance than phenylpropanolamine. Tolerance to ephedrine's thermogenic effects during 7-week-long experiments was not reported, although tolerance to the anorectic effects of theophylline was noted. (Dulloo, 1984)

Although tolerance to the anorectic, central-nervous-system stimulant, and cardiovascular effects of ephedrine occurs within a few weeks, experiments on the chronic long-term use of ephedrine in humans show that the thermogenic effects are actually enhanced by its extended use over a 12-week period. These experiments were conducted on women having body fat percentages of 30 to 39 percent, all of whom had a family history of obesity, but none of diabetes mellitus (insulin-sugar diabetes). A 20-mg dose of ephedrine was taken 1 hour before each of 3 daily meals. After 12 weeks, their body fat percentages were reduced by an average of 5 percent, with an average weight loss of 12 pounds. Their oxygen consumption (an indirect measure of calories burned) increased for hours after taking the ephedrine. There was no significant difference between this increase at 4 weeks and at 12 weeks. A slight hand tremor was reported by 2 of the 5 subjects during the first 2 to 5 days of drug use. There was no significant effect on the pulse rate. Initially blood pressure was slightly elevated (by an average of 23 mmHg) 1 hour after taking the drug. After 4 weeks of continued treatment, however, there was no longer a significant blood pressure elevation. Weight regain averaged 1 pound, 2 months after the end of the experiment. (Astrup, 1985)

Due to ephedrine's close chemical, physiological, and structural similarity to phenylpropanolamine, we would also expect that there would be a synergistic thermogenic effect with caffeine or theophylline, just as there is between caffeine and phenylpropanolamine.

(Wellman, 1985) Ephedrine can be more convenient to use than phenylpropanolamine because it's mentally stimulating effects wear off quicker after one takes a dose. This means that a before-dinner dose of ephedrine is less likely to cause insomnia than an equally stimulating dose of phenylpropanolamine.

Herbal diet preparations sometimes contain ephedrine as an anorectic, though they are rarely labeled as such. The label may tell you that the product contains Ma Huang or horsetail, or if the scientific names of the herbs are given, they will usually contain the name *Ephedra*. Although we think that the use of ephedrine or ephedrine-containing herbs as diet aids is an option worth considering for most obese but otherwise healthy adults, we strongly oppose their use in products without an appropriate quantitative contents statement and safety warnings. Moreover the amount of ephedrine in one batch of herbs can be ten times as great as in another batch. *This is enough variation so that one batch of unstandardized* Ephedra *herb product could be ineffective and the next batch of product potentially lethal. Each batch of herbs should be quantitatively analyzed for ephedrine content, and the amount of herbs used adjusted to standardize the ephedrine dose. This dose should be stated on the label. Unfortunately this is rarely done in nonprescription herbal products.*

Warning: Before using ephedrine or an ephedrine-containing herb, be sure to see the Safety Appendix! Do not take phenylalanine or tyrosine supplements while using ephedrine. Persons with cardiovascular disease or thyroid disorders should not use ephedrine or herbs containing it.

Many compounds related to adrenaline can stimulate brown fat thermogenesis. That includes the above-mentioned ephedrine, phenylpropanolamine, and many other sympathomimetic (adrenaline-like) drugs.

Warning: There are a number of important precautions to observe when using ephedrine, phenylpropanolamine, or any other adrenaline-like drugs. Blood pressure may be substantially increased in some sensitive persons, and it is prudent to monitor it, at least during the first week of use. Do *not* use these drugs if you have high blood pressure or cardiac arrhythmia, which are also possible side effects in a few sensitive individuals. It is advisable to have a heart checkup by your doctor before using these drugs, particularly if there is any history of cardiovascular disease in your family. Do not use the drugs if you have a thyroid disorder. Do not take phenylalanine or tyrosine supplements while using an adrenaline-like drug unless directed to do so by your physician, due to the theoretical possibility of hypertension or even cardiac arrhythmia. Phenylpropanolamine and caffeine have been used as anorectics by millions of dieters, *Ephedra* herb teas have been used by millions of people for thousands of years, and ephedrine and theophylline have been used by millions of asthma sufferers for many years with a good safety record, but that does not mean that they are safe if used carelessly! See the Safety Appendix for further precautions, dosage, and use instructions.

Nicotine is another popular recreational drug that increases thermogenesis. That, along with a possible effect on appetite, may be why so many people gain weight when they quit smoking. Nevertheless we don't recommend smoking or the safer nonsmoked forms of tobacco due to problems of addiction, cancer, and cardiovascular disease. See the Safety Appendix for a discussion of these problems and for how nutrient supplements may be used to reduce these risks if you choose to continue to use tobacco or nicotine.

Tobacco smoking is highly addictive (more so than heroin!) and causes over 250,000 deaths per year in the United States. (Brecher, 1972) Nevertheless a serious discussion of the nicotine use option is in order since many people are strongly addicted to nicotine and since many people exhibit such great weight gain when withdrawn from nicotine, presumably due to its thermogenic properties and perhaps also due to a possible anorectic effect. See the Safety Appendix for further data.

Thyroid hormone is required for normal thermogenesis. If you are hypothyroid, you will probably feel cold when normal people feel comfortable, and you will not be able to effectively use thermogenic techniques. In most cases of hypothyroidism, there is a decrease in blood T3 or T4, which are two forms of thyroid hormone, leading to a decrease in fasting metabolic rate. This decline in metabolic rate results in a decrease in heat energy output, so that obesity can occur at a lower level of dietary input than would otherwise be the case.

Thyroid hormone may enhance the sensitivity of the peripheral tissues to the thermogenic effects of the catecholamines (adrenaline and noradrenaline), possibly by altering the adrenergic (adrenaline or noradrenaline) receptors. Cafeteria-style overfeeding in rats increases the blood plasma level and production rate of T3. (Danforth, Horton, 1981) T3 levels also increase in overfed humans, regardless of whether carbohydrate, fat, or protein was eaten, but the carbohydrate content of the diet may be a particularly important modulator of thyroid-hormone metabolic changes in response to diet. (Danforth, 1975; Danforth, Horton, 1981) Thus thyroid hormone may play a role in diet-induced thermogenesis. It is believed, however, that the major control of thermogenesis is exerted by the catecholamines (adrenaline, noradrenaline, and dopamine) rather than by thyroid hormone, even though normal thyroid hormone function is necessary.

Under a doctor's supervision, thyroid hormone is sometimes used as an adjunct in the treatment of obesity. This is a potentially risky procedure, however, and should never be attempted by a layperson without a physician's direction. We recommend *against* the use of thyroid hormone as a weight loss drug in persons with normal thyroid hormone function. Although increasing subnormal thyroid hormone activity to normal is very desirable, be warned that increasing it further is likely to indiscriminately burn lean body mass too. *Warning: excess thyroid hormone can be extremely dangerous to your cardiovascular system when combined with adrenaline-like compounds such as ephedrine and phenylpropanolamine.* Brown fat thermogenesis requires normal thyroid hormone function, but excessive thyroid hormone can actually decrease brown fat thermogenesis.

A person who is overweight may have hypothyroidism, a deficiency of thyroid hormone. He or she should be tested by a doctor. This is very important because thyroid hormone has many functions, including maintenance of your immune and central nervous systems. The two commonly used clinical measures of thyroid hormone are blood levels of T3 (L-triiodothyronine) and T4 (L-thyroxine). However, the thyroid functions T3 and T4 may be measured as normal by a clinical laboratory test in a person who still has functional hypothyroidism. The T3 and T4 just measure the amount of thyroid hormone in the bloodstream, not how effective that hormone is. As some animals and people age, they become less sensitive to their thyroid hormone. This can occur, especially in women, when one's immune system makes the error of producing autoantibodies (antibodies against one's own tissue) which destroy or block one's own thyroid hormone receptors. Your physician can test you for this by sending a sample of your blood to a good clinical immunology-testing laboratory. If your T3 and T4 are normal but your body temperature is too low, you may have inadequate thermogenesis, a problem with the body temperature control system in your hypothalamus, or thyroid receptor autoantibodies which cause you to be functionally hypothyroid by partially blocking the effects of your T3 and T4 thyroid hormones.

Some physicians have observed that Armour thyroid extract, rather than pure L-thyroxine (thyroid hormone), seems to be more effective in some people. You can ask your doctor to prescribe thyroid extract rather than L-thyroxine, the pure thyroid hormone, if you are deficient. Both drugs are FDA-approved for this purpose.

Warning: Be sure not to exceed your doctor's prescribed dose of thyroid! Do not borrow thyroid pills from a friend. Side effects of overdoses may be severe. The 1984 *Physicians' Desk Reference* contains the following warning: "In euthyroid [normal thyroid] patients, doses within the range of daily hormonal requirements are ineffective for weight reduction. Larger doses may produce serious or even life-threatening manifestations of toxicity, particularly when given in association with sympathomimetic amines [amphetamine-like and adrenaline-like compounds] such as those used for their anorectic effects."

EFFECTS OF OBESITY ON THE EFFECTS OF THERMOGENIC DRUGS

The effects of adrenaline-like drugs on thermogenesis apparently depend both on environmental temperature and on body fat percentage. In one experiment, human subjects were put in a warm room (81° F), and given noradrenaline to stimulate thermogenesis. All subjects had normal thyroid function. The increase in resting heat production was twice as great in lean subjects as in obese subjects, with formerly obese subjects being a little closer to the lean subject's responses than to the obese subject's responses. (Jung, 1979) A similar experiment was performed (without mention of elevated environmental temperatures) by another group of scientists. They found that under their conditions there was no reduction in noradrenaline-induced thermogenesis, even in massively obese subjects. Indeed they found that their very obese subjects had a stronger thermogenic response to noradrenaline than lean normal subjects. (Finer, 1985) This agrees with the results on a variety of obese mouse and rat models where the best results were obtained in the obese animals. (Dulloo, 1984) A third group of scientists found that genetically obese Pima Indians had an unimpaired thermogenic response to noradrenaline. (Danforth, Daniels, 1981) These results suggest that the optimum induction of thermogenesis in the obese with adrenaline-like drugs (such as noradrenaline, ephedrine, and phenylpropanolamine) may require a cool environment. Remember that your clothing is part of your personal environment; warm clothes help defeat the effects of thermogenic drugs.

EFFECTS OF THERMOGENIC DRUGS
ON GH-RELEASER USE

Warning: Do not use adrenaline-like drugs with clonidine and/or propranolol, or severe hypertension may result. (Mann, 1984) There have also been reports of severe hypotension under these conditions. Simultaneous use of L-Dopa and adrenaline-like drugs may also cause unpredictable changes in blood pressure.

Thermogenic drugs do not interfere with the effects of arginine. (Boyd, 1970) This will be true for ornithine, too, since it works by the same mechanism. Thermogenic drugs should not have an adverse effect on the GH release of niacin, methionine, or tryptophan, and should not complicate their use.

EFFECTS OF MEAL SCHEDULE ON THERMOGENIC DRUG USE

The thermogenic drugs may work best in conjunction with diet-induced thermogenesis (Dulloo, 1984) since the underlying mechanism is the same. (Himms-Hagan, 1984) Take them about 1 hour before each meal. Ephedrine-theophylline taken before dinner is less likely to cause insomnia than a thermogenic product containing phenylpropanolamine and/or caffeine. One rapidly develops tolerance to the insomnia-promoting effects of ephedrine-theophylline. This rapid development of tolerance does not apply to the thermogenic effects. To avoid possible insomnia, use the thermogenic drug only before breakfast and lunch for the first few days, then add a third dose at dinner.

EFFECTS OF EXERCISE

Exercise not accompanied by a rise in body temperature (such as swimming in cool or lukewarm water) increases the amount of brown fat in experimental animals. Exercise in body temperature water suppresses brown fat formation. (Leblanc, 1982; Hirata, 1981) If you decide to use the optional 5-minutes-per-day peak output exercise technique (see Chapter 14), consider doing it in a cool shower or a cool tub. You do not need to be shivering; water at 72° F is plenty cool. Do not use cold water; a few sensitive individuals may have an excessive blood pressure rise. (People have died of strokes and heart failure after a plunge into cold water from a hot sauna.) Unless you monitor your blood pressure, we recommend that you do not engage in peak output exercise during the first week of phenylpropanolamine or ephedrine use; a few sensitive individuals might have an excessive blood pressure rise.

EFFECTS OF REDUCED ENVIRONMENTAL TEMPERATURE

Cooler environments stimulate thermogenesis. A cooler environment is also known to increase adrenaline and noradrenaline levels in both animals and humans. (Landsberg, 1981) These natural amphetamine-like hormones have both thermogenesis-facilitating and appetite-reducing effects, which may help to explain why exposure to reduced temperatures does not result in a big enough increase in hunger in free-feeding experiments to cancel the net thermogenic fat loss.

Cold acclimation in lab animals leads to a marked growth in brown fat and in the rate at which calories are burned in nonshivering thermogenesis. Cold acclimation and its increased thermogenesis definitely occurs in man. (Landsberg, 1981) Nevertheless who wants to trade the discomfort of caloric restriction for the discomfort of cold? Fortunately cold acclimatization does not require a degree of cold that is really uncomfortable for most people. In normally clothed humans, 22° C, which is 72° F, increases thermogenesis. (Dauncey, 1981; Himms-Hagen, 1984) Human thermogenesis increases rapidly at temperatures that are only slightly cooler than your normal room temperature.

How can you thermally induce thermogenesis? You can simply turn down your heating and air-conditioning thermostats a few degrees. If you lower your home's temperature by 1° F per week, most people will acclimate to the reduced temperature with increased thermogenesis and not even notice the falling temperature until it is about 10° F cooler. This thermally induced thermogenesis may burn off 25 pounds of fat per year. If you turn the temperature down suddenly, you will be unnecessarily uncomfortable. Your fat has been with you a long time. Make things easy on yourself; turn down the temperature gradually, and give yourself time to cold-adapt.

EFFECTS OF CLOTHING

The type of clothing that you wear has a great effect on thermogenesis, since clothing insulates you from heat loss to the environment. Heavy warm clothes suppress thermogenesis, whereas light cool clothes facilitate it.

You can also wear less clothing, or clothing that retains less heat. Get rid of your underwear, and you will get rid of some calories. Wear fewer clothes at home, just as you would at a gym. You can lose hundreds of calories every day just sitting on your tail and watching TV—if all you wear is shorts and if you have the room temperature set at 72° F or cooler.

Warning: Ultraviolet light from the sun is the number one cause of human cancer, and (with tobacco smoking and excessive use of alcohol) is a major cause of premature skin aging. If you wear fewer clothes outside, you should protect yourself from these damaging rays with either external or internal sunblocks. We recommend *PABA ester sunblocks* for external use. *The nutrient PABA (a B vitamin) itself can be taken orally with the nutrient beta-carotene for good solar UV protection.* Taking these two nutrient supplements for ultraviolet light protection has three big advantages over externally applied sunblocks: they don't make your skin sticky or oily, they don't wash or rub off, and you are significantly protected at all times without the bother of smearing a sunblock on all your exposed skin every time that you go out. See the Safety Appendix for doses.

But you can't wear athletic shorts to work or to a gourmet restaurant, can you? Well, unfortunately you can't in most places—except for Southern California, which is like a different country—but a tropical weight suit can help you lose hundreds of calories per day compared to a wool three-piece suit.

We think that there is a real use for "thermogenic" clothing—clothing that appears conventional and socially acceptable but which is made of thermally leaky material and contains cleverly hidden vents to allow warm air to escape. The difference between a typical wool three-piece business suit and a properly designed three-piece thermogenic business suit of identical appearance should be equivalent to the calories consumed by jogging *one to two hours* per day! If you have ever seen us on TV, you have certainly seen some rather unconventional appearing thermogenic clothing!

Thermogenic clothing should include heat loss mechanisms that increase in effectiveness with an increase in physical activity. This will make the clothing comfortable and thermogenically effective over a wider range of environmental temperatures and levels of activity. The jogger who is wearing a sweat suit will lose a lot of sweat (electrolytes), but this is not a loss of fat and is very temporary. *The jogger wearing nothing but light shorts will lose a lot more calories for the same amount of physical exertion, especially on a cool day.* With clever thermogenic design, a jogging suit could be almost as cool as shorts while one is running and as warm as a sweat suit when one rests. Good thermogenic clothing design will require physicists, aerospace material scientists, and biochemists as much as stylists. (See Carlson, 1970, for some of the technical complexities involved in clothing heat transfer engineering.)

Remember that exercise which does not involve a body temperature rise increases the amount of thermogenic brown fat in experimental animals. The jogger in the sweat suit is cheating himself of this advantage too, as well as putting an unnecessary additional stress on his cardiovascular system.

Good thermogenic design also requires particular attention to cooling the patches of brown fat that are near the surface of the skin, particularly those at the back of the neck, along the spine and upper back between the neck and shoulder blades, the armpits, and the groin. There is an additional advantage for men who wear thermogenic clothing that keeps their groin cool: they will make more testosterone! Testosterone production in the human testes is very temperature-sensitive and is maximized at well below body temperature. This is why the testes are in a scrotum which elongates when too warm and contracts against the crotch when too cool. The pants and underwear worn in western societies keep the testes well above their optimum temperature, a problem that would be corrected by good thermogenic clothes design. The effect of testes overheating is so great that an athletic supporter lined with about 1/3 inch of cotton has been used as a male contraceptive in India! Testosterone production, sperm count, fertility, and sex drive were all greatly reduced. In fact, only a few of the men were willing to continue using this method, due to loss of libido and potency.

Increased production of testosterone in men who wear properly designed thermogenic clothes will have anabolic (muscle-building and anti-fat-deposition) effects, like the hazardous synthetic anabolic steroids used by many athletes but without their risks. More testosterone can also increase male aggressiveness, sex drive, and potency.

You don't have to be shivering cold to induce thermogenesis; cool and crisp is good enough. In fact, if you get too cold, your body will conserve heat by reducing blood flow to your skin and extremities; although you will lose more heat than if it were warmer, the additional heat loss is rarely worth the discomfort brought about by this condition.

Who is burning calories faster—a jogger or someone in a cool bath? The cool bather is probably burning calories faster. You can lose calories rapidly with a cool tub and a little more quickly with a cool shower. Cool water carries away calories fast! How fast you lose calories depends primarily on the water temperature and your body fat percentage. For the same water temperature and body surface area, a person with twice the skin-fold fat thickness will usually lose calories at about half the rate of the leaner person. Blubber is a good insulator. An athlete with a low body fat percentage may lose calories 4 times as fast as someone who is mildly obese, but the mildly obese person can often tolerate cooler water for longer.

Due to the excellent insulating properties of fat, this technique will not be of much use to the hyperobese, some of whom also have a defect in their cold-stimulated thermogenesis that allows their core body temperature to drop substantially rather than burn more fat. It can work well on persons who are mildly obese.

Typical U.S. Army men burned about 360 to 540 extra calories per hour, depending on their build, in a tub of water at 22° C (72° F). (Strong, 1982) This is as cool as Durk or Sandy can comfortably stand since Durk is tall and slim, and both have a low body fat percentage. To put this caloric expenditure into perspective, freestyle gymnastics requires 290 calories per hour, rowing at 80 meters per minute takes 365 calories per hour, and carrying a load of 96 kg (211 pounds) takes 520 calories per hour. (Minh, 1980; Yakovlev, 1967)

If you have to commute to work, you might as well lose a few calories while you are doing it. You don't really need to wear your suit jacket while driving. The gas station attendant isn't going to think less of you. If it is cool, open your window and let in as much cool air as is possible without discomfort. If it is a warm day, turn down the air conditioner to as cool a temperature as is still comfortable. Driving along in an open car on a delightful 75° F day wearing jogging shorts can help you lose energy about as fast as that poor jogger struggling along behind you in his heavy sweat suit. Of course these thermogenic weight loss techniques do not give you the cardiovascular conditioning that exercise provides, but cardiovascular conditioning is done more rapidly by relatively brief peak output exercise rather than jogging. See Chapter 14 for more information on cardiovascular conditioning and peak output exercise.

Now that you understand the principles of thermogenesis, go to "Designing Your Own Personal Program," Chapter 15, and write down as many ways as you can to play it cool. Thermogenic clothing is one of the most universally applicable techniques. Remember that it's good to be cool, but you don't have to shiver.

Warning: Thermogenic techniques work by making you burn more calories. Thermogenic clothes and thermogenic drugs increase your rate of burning calories. Free radicals are produced whenever you burn any kind of calories, and the more calories you burn, the more free radicals you produce, whether that burning is promoted by exercise, thermogenic drugs, or cool weather. Inadequately controlled free radicals can cause cardiovascular disease, cancer, and aging. (See our *Life Extension: A Practical Scientific Approach* and *The Life Extension Companion* for further data.)

Anything that increases the rate at which you burn calories requires added free-radical-scavenging protection. Do NOT take phenylpropanolamine or ephedrine-containing drugs unless they also contain properly formulated free-radical-scavenging nutrient supplements. Several essential nutrients such as vitamins E and C and the mineral selenium are needed by your body to control free radicals. See the Safety Appendix for our suggested free-radical-scavenging multivitamin-mineral supplement.

13

Changing Your Behavior: How to Act Slim, or It's All in Your Mind

If you have a bad relationship with food, you can help change it by behaving differently. By behavior change, we do not *mean forcing yourself to be hungry when you want to eat.* These behavioral changes do not require a lot of will power, but they do require learning a few new *habits.* These may be as simple and enjoyable as paying more attention to your food. Wouldn't you like to get *more* pleasure out of your food while at the same time getting *fewer* calories?

It's possible to obtain a significant degree of weight control by following some simple practices that act as biofeedback to your brain's own biochemical feeding and weight control mechanisms.

Much of the satisfaction of eating food is caused by the release of a hormone called CCK in the hypothalamus in your brain. Rats given CCK brain injections will starve themselves to death next to a pile of their favorite food. Rats with brain damage to the CCK-sensitive areas will literally kill themselves by overeating.

The satisfying effect of the CCK that stimulates your brain depends on your perceptions *of eating, and on your* perceptions *of your body's fat stores, as well as on your actual caloric intake.* Your body has natural built-in mechanisms to tell you when you should eat and when you should stop. The trouble is, you may be so involved with a television program or the newspaper that you hardly notice you're eating at all. Eat like Durk and Sandy, both of whom are devoted gourmets.

Pay attention to your food. Don't let the TV or a newspaper compete for your attention while you're eating. If you watch the news or read a newspaper while eating, your lack of attention to the food may cause you to consume considerably more food before feeling satisfied. When you pick up your newspaper, you should put your fork down. When you put down your newspaper, you can pick up your fork again. *Using our program, most people can eat all they want, but they should not habitually eat food that provides no satisfaction.* Turn off the TV when you eat and put that newspaper away until you are done. Food should be one of the finest sensual pleasures of life, not an ignored side activity while you do something else. *Even if it is a TV dinner instead of a gourmet feast, you must pay attention to your eating if you expect to feel satisfied with the number of calories that your body really needs.*

When you eat, CCK (cholecystokinin, a polypeptide hormone) is released in the hypothalamus in your brain to make you feel full and satisfied. If you do not pay attention to the sensory qualities of your food and the act of eating itself, you may get less CCK released per calorie. This CCK release and the resulting satisfaction takes time. *You can facilitate the effectiveness of your CCK satiation mechanism by eating slowly, savoring your food, and allowing adequate time for the CCK release to occur and make you feel satisfied. When you wolf down your food, you don't give the mechanism a chance to stop you. You eat more than is really necessary to make you feel good and full.*

You can increase your eating satisfaction without increasing the amount of food that you eat. One thing you can do is make the food look good on your plate. Use slightly smaller bowls, plates, forks, and spoons if you want to eat less. The plate won't look so empty, as if there were a food shortage, and you can clean your plate without feeling guilty. Sandy is a creative gourmet cook and arranges the food artistically on the plate so that it is visually beautiful as well as delicious. This helps focus attention on food and eating, which in turn facilitates CCK release. The smaller spoons and forks also give you the time that you need to get that satisfying CCK release before you go on to overeat.

Unless you are on a very unpleasantly restrictive diet such as the Pritikin program, you will be *cafeteria-feeding.* This means that you will be tempted by unlimited quantities of a wide variety of foods. As we mentioned previously, cafeteria feeding leads to obesity in experimental animals which do not become fat even when allowed to eat all the lab chow they want.

It is possible to eliminate unnecessary food consumption and eliminate obesity in normal laboratory animals simply by eliminating all variety and giving them unlimited supplies of just one nutritious lab chow. This is a very boring diet, and we don't think you'd want to do that any more than we do. If you are interested in trying this type of diet, we highly recommend Ralston Purina High Protein Monkey Chow. It is ideal for this type of diet; it is extremely nutritious and exceedingly boring. If you try this experiment, please write us and let us know what happens. Our address is in Appendix 2, "How to Join Our Research Program."

Since you are going to be eating cafeteria style anyway, you might as well make the best of it. *Learn to use spices and herbs to make food taste more interesting and to hold your sensate focus.* It is not much fun to eat boring, bland food, and it is difficult to pay close attention to it continually. Try to detect all the different flavors in the food as you eat. The human gustatory system is really quite sensitive. Savor every bite of your food.

Don't eat food that you aren't really enjoying. You should be delighted with each and every calorie. When you aren't, it's time to stop eating and find something else to do with your time. *Never eat automatically.* When you are hungry, you will have no trouble at all focusing on your food. If you are having trouble paying close attention to your food, you are either simply not hungry or your food is terribly boring and bland, such as an ulcer patient's diet.

Don't talk with your mouth full; that is simply another way to ignore your food and the satisfaction of eating. Eat with someone else whenever you can and talk as much as you like; this will give more time for your CCK release and satiation to occur. If chewing and swallowing a big mouthful of food takes too long for you to keep up with the conversation, don't talk with your mouth full; take smaller bites instead. Whether talking with your mouth full in your home is acceptable etiquette or not is irrelevant; talking with your mouth full can help make you fat. Perhaps someday that will be a new old wives' tale.

Try taking about 85 percent of your normal serving size and eating slowly. If you still feel hungry, wait 10 minutes before taking more.

Keep the extra food out of sight until the 10 minutes is over or your famine insurance behavior genes will try to get you to eat every bit of it by keeping you hungry when you would otherwise feel satisfied. This 10-minute delay gives your body's satiation signals, such as CCK release, more time to take place. It's all right to read or watch TV while you're not eating.

Eat just as much as is necessary to satisfy you, not more. When you stop enjoying the food and are just going through the motions, remember that it is time to stop eating. Frankly we sometimes have trouble with this one ourselves; it is awfully easy for us to continue to munch away automatically when our minds are absorbed by some fascinating scientific data.

Never eat because there is nothing else to do! Wait until you feel at least a little hungry so that you can really enjoy it. Don't make your eating a slightly less boring alternative to being bored!

Take charge! You can decide in advance just how much food you will eat. Be reasonable. You neither want to deprive yourself nor eat beyond what is really needed for satisfaction. *Try portion control.* An excellent way to do that is to eat the low-calorie, high-quality, good-tasting "gourmet" TV dinners. A wide variety of them is now available at supermarkets. Sandy, although she is an excellent cook, often has one of these for lunch. It is amazing how much food satisfaction you can get with only 300 calories. Nutrition is generally very good. Besides, the plates that come with these frozen microwave-oven meals are reusable and make excellent plates for home-made controlled portions, since they are relatively small.

Don't eat a liquid food when you are just thirsty. You can consume a lot of calories without really quenching your thirst. If you are *thirsty,* don't reach for that high-calorie, sugar-filled soda pop. That lingering sweet taste will leave you thirsty anyway. You can quench your thirst even better without the calories by drinking good-tasting activated charcoal-filtered water. Many people may be eating a liquid food when they are thirsty simply because their tap water tastes so bad. There is no reason to put up with that yucky taste when inexpensive activated charcoal filters are so easy to get. The best type mounts under your sink and provides another tap for the treated water. It uses a disposable activated charcoal cartridge that is about 10 inches long and 3 inches in diameter, lasts about 6 months, and costs less than $10.00 to replace. Beware of small units that attach directly to your tap; they are not big enough to hold much of the activated-charcoal purifying agent, so they must be replaced quite frequently.

You can help control the complaints of your empty stomach by drinking plenty of water, especially when you feel like snacking. We aren't suggesting that you drink ordinary tap water, which usually tastes terrible and often contains small amounts of mildly carcinogenic (cancer-causing) chlorine and chlorinated organics. A simple inexpensive activated-charcoal filtration unit (see the Suppliers' Appendix) can remove these pollutants while leaving in the healthful minerals. This filtered water tastes as good as bottled water, at a greatly reduced price and with greater convenience.

For a real treat, drink club soda (carbonated water) when your stomach needs something to do. It tastes delicious, and Sandy thinks the fizz really feels good on her tongue. Sandy is a full-fledged club sodaholic and drinks about a liter a day. We wonder whether the physiological effects of carbon dioxide might be responsible for the great popularity of carbonated drinks. Carbon dioxide is known to open up the blood-brain barrier, allowing migration of substances into the brain that would otherwise take place more slowly or not at all. Carbon dioxide also increases brain blood flow. In any event it is a delightful snack. Soda water doesn't have to be expensive. Sandy once believed that she could tell the difference by taste between Perrier water and a less expensive club soda (Schweppes). In a double-blind taste test (neither Sandy nor Durk knew what type of water was in the glasses she drank from until the experiment was over), Sandy was unable to distinguish between them.

You can help control your figure and fat stores with biofeedback, by measuring your size, body fat percentage, and weight regularly.

Many types of physiological functions can be controlled by biofeedback, including pulse rate, blood pressure, body temperature, and brain waves. Both Durk and Sandy have been able to reduce their pulse rate by at least 10 beats a minute with as little as 15 minutes of practice using a pulse rate meter and have learned to alter their brain waves with EEG (electroencephalograph) biofeedback. Many studies have demonstrated biofeedback control of body temperature. Some people have even learned how to control their migraine headaches by biofeedback reduction of their scalp and fore-head temperature. (Migraine headaches are due to abnormal dilation of blood vessels in the brain, and dilation increases the temperature of the skin over blood vessels.) In a study of people with high blood pressure, 43 percent of them were able to reduce their blood pressure by at least 10 mm of mercury systolic pressure (blood pressure when the heart contracts) or 10 mm diastolic (blood pressure when the heart relaxes) by simply measuring their blood pressure twice a day for a month. (Laughlin, 1979)

In the same way, if you tape-measure your fat problem areas and weigh yourself daily, you can help your brain's weight setpoint center to stabilize your weight. Both Durk and Sandy have found that if they neglect to weigh themselves daily, their weights tend to creep up by as much as fifteen pounds! It is best to weigh yourself at the same time of the day on the same scale. We are not suggesting that you look at your weight and tape measurements and say, "Aaargh! That's awful! I've got to force myself to go hungry!" That is not the purpose at all. The purpose is to provide you with an up-to-date accurate perception of your figure and weight, which in turn will unconsciously affect how much you *feel* like eating.

A person's perception of his or her fatness or lack of it is extremely important. People may erroneously believe that they are fat and may be constantly dieting (which could cause severe nutritional deficiencies and cardiovascular problems) and, of course, may never reach their goal because of their misperceptions. Anorexia nervosa and bulimia are extreme examples. These are bizarre, potentially fatal diseases in which there are pathological misperceptions of fatness that cause people to starve themselves or to binge-eat and then use laxatives or purgatives to get rid of the eaten food.

For the purpose of maintaining an accurate perception of your body, you should:

1. Use a tape measure to measure your fat problem areas once per day. Good accurate hip and bust measurements on women are easy to make, but be careful to make abdominal measurements the same way each time. Don't suck your belly in for one measurement and let it hang out for another. We suggest that you make your abdominal measurement while you are standing and relaxed since you don't really plan to go around for the rest of your life laboriously pulling

your abdomen in. The best time to do this is before your biggest meal of the day. Write your daily measurements down on the chart in Appendix 1, "Your Own Case History."

2. Look at yourself nude in a good mirror at least once a day. Use a flat mirror which does not produce "waves" in your image; that would not be an accurate self-perception and might not be credible to your weight control center. Either plate-glass or the less expensive float-glass mirrors are suitable. We think that the cheapest window-glass mirrors have too much distortion to be acceptable. Focus your attention on those areas of your body that you would like to reshape or reduce. Look at them, touch them, think of how they are now and how you would like them to be. It is difficult to have a realistic perception of your body if you keep it covered with loose clothes and never look at yourself nude in a mirror. A three-piece suit can hide the difference between an athlete and someone who has 30 extra pounds of fat. In that sense, a three-piece suit can help make you fat!

3. Use an accurate electronic scale or doctors' beam balance. Using an inaccurate "cheapo" scale or using different scales rather than the same one can give you an inaccurate picture of what is happening to your body. Different scales can give widely differing readings for the same person, and an inaccurate one can be off by several pounds. Weigh yourself at the same time each day while wearing the same clothing, or circadian (day-to-night biorhythm) weight variations and clothes weight variations may just confuse your weight control center. (It is best to weigh yourself nude in front of a mirror.) You can expect a significant day-to-day variation in your weight; pay attention to the weekly trend, not just today's latest number. Plotting the data on a weight-trend graph can help you do this. This technique is explained in Chapter 16, "Measuring Your Progress."

Ideally we suggest tape-measuring and weighing yourself, and looking at your nude reflection when you wake up in the morning, just before dinner, and when you go to bed at night. A taping, weigh-in, and look-at just before your largest meal of the day can really alter the amount of food that it takes to make you feel satisfied. If you don't pay regular attention to the shape of your body, is it so surprising that it isn't what you want? See Chapter 16 for further information.

Medically supervised behavior change weight loss clinics can be very helpful in producing and consolidating changes of habits. Many people have trouble ridding themselves of old, undesired habits because those habits have become invisible to them over the years. It is very difficult to change something when you are not aware of it. Forming new habits can be difficult too, since it is easy to forget to incorporate a new desired habit into an old, well-consolidated behavior pattern. In a way these clinics supply biofeedback about your eating habits, thereby helping you to change them. The peer groups at these clinics play an effective role in helping an individual to become fully aware of his or her habits. If you need help in changing your habits, one of these clinics may be right for you. (Blackburn, 1978; Bray, 1970; Bray, 1983; Brownell, 1983; Clausen, 1980; Johnson, 1979; Steffee, 1982; Stuart, 1978; Stunkard, 1983; Stunkard, 1979; Volkmar, 1981)

How do you pick a good clinic? It isn't easy. A lot of them are full of expensive nonsense. First look for a clinic with real medical supervision. Do they have a physician or registered nurse on duty? Do they draw blood for an initial panel of clinical laboratory tests and for subsequent follow-up tests? Are the results of these tests explained to you by a physician? Does their sales literature cite any real scientific papers? *Important Note: the FDA will not permit them to give you scientific literature references which deal with uses for foods and drugs that have not been approved for those specific purposes by the FDA. They can give you copies of papers on behavior therapy, however, since this is not FDA regulated.* Do they have documented proof of the effectiveness of their techniques? Do they give you a nutritional supplement that is something like our suggested supplement, or is it more like the FDA's frequently less-than-optimum Recommended Daily Allowances? (For details see "The FDA's Recommended Daily Allowances" in *Life Extension.)* Do they measure your fat loss progress with a tape measure and a skin-fold caliper (or by underwater weighing), or are they only interested in your weight on a scale? Do they provide free follow-up visits? Behavior change frequently requires occasional follow-up visits to the clinic to thoroughly consolidate the new habits. If these additional visits cost extra, you are unlikely to use them as often as is required, and the new habits are likely to fade away, leaving you with your old habits and a substantially smaller bank account. See Appendix 4, the supplier section, for firms with effective programs.

Incidentally, do not expect existing weight loss clinics to be using many of the techniques described in this book. Very few clinics are biochemically oriented. They will put you on a low-calorie, highly restrictive diet and make you stick to it, but they will teach you some good habits and will make sure that you unlearn some old bad habits. *We look forward to the day when professionally medically supervised weight loss clinics will be using the advanced biochemical techniques described in this book.*

Warning: See the warning in Appendix 4, the Suppliers' Appendix, before assuming that any organization's implications or explicit claims that we are associated with them are true. Most likely they are misleading you. While we would be delighted to help develop a program of this sort, it has been our experience that there are a lot of fly-by-night outfits that are not interested in our information and just want to illicitly appropriate our names and the trust that people have in them.

Dr. Ronald Klatz has had a lot of clinical experience with behavior modification as part of weight reduction programs. He writes about some of his own experiences and makes some very useful suggestions in the remainder of this chapter.

CLINICAL BEHAVIOR MODIFICATION

Get a Good Start

A wise man once said the journey of 100 pounds starts with the first ounce, or something similar. Losing weight, like any other worthy project, requires a certain amount of thought, dedication, and energy.

I recommend that my patients don't even start their weight loss program until their personal and professional lives are straightened out so that a sudden unexpected upset will not drive them back to their friend and comforter . . . food.

Give yourself 3 weeks to get a good start on your weight loss program. *Make it your number one priority.* Nothing else succeeds like success, and three solid weeks of successful weight loss will help you not to quit when the novelty of this new life-style wears off.

Lock Up the Kitchen at Night

Mrs. W. was a late night snacker. As a child she would have milk and cookies before bed. On occasion her mother would punish her by sending her to her room without dinner; going to bed without a snack meant being unloved. Unfortunately the midnight snack behavior initiated in childhood contributed significantly to Mrs. W.'s being 126 pounds above her ideal body weight. Food ingested before sleep is usually deposited as fat because the body is at its lowest level of metabolism at night, and bowel motility is similarly slowed.

Following the proper therapy, Mrs. W. has in the last 6 months been able to obtain a 62-pound weight loss with the aid of her husband, who padlocks their refrigerator at night and also leaves out a plate of high-fiber low-calorie foods such as celery, lettuce, radishes, and plain popcorn.

The added advantage to her new late snack is that these high-fiber foods can decrease the risk of gastrointestinal tract cancer by 75 percent and also speed bowel transit so that less food is absorbed.

Feeding Frenzy, Not Just for Sharks

If your eyes roll back in your head and your ears seem to disconnect when eating your favorite meal in 3 minutes or less, you suffer from this maladaptive behavior.

Most afflicted don't even know that they have it. It requires the loving interest of someone nearby to alert you to this problem. Chances are you won't believe them until they perform the ultimate test: *take away your plate in midmeal and try to have a five-minute conversation with you.* If you find yourself threatening your loved one's life with your butter knife, you do indeed suffer from feeding frenzy. Feeding frenzy is a problem because higher centers of consciousness are disconnected during the meal so that they are unable to monitor the number of calories you are busily stuffing into your face. Also the biochemical clues which tell your body that you have eaten enough can require 20 minutes to be liberated from the glands of your digestive tract and reach the brain. This rapid unconscious eater can eat hundreds of calories more than necessary to achieve the same level of satisfaction.

This is the most effective and possibly most dangerous technique to stop feeding frenzy. Have someone you love and will not hurt even in anger help you stop eating by disfiguring your meal with unpalatable combinations of condiments on your food. Have them pour salt on your hot fudge or pour mustard on your pancakes, etc. This technique is immediately successful in stopping the feeding frenzy behavior; however, it should be handled with caution as rage and violence often erupt. It may even be good to try this technique on yourself as a test of your own willpower.

Put a Bug in Your Ear

Subliminal training of the subconscious mind is a fast and powerful technique. Just remember that your sweet tooth and your urges to binge-eat are all programmed at a subconscious level, and reinforced by years of habit.

Psychological studies of the sixties conducted by the CIA for brainwashing and later adopted by advertising executives trying to sell cola at the movies, involved flashing subtle cues on the movie screen faster than the conscious mind could register the message (approximately 1/60 of a second) . . . too fast for the conscious mind but not too fast for the subconscious mind to understand: *Thirsty? Have a cola.* Fortunately for consumers, to be effective these techniques had to be right on the borderline of consciousness; this made detection fairly easy for those whose visual perception was a little quicker than average. Public outcry forced the mind games to stop.

A similar method of subliminal training is available to anyone with an auto-reverse tape recorder. You can, for about $45.00 (including tapes), make your own training cassettes. The suggested tape is a C-20 dictation tape with 10 minutes of playing time per side. Play a soothing instrumental, or natural sounds such as rain or a waterfall—any sound you will find soothing and wouldn't mind listening to repeatedly.

While your background music is playing (approximately 6 inches from the microphone), speak in a soft, distinct monotone voice (place the microphone about 12 inches from your mouth). You may say something like: "I will sleep a sound and restful enjoyable sleep tonight for I know that every day I am becoming thinner, more vital, and more energetic than before. I feel great and look great. I enjoy eating healthful foods but I don't eat excessively. I enjoy a 30-minute aerobic workout each day. I feel alive and healthy, better in every way than the day before."

You may pause for a few minutes and repeat this three times on each side of the tape. Now if all has gone well you should have your own custom subliminal tape. Play back your tape, and you should have a soft instrumental background with a barely audible voice urging you on to a happier and healthier life-style. Now tonight, when ready to retire, put the tape recorder under your mattress to dull the click of the auto-reverse mechanism and play your tape. It will run throughout the night delivering over 144 inspirational messages to your subconcious at the end of 8 hours sleep.

To avoid boredom and the occasional side effect of hearing that melody play on in your head throughout the next day, I recommend making 3 or 4 tapes and rotating them.

You will soon find that you have successfully programmed your inner self with new beliefs which will beget healthier behaviors . . . and as your inner self changes for the better, the external you will soon follow.

How Would You Like to Lose an Extra 20 Pounds a Year?

My patients' favorite behavior-modification trick is to carry a pedometer; just like Jiminy Cricket on Pinocchio's shoulder, your friendly pedometer will click off each step you take every day and record it on its dial.

I was amazed to see the miles expended daily by my patients increase from an average of 2 miles per day to 7 miles per day. This increased low-level exercise can mean an additional 200 calories spent each day, or 73,000 calories per year, or 20 pounds a year! An easy victory in the course of life-long weight control.

Weight Loss Log

Perhaps the best and most effective behavior modification technique is the personal weight loss log. By your daily tracking of calories in and calories out, you begin reprogramming your subconscious as to just how many calories your body really requires to maintain your ideal body weight.

First decide on your approximate daily caloric requirements. For example, you may wish to use this formula: 10 calories a day for each pound. For example, a 150-pound man may have a resting metabolic level of 1500 calories a day to maintain his metabolic needs. If that person ate 1500 calories and exercised 300 calories per day, that would result in a net loss of 300 calories a day or 1 pound per week. (Remember that this is an approximation, and your metabolic rate will vary according to many factors, including time of day, temperature, age, activity level, etc.)

Suppose you are a 150-pound female who currently expends 400 calories of aerobic exercise daily. Your estimated daily caloric need is 1900 calories per day or 13,300 calories per week. You decide to cut your dietary intake to 1400 calories, leaving you 500 calories a day low, or a 1-pound weight loss per week.

Keep your calorie log with you at all times. Write in how many calories you're about to eat. This alone may dissuade you from snack eating when you must count up the cost prior to the meal.

Keep a record even when you blow it. A page or two of 3,000 calorie plus days may encourage you to make up for it with a few lower-calorie days.

Most important of all, it will give you a true sense of responsibility regarding your weight. If you develop the habit of recording caloric input and output, the numbers will start to speak for themselves. If you are not losing weight at 1200 calories per day, then your log book will tell you that you must decrease your daily caloric intake to

1000 calories per day or increase your daily calorie output by additional exercise.

Without this method of calorie tracking, you're a millionaire without an accountant; you can spend yourself into the poorhouse of massive obesity and not even know why.

The Belly Belt

Scales lie! (Isn't that great news . . . ?) In a fat loss and muscle-building program, it is quite possible that you might put on more pounds of lean body mass (in the form of muscle) than you lose of fat. Remember that muscle weighs considerably more than the same amount of fat; thus you might lose significant amounts of fat without the scale budging a pound.

To help prevent my patients from becoming discouraged and drowning their sorrows in a 4000-calorie super hot-fudge sundae, I give them a belly-measuring belt. It is a military issue brass buckle cotton web belt that is infinitely adjustable.

Every day, or at least once a week, my patient can measure his or her progress by tightening the belly belt to a new leaner mark, showing the patient positive improvement toward a slimmer body regardless of what the scale has to say. Do it at the same time of day each time. Mark the belt each time with a pen, and every 7 days write the date next to that day's mark.

Mind Training

Amazing new discoveries in the areas of peak performance athletics are showing that mental training is of even greater importance than physical conditioning to world-class athletes. As a sports medicine consultant to several top elite world champion athletes, I have seen how important concentration and mental conditioning is to a winning performance at the tournaments and on the training floor.

These same techniques can now be used by you to help recondition your eating behavior. New research shows that our subconscious thoughts can alter insulin release, growth hormone secretion, body temperature, heart rate, and metabolism. *The correct mental attitude toward weight loss can also help you to reset your metabolism.*

Always concentrate on a positive image. You may tell yourself, "I am getting stronger, healthier, thinner, and more vigorous every day." Never tell yourself, "I am a fat pig, and if I don't shape up soon, I'm going to die a horrible death." Your subconscious mind just might believe you and make your wish come true!

Write down your positive self-image itinerary on 3 × 5 cards and put them on your bathroom mirror to read first thing every day. Put them in your top desk drawer at work; put them on the dashboard of your car. Soon you'll come to believe it yourself and will start taking steps to make it your reality.

Send yourself a letter, just so you won't forget.

Cut out a picture of someone whose body you'd like to have and then cut your face from your own picture and stick it on the body you would like to own. Take this new hybrid photo and stick it to your refrigerator to give yourself a clear-cut mental image of the person you will become.

It is amazing how many of my overweight patients have no sense of a positive self-image. They are afraid to take a really good look at themselves in the mirror for fear of what they would see. I suggest that you invest in a full-length mirror so that you can see yourself every day. Many overweight individuals have difficulty finding clothing that fits well; this compounds their appearance problem, leading to an even worse sense of low self-esteem. A mirror will let you check your progress toward a firmer, thinner body, which can be a tremendous reward. Beyond that, it will also encourage you toward better posture and a more attractive appearance.

The Spoilers

Chances are that if you are overweight, you have tried to reduce many times in the past. The grim statistics are that over 95 percent of all persons who attempt permanent weight loss fail. Your chances are much better in beating cancer . . . ever wonder why?

Of course many overweight persons have a slower metabolism, but how many weight reduction programs have been sabotaged by an Old World mother saying "Eat, eat, eat," or "You're too thin, you'll get sick," or by a friend who just can't stand to drink those 200-calorie beers alone . . . Or perhaps it's the girlfriend or boyfriend trying to win your heart through your stomach and who loves you just as you are.

The sad reality of many failed weight reduction programs is that many times those you care about most are helping to ensure the failure of your diet program. They may have a psychological commitment to your staying overweight. If you slim down, you might change your behavior to suit your new body, you might change your friends, you might be more attractive to the opposite sex, and you might not love them anymore . . . so it's simply not safe for them to allow you to change.

This is a very difficult problem to handle. The best result I have seen in my medical practice has been to include family and friends in an initial weight loss counseling session to tell them all that it was of urgent medical importance for the patient to lose weight, and if they loved the patient, they would do all that they could to encourage the weight reduction program.

Sadly even this intervention was only helpful about half of the time, and even then the effect of my "sermon" usually lasted for only about two months; knowledge of this phenomenon may help you to handle this pitfall.

Can a Full Life Take the Place of a Full Belly?

Here are some tips which seem to work well for my patients:

1. Try not to eat alone; being with others usually requires conversation, which slows eating.

2. Try to eat bites no larger than your thumbnail.

3. Take a 2-minute break sometime in the middle of your meal to allow your mind to catch up with what you've eaten.

4. Count calories before eating them so that you won't overeat.

5. Have a meal with yourself; take a full-length mirror and put it

across the table from yourself! *Watch yourself as you eat.* Do you rush to empty your plate, or do you eat with a slow, dignified confidence? What are you afraid of . . . that somebody bigger will come along and eat your food? Two weeks of this psychological feedback can change your eating habits forever.

6. Plan your meals for each day by placing the foods that you will eat today in a minirefrigerator or an ice chest. Then bolt the doors shut on your main refrigerator and give the key away. This will force you to make do with what is in the small refrigerator and end high-caloric nighttime food raids. This technique works very well for those with *no willpower.*

7. Take a 20-minute brisk walk after dinner; it will speed digestion and burn a couple of hundred extra calories.

8. Take multivitamin and antioxidant nutrients daily with any weight loss program to compensate for lost nutrition due to your calorie restriction.

9. As we age, metabolism slows approximately 7 percent for each decade of life past age 20. So you must eat less just to maintain your ideal body weight.

10. Twenty minutes of exercise a day will add up to a 20-pound loss in one year, provided you don't compensate for the added exercise with extra food.

11. Always leave something on your plate; it may save you 50 calories a day, which can add up to a 5-pound weight loss at the end of one year. Victory over weight comes from winning many small battles. These techniques also help to break the habit of eat, eat, eat . . .

14

Peak Output Exercise: The Astronauts' Fast Exercise Method

There are different types of exercise. You need to understand the different benefits conferred by different types of exercise and have a clear picture of your own personal goals before designing your exercise program. What is your principal goal? Is it improving your figure and/or building your muscles? Is it cardiovascular conditioning? Is it improving your stamina for endurance sports? These different goals require different approaches.

The type of exercise that is touted the most in the popular press is aerobic exercise, which is subpeak exercise (you aren't working almost as hard as you can) done for long periods of time to increase stamina and endurance. You need this type of exercise to be competitive in an endurance sport such as tennis. We do not yet have a quick replacement for all that time-consuming hard work.

Most people reading this book are not competitive athletes. They are very interested in their figure; they want to know how to slim their fat deposits and perhaps build up some of their muscles. They want a better body shape. If this is your goal, we do have a quick replacement for a lot of time-consuming hard work.

We also hope that our more sedentary readers will be interested in cardiovascular conditioning, especially since worthwhile results can be obtained without lengthy exercise.

These latter two goals are appropriate applications for peak output exercise. Peak output exercise involves working nearly as hard as you can for a short period of time, whereas aerobic exercises such as jogging involve working at much less than peak output for a long period of time. Since this is not an exercise manual for endurance sports athletes, we will be focusing on the fast results that can be obtained from peak output exercise.

Exercise is capable of delivering certain health benefits to those who do the right type and the right amount. Yet many myths prevail about the efficacy of exercise. For example, many people believe that exercise is a good way to burn up excess calories. *It takes about* 10 *hours of jogging to burn one pound of fat!* That is a lot of time and effort, more than many people are willing to expend.

A 70-kg (154-pound) person would use up the following calories per hour for the designated activities: sitting, 100; typing, 139; rowing (50 m/min), 180; fast rowing (80 m/min), 365; very fast rowing (100 m/min), 680; driving a car, 112; cycling (10 km/hr), 300; sawing wood, 480; carrying a 211-pound load, 520. You can see that you have to do a lot of work to burn off a significant amount of fat. While exercise can provide you with valuable benefits, we do not recommend exercise as a quick and easy way to lose fat.

GH RELEASERS AND EXERCISE

The muscle-building and fat-mobilizing effectiveness of exercise can be increased, however, through the proper use of growth hormone releasers. (See Chapter 5, "Growth Hormone Releasers and Your Muscle-to-Fat Ratio.") A major finding of the Baltimore Longitudinal Study of Aging (sponsored by the National Institute on Aging) is that adults over about 30 years old no longer release growth hormone in response to exercise. (Muscle, 1980) Most teenagers respond rapidly to exercise by building muscle and losing body fat because they release GH when they exercise. We think that unless the exercise is very lengthy, the fat-mobilizing, anti-fat-storage effects of the exercise-induced GH release are likely to be more important than the number of calories burned by the exercise.

Many scientists think that this decline of growth hormone output is responsible for much of the loss of lean body mass which usually occurs as you age. Our GH-releaser supplementation program is capable, in the average healthy adult, of restoring peak GH levels back to that of a vigorously exercising young adult or someone in their late teens, thus restoring the ability of your body to build and maintain lean body mass, mobilize stored fat for burning, and retard fat storage.

Growth hormone from our use of GH releasers has a lot to do with our relatively large ratios of lean body and muscle mass to fat. However, another biochemical system controls muscle tone.

MUSCLE TONE AND CHOLINE

Poor muscle tone can make a fairly lean person look fat. A sagging stomach may not be due to fat at all but to poor muscle tone in your abdominal muscles, which fail to hold your gut in. Exercise is certainly capable of improving muscle tone, but only when you do specific exercises for the sagging muscles. Doing biceps exercises will not tone your stomach, no matter how many of them you do. There is another method of improving muscle tone which does not require exercise but does require taking a nutritional supplement regularly.

The natural biochemical responsible for maintaining muscle tone and making your muscles contract is acetylcholine. Acetylcholine has other functions as well. It also plays an important role in verbal activity, memory, and sex. Choline, a nutrient that you can buy at a health food store, is used by your body and brain to manufacture acetylcholine. A good natural source is fish.

Most people can improve their muscle tone simply by taking choline supplements. Your choline supplement should include vitamin B-5, also called pantothenic acid or calcium pantothenate, since this is a necessary cofactor your body needs to transform choline into acetylcholine. If you take too much choline, however, your muscle tone can become too high and you can get a muscle tension headache or a stiff neck. If you take the wrong type of choline, it can cause diarrhea. See the Safety Appendix for recommended dose and details.

If you take the recommended dose of choline every day for muscle tone, you may experience a beneficial side effect because this dose of choline per day has been shown in humans to improve memory! MIT students taking choline (the same amount that we suggest in the Safety Appendix) in a scientific study had improved memories and improved abilities to learn a list of words. (Sitaram, Weingartner, Caine, Gillin, 1978; Sitaram, Weingartner, Gillin, 1978) Anecdotal reports by people we know who are taking the supplement include increased vocabularies and improved verbal abilities. The "Mr. Smith" in the case histories section of our *Life Extension: A Practical Scientific Approach* (who we can now admit is really Clint Eastwood) experienced dramatic benefits of this sort. Other frequent anecdotal reports are of increased sexual activity and capacity, particularly in subjects in their sixties and seventies. (We have not heard of this effect on sex from people under fifty.) For more details see the brain biochemistry and case history sections of our *Life Extension: A Practical Scientific Approach.*

Note, however, that while this method of improving your muscle tone may quickly and easily improve your appearance by helping to hold your tummy in, it does not build muscles or improve your cardiovascular conditioning, unlike exercise.

SOME RISKS AND BENEFITS OF EXERCISE

Exercise, like other activities, has both potential benefits and potential risks. Prolonged heavy exercise may be addictive. Natural opiate-like compounds, such as the endorphins, are increased in the bloodstreams of joggers. Dedicated joggers who cannot jog due to injury or bad weather can experience "withdrawal" symptoms. These withdrawal symptoms are similar to those of heroin withdrawal and can be medically treated in the same way with clonidine. The "high" of exercise may be due to these natural substances, at least in part. The risk of injury (particularly when you are filled with pain-deadening endorphins) is also part of exercise and should be considered when choosing the type of exercise you want to do.

Reports of sudden death from cardiovascular incidents, even in apparently healthy young individuals, are common enough so that anyone who intends to do strenuous exercise would be foolish not to have a complete physical exam performed prior to such exercise.

Some types of heart problems do not have symptoms, and being young is no guarantee that your heart is sound. The closest thing to a guarantee that you will get is a resting vector electrocardiogram followed by a cardiac stress test, both performed by your physician. In the latter test, your electrocardiogram is taken while you are exercising strenuously. This test is not entirely risk-free. There is a small chance that you will have a serious cardiac problem while exercising on your physician's treadmill before the EKG gives any warning. Nevertheless if you are going to have an exercise-induced heart failure, your doctor's office is certainly the best place for it! If these tests yield equivocal results, your physician will order further diagnostic tests.

Scientific reports have found that exercise is capable of decreasing cardiovascular risk factors such as blood triglycerides, and low-density lipoprotein (LDL) cholesterol levels. High-density lipoprotein (HDL) cholesterol, widely believed to be protective against cardiovascular disease, can be increased by exercise. (Ollivier, 1981) Some studies have indicated that a considerable amount of exercise may be required to obtain these benefits. For example, one study found that plasma concentrations of HDL and LDL did not begin to change until a threshold exercise level of running 10 miles per week was maintained for at least 9 months. (Williams, 1982) It is interesting to note that vitamins C and B-3 (but only as niacin, not niacinamide) have both been shown in human studies to greatly reduce serum triglyceride and VLDL cholesterol levels, without either exercise or changing diet. For more on this, see our *Life Extension: A Practical Scientific Approach,* and *The Life Extension Companion.* Note, however, that although nutrient supplements can improve your blood lipid levels and reduce your cardiovascular risk factors, they do not provide cardiovascular conditioning.

FREE RADICALS AND EXERCISE RISKS

During exercise the mitochondria (microscopic sugar- and fat-burning power plants) in your muscle cells are working overtime. While they are in the process of doing this, they create a lot of *free radicals,* promiscuously chemically reactive entities that are a natural part of mitochondrial metabolism. Unfortunately some of these free radicals escape the elaborate defense mechanisms in your mitochondria. Free radicals have been shown to be major causes of cancer, abnormal blood clots (leading to strokes and heart attacks), atherosclerosis, and aging processes. Free radicals are even responsible for all of the damage caused by X-ray radiation. (For a review of hundreds of scientific papers on this subject, see our *Life Extension: A Practical Scientific Approach.*) While we all have protective enzymes to help prevent these free radicals from getting out of hand and damaging our DNA, RNA, enzymes, structural proteins, fat-rich membranes, and other cellular components, our protection is not perfect and some damage does occur.

Several scientists, such as Dr. Lester Packer (professor of physiology and anatomy at the University of California, Berkeley) have proved that a considerable amount of free radical damage can take place during exercise. (Packer, 1984; Davies, 1982; Dillard, 1978) Older animals and older humans are particularly susceptible. Also extra susceptible are people who engage in behavior that generates unusually large amounts of free radicals, such as smoking and drinking too much alcohol. Free radical dangers are magnified if you exercise in air that contains elevated levels of ozone and nitrogen oxides (common constituents of smog) because these gasses cause free radical lung injury. The danger is especially severe if you are deficient in the antioxidant (anti-free radical) nutrients such as vitamins E and C, and the mineral selenium. (Too much vitamins and minerals can be dangerous too. See the Safety Appendix for suggested doses.)

Engaging in exercise causes your body to make more of some anti-free radical protective enzymes. This is called enzyme induction. Unfortunately not nearly enough of these protective enzymes are created to handle all the additional exercise-created free radicals. (Higuchi, 1985; Gyore, 1981) That means that you are somewhat better protected after exercise, but you are still at considerably greater risk of free radical damage while exercising. In one experiment, prolonged exercise increased the free-radical-scavenging enzyme superoxide dismutase by 14 to 37 percent in the mitochondria of exercised muscles, but there was no increase in two other important protective enzymes, catalase or cytoplasmic superoxide dismutase. Very vigorous exercise can increase your free radical production by as much as 10 times! Excess free radicals in your body can increase your risk of abnormal blood clots, which can result in heart attacks or strokes, and they may also sensitize the heart to cardiac arrhythmias.

These increased risks of free radical pathology can be reduced by taking anti-free radical antioxidant nutrients such as vitamins C, E, B-1, B-5, B-6, and the minerals zinc and selenium. It is important to take these antioxidant nutrients at least 3 times and preferably 4 times a day because most of the water-soluble ones are quickly eliminated via your urine when they are taken in large doses. The high serum levels you have a short time after taking them are back to your normal low levels within several hours. (For very detailed information on how and why to use these nutrients and how they work, see *Life Extension: A Practical Scientific Approach* and *The Life Extension Companion.*) See the Safety Appendix for our suggested multivitamin-mineral free-radical-scavenging formula and dosages.

Some of the incidents of sudden death during exercise (particularly after alcohol use) documented in the scientific literature may be due to the effects of increased numbers of these inadequately controlled free radicals. (There are other causes of course. A congenital heart condition called ideopathic hypertrophic subaortic stenosis is an important killer of exercise devotees. Your physician can test you for this condition.) We believe that this death toll might have been reduced if these people had been taking free-radical-controlling nutrients.

Caution: If you plan to engage in any exercise program, you should be aware of these precautions:

1. *Exercise and alcohol don't mix.* Even amounts of alcohol as small as a single drink cause damage to muscle fibers which can be seen with an electron microscope, and nerve damage in an injury is greatly increased. (Song, 1972; Flamm, 1977; Luck, 1983) Remember that your heart is a muscle and that its beating is neurally controlled. A frighteningly high percentage of sudden cardiovascular deaths in exercising apparently healthy young adults occur within 24 hours after using alcohol. You don't have to be drunk or even to have been drunk the night before for your risk to be significantly increased. The effect is statistically very significant; it is not due to

mere coincidence. Alcohol, especially when taken rapidly on an empty stomach or in large quantities, can be metabolized by a route involving the production of a lot of undesired free radicals.

2. *You should monitor your heart rate.* There is a heart rate that you should not exceed; it depends on your condition and age. We will have more to say about this later in this chapter. Inexpensive electronic pulse rate monitors are readily available, but most of them will give false readings if you move violently during the measurement. You can, however, use them to make a pulse rate measurement within a few seconds after you stop moving. There are even some pulse rate monitors that are designed to be used while exercising. One of the best units is actually a simple microminiaturized EKG that clips to your belt, with electrodes that are taped to your chest. This unit even has two adjustable pulse rate alarms—one tells you when you are not working hard enough; the other warns you when you are going too far. A similar EKG pulse rate monitor and alarm is available on some advanced exercise bicycles; the bicycle's handlebars are the EKG electrodes. See the Suppliers' Appendix.

3. *You should monitor your blood pressure.* Although many scientists believe that over a long period of time exercise may decrease blood pressure, your blood pressure is increased while you are doing the exercise and for a short period afterward. There are many inexpensive electronic blood pressure gauges on the market. You will probably have to make the measurement immediately after you stop exercising, since these devices can be confused by movement. The easiest to use, the least likely to give you a false reading, and the only one that may work while exercising (but only if one of your arms is reasonably still) uses what is called an oscillometric measuring system. There is no microphone in the pressure cuff; hence cuff placement is far less critical, and movements are much less likely to cause errors. Surprisingly an oscillometric instrument costs no more. See the Suppliers' Appendix.

4. *You should consult with your physician, letting him or her know of your exercise plans, and seek advice as to your personal maximum safe heart rate and blood pressure for short exercise periods.*

5. *Cardiovascular patients* must *have a cardiac stress test before attempting to engage in exercise, especially if it is of the highly stressful peak output type.*

6. The more exercise you do and the greater its intensity, the more free-radical-controlling nutrient supplements you will require.

7. We also suggest that during exercise you pay close attention to your body and what you are doing with it. We have noticed that many people who exercise, such as joggers, are actually listening to a radio rather than being focused on their body and their actions. *This inattention undoubtedly contributes to a lot of joggers being run over by cars. The risk of accidents during exercise is much greater for someone in normal health than all the other risks combined. Most accidents are caused by inattentiveness. Pay attention to what you are doing!* There may be another benefit from paying close attention to your exercise. Although we have no scientific proof of our contention, it is our unsubstantiated opinion that better results seem to occur with exercise when you pay close attention to your body. Perhaps it helps form more mind-body neural connections. We called a friend of ours who is a weight trainer at Gold's Gym in Venice, California. He said that although some bodybuilders listen to radios while they exercise, the serious ones usually don't; they pay close attention to their bodies.

PEAK OUTPUT EXERCISE AND CARDIOVASCULAR CONDITIONING

We promised you a fast approach to improving your figure, building muscles, and cardiovascular conditioning. It is a peak output exercise technique that was used in NASA's manned space flight program.

The Case of the Collapsing Astronauts

When man first ventured into space for periods of weeks rather than hours, the returning astronauts would be so weak that two strong men were assigned to each hero to hold him up so that he wouldn't collapse in front of the cameras. Living in the zero gravity of an orbiting space capsule is the ultimate in a sedentary life-style. With no physical exertion the muscles of the initially physically fit astronauts—including their heart muscles—rapidly deteriorated until they became too weak to walk on Earth. If this process of sedentary muscle deterioration continued, man would never go to the moon, and there would be no space stations, for who would become an astronaut if return to Earth meant death due to cardiovascular insufficiency?

NASA and its Gemini program contractor Douglas Aircraft selected exercise physiologist Dr. Lawrence E. Morehouse to do research to solve the problem of muscular and cardiovascular deconditioning in space, the most sedentary imaginable environment. To make the problem even more difficult, there was a serious time constraint. The astronauts had very full schedules, and time in orbit is precious. The astronauts could no more afford to spend hours a day working out than the most harried 80 hours of work a week business executive.

Dr. Morehouse and his colleagues succeeded. Man did go to the moon, and men can live in space stations. You can benefit from these techniques just like the astronauts.

Dr. Morehouse found that 10 minutes of *peak output* exercise every other day would give you most of the cardiovascular conditioning that could be obtained by an hour or more of conventional aerobic exercise every day. The peak output technique does not increase your stamina (a lot of aerobic exercise is still required to do that), but it does rapidly strengthen your heart muscle.

When Dr. Morehouse's peak output exercise techniques are combined with our growth hormone releaser techniques, the results can be amazing. With GH releasers and just *5 minutes per day* of peak output exercise, many people can see the difference in their muscles *in 2 weeks.* A total of 35 minutes of exercise a week makes a visible difference in many people. *Sandy's experience with GH releasers and 2 or 3 minutes a day of peak output exercise took off 25 pounds of fat and put on about 5 pounds of muscle in 6 weeks—with a grand total of less than 2 hours of exercise.* Peak output exercise alone does not have these dramatic results, although even alone it certainly improves your cardiovascular conditioning faster than jogging.

We do not have to write several long chapters or even an entire book on this subject because this exercise physiologist has already done the job. The book is well written, easy to understand, and designed for the layperson, not for other scientists. It is also inexpensive and available in paperback.

Dr. Lawrence A. Morehouse and Leonard Gross's book Total Fitness in 30 Minutes a Week *(hardback from Simon and Schuster, 1975; paperback from Pocket Books, 1975) is a good source of information for the layperson on the proper way to do peak output exercise.* (We should comment, however, that the title was probably chosen by the publisher; peak output exercise is not a substitute for prolonged aerobic exercise in sports requiring endurance.)

Dr. Morehouse not only designed the peak output exercise program for the NASA astronauts, he founded and directed the Human Performance Laboratory of the University of California at Los Angeles and has coached many Olympic gold medal winners. (For more on this subject, see his popular book *Maximum Performance*, Pocket Books, 1977.)

Peak output exercise is not easy, but your misery will be over fast! For healthy people, we suggest 5 minutes per day of peak output exercise and more for those who are willing. You can prepare yourself by taking your GH releasers 90 minutes in advance. You should be working hard and end up sweating and breathing heavily for a minute or two afterward. If you aren't, it is not peak output exercise. How hard is hard? This is measured by your pulse rate.

Total Fitness in Thirty Minutes a Week includes a simple do-it-yourself cardiovascular condition test that healthy people should take before embarking on a peak output exercise program. This book tells you how high *healthy* persons of various ages and cardiovascular conditions should push their heart rates during the peak output exercise. We want you to read this short, simple book before doing peak output exercise, so we have not included the heart rate information here.

You can use your pulse rate and blood pressure monitors to give you a rough appraisal of your cardiovascular conditioning improvement. How rapidly your heart rate and blood pressure return to normal after vigorous exercise are two useful measures of your cardiovascular conditioning. Generally in a healthy person, the time that your pulse rate and blood pressure take to return to normal after heavy exercise decreases with improved cardiovascular conditioning. Dr. Morehouse tells how you can relate the time it takes for your pulse rate to return to normal after peak output exercise to your degree of cardiovascular conditioning.

Caution: Read Dr. Morehouse and Gross's inexpensive paperback book before starting a program of peak output exercise. Have your doctor give you a complete physical exam too, like the astronauts, before you start exercising like the astronauts. You might have an unhealthy heart and not know it.

Warning: Anyone with cardiovascular disease or a family history of cardiovascular disease MUST *consult their physician before starting a peak output exercise program. Ask him or her about a cardiac stress test. This test has a degree of risk, but a lot less risk than unsupervised peak output exercise by a cardiovascular patient!*

In order to work your heart hard enough to get rapid benefits, you will have to exercise major muscles. The muscles in your arms are not massive enough to do this alone, but your leg and thigh muscles are much larger. The step exercise is a simple standard cardiovascular exercise stress technique. It is very simple; you rapidly step up and down one or two steps of any comfortable height between 7 inches and 1 foot. You adjust your rate of stepping to give you the prescribed pulse rate, or alternatively you adjust the single step height to give you the prescribed pulse rate of 24 steps per minute. (Nagle, 1965; Master, 1967)

The step-test exercise has 97 percent of the cardiovascular workout efficiency of running up a 3° hill. (Astrand, 1977) This is hard work, like running uphill, but you won't get run over by an automobile while doing it. Although relatively safe, this is certainly boring, though it doesn't take very long. We like to run up stairs two at a time (definitely a lot more dangerous), or dance extremely vigorously to hard rock music (a little more dangerous than the step-test exercise, but a lot more fun). What counts is achieving the proper heart rate; the type of exercise you do is of secondary importance. Popular aerobic exercise is generally not nearly intense enough for this purpose.

Your oxygen consumption (a measure of your metabolic rate) will increase very rapidly with heavy work, reaching steady-state conditions within about 2 minutes. (Astrand, 1977) After 2 minutes, your heart should be working at its prescribed pulse rate. If it is not, you will have to alter the intensity of your exercise.

Peak output exercise is a rapid method for cardiovascular conditioning, and it is excellent for quickly stimulating muscle growth in teenagers, young adults in their early twenties, or healthy people at any age who are properly using GH releasers. Your heart is a muscle, and it will respond to GH (Murad, 1980) and peak output exercise by growing bigger and stronger, just as it does in an exercising teenager.

Peak output exercise will increase your peak strength and the size of your muscles. It is not necessarily a replacement for aerobic exercise, however. Aerobic exercise does not generally increase muscle mass in adults, but it does increase the number of power plant mitochondria in each skeletal muscle cell and the amount of certain enzymes that are required for aerobic metabolism and sustained muscular output. Peak output exercise does not do this. If you are an athletic competitor in a sport which requires stamina, such as tennis or marathon running, you will still have to do prolonged aerobic exercises to get the increased number of mitochondria and elevated levels of respiratory enzymes required for skeletal muscle stamina. (Skeletal muscles are muscles, such as your biceps and calf muscles, that are attached to your bones. These are the muscles that are normally under your voluntary control.)

One of the reasons that peak output exercise is appropriate for cardiovascular conditioning is because the heart muscle does not exhibit this mitochondrial proliferation and respiratory enzyme induction, even with prolonged endurance exercise. (Oscai, Mole, Brei, 1971; Oscai, Mole, Holloszy, 1971) Prolonged strenuous exercise does increase the size of the heart muscle, unlike skeletal muscles. (Holloszy, 1977) In our opinion peak output exercise combined with GH releasers is a much faster way of building your heart muscle. In healthy people there appears to be a good correlation between heart size and maximum cardiac output, and this is thought to be a major factor in cardiovascular conditioning. (Grande, 1965) Nevertheless there is evidence that an endurance-trained heart is more resistant to the effects of severe oxygen deprivation such as occurs in a heart attack, and endurance training may also increase the strength of the heart's contraction. (See Holloszy, 1977, for a review of adaptations of muscular tissue to training.) While peak output exercise may not provide all of the cardiovascular-conditioning advantages of prolonged aerobic exercise, it does provide a far larger payoff per minute of time invested.

BIGGER MUSCLES

Bodybuilders know that peak output exercise is the fastest way to enlarge their muscles. Muscle growth occurs when the muscle is stressed to near its strength limit. For fastest results each major voluntary muscle group that you exercise should be really *exhausted,* usually with between 8 and 12 exercise repetitions. If it takes less than 8, you may be overstressing your muscles and tendons and are unnecessarily risking injury. If it takes more than 12, your muscles are usually not working close enough to their limits to stimulate rapid growth. (Of course one dares not exhaust the heart muscle in 8 to 12 beats, so the bodybuilder's approach to exercise is the ultimate in the peak output technique.) By using GH releasers along with this exercise technique, you can get the very rapid muscle growth of a bodybuilder in his or her late teens.

Dr. Morehouse, an exercise physiologist, is well qualified to tell you how to improve your cardiovascular conditioning. When you want to use more extreme peak output techniques to build up your visible muscles, we suggest turning to a different type of expert, Arnold Schwarzenegger, a world champion bodybuilder. For a richly photographed and detailed description of body-building techniques, see *Arnold's Body Building for Men* (Simon and Schuster, 1981) by Arnold Schwarzenegger and Bill Dobbins, *Arnold's Body Shaping for Women* which he wrote with Douglas Hall, and *Gold's Gym Weight Training Book* by Bill Dobbins. These books even help you to define what specific muscles you want to build and include fill-in forms for recording your workouts and progress.

Sandy would like to have big muscles like some beautiful muscular professional women bodybuilders, such as Bev Francis. Many women do not want big muscles; they think that muscles are unfeminine. Bodybuilding does not necessarily mean bulging muscles. We suggest that you take a look at the women in *Arnold's Body Shaping for Women;* they are very attractive and do not look at all like male bodybuilders. Part of this difference is anatomy; male and female skeletons and muscle geometry differ. Part of this difference is biochemical; male testosterone and female estrogen both have a powerful influence on body shape. Another part of this difference is in the type of exercises used to work on different muscle groups.

If you are a woman who wants to look like a *Playboy* model, bodybuilding has a lot to offer you! If you lose body fat, your breasts will shrink because they are mostly fat. You can be very lean and still have big breasts by building up the pectoral and other muscles under your breasts. This will push your breasts upward and outward. Unlike large breasts containing a surplus of fatty tissue, this approach to big breasts will not increase your risk of breast cancer. Moreover this approach to big breasts is a real winner in the long run; heavy fatty breasts will inevitably droop with age, and the bigger they are, the sooner and more seriously they'll droop. A big breast that is only a couple of inches of fatty tissue over large muscles is droop-proof!

Sandy has nice round upstanding breasts in spite of her Olympic-range body fat percentage and 42-year age. They look good and feel as soft as any other woman's breasts. The secret is in the muscles behind her breasts. You may have seen the way that Sandy bends steel horseshoes on TV; guess where most of those muscles are hiding!

15

Designing Your Own Personal Program

We present a great deal of information on how to lose fat and keep it off in this book, but we don't expect anyone to use all of these new experimental techniques. You have your own unique combination of goals, physiological limitations, and personal tastes, so you will prefer some of these techniques to others. Before you actually tackle any of these methods, you should clarify what you are looking for and what you are willing and able to do about it. *You should also check our Safety Appendix before taking anything.*

LIST YOUR GOALS.

If you want to lose 5 pounds, you will probably plan your fat loss program rather differently than if you want to lose 50 pounds. If you are trying to reduce your body fat to that of an athlete, you will need to use more of our techniques and apply them more vigorously than if you are trying to reduce your body fat to an attractive though not necessarily athletic level. Women should remember that menstruation becomes irregular or stops when their body fat drops below about 17 percent.

Don't confuse medical necessity with personal preferences. Most people who want to lose weight do not *have* to do so from a medical point of view. (Andres, 1980; Thomas, 1977) Unless your physician says otherwise, we personally think that if you are in good health and don't have any relevant genetic problems, you probably do not have to lose fat for medical reasons unless your body fat percentage is over about 25 percent for a man and 30 percent for a woman. Looking good and feeling fit should be sufficient incentive unless your physician says that your body fat percentage puts you at medical risk.

If you want to look better and be leaner than average, you have to know what that average is. You also need to know how much, on the average, a given amount of extra fat increases your risk of dying. The following tables are based on data from millions of insured men and women, gathered by insurance companies. Remember that these are average weights, not desirable target weights for optimum health or appearance. Remember too that if your extra weight is muscle and not fat, that weight is not "excess."

The lowest mortality rate for men was for those who were 5 to 15 percent below average. Quantitative data is not given in these tables for the potentially decreased mortality risk of weighing less than these averages. This is because interpretation of this data is very difficult, due to confounding factors that are associated with being under the average weight. These factors tend to make being less than average weight look less healthy than it really is. For example, terminal cancer patients often lose a great deal of weight before dying, contributing excess deaths to the lean group which are not caused by leanness.

Smoking is an even bigger confounding factor. In the Framingham Heart Study, 80 percent of those who were under average weight for their heights were smoking at the time of their first examination, and only 5 percent of those who were under the average weight for their heights had never smoked! (This may be due, at least in part, to the thermogenic effects of the nicotine.) As a result the high proportion of smokers in the lean group makes being lean look less healthy than it really is. The American Cancer Society's 1959 study found that among nonsmokers the lowest mortality rate for all persons occurred at between 80 and 89 percent of average weight. (Simopoulos, 1984)

Based on the shape of the mortality versus excess weight curves for people of above average weight, we are willing to hazard an educated *guess* as to what the curves would look like for people of below average weights if the confounding factors were removed. Our best guess for healthy men would be about 10 percent less mortality than normal at 10 percent under average weight, and 15 to 20 percent less mortality than normal for 20 percent less weight, with the risk of death usually increasing again for even lower weights. Our best guess for healthy women would be about 5 percent less mortality than normal at 10 percent under average weight, and 7 to 10 percent less than normal for women 20 percent under average weight, with the risk of death usually increasing again for even lower weights. Remember though that this is based on the aggregated data from millions of people and that your own genes may not be average. For example, if you are a Pima Indian, you will almost certainly be healthier at a weight that is over 50 percent above average for your height.

Finally, remember that you should really be concerned with your body fat percentage, not with your weight per se. Unfortunately the insurance companies, the American Cancer Society, etc. did not make body fat percent measurements during these studies. We strongly urge them to do so in the future. A person with large bones or more muscle than average will weigh more for the same height and same body fat percentage. Arnold Schwarzenegger is way over the average weight for his height, but he certainly isn't fat!

How to use the height and weight tables

Do not be discouraged by the large number of tables that follow. Only four of them apply to you. Just ignore the others. There are a lot of tables because there are a lot of physiological differences between people. There are tables for males and tables for females. There are tables for each age group. Some of these tables are further divided into height-versus-weight relations for small, medium, and large frame size. Your frame size is how thick your bones are compared to your height. If you have thin delicate bones, you have a small frame size. There are even tables for men's and women's frame sizes; by measuring the width of your elbow and your height, you can determine your frame size from these tables.

All tables are for heights measured barefoot and weights measured nude.

Remember that these weight-versus-height tables do not apply to athletes and bodybuilders, who may be well above average in weight for their heights, yet have less than average body fat.

The first set of six tables will give you a rough relationship be-

INCREASED MALE MORTALITY DUE TO ABOVE AVERAGE WEIGHT
For men 30 to 39 years old

Risk factor:	less	less	normal	+11%	+20%	+33%	+50%	+71%

height (in feet and inches)	WEIGHT (in pounds)							
	below average		average	above average				
	−20%	−10%		+10%	+20%	+30%	+40%	+50%
5 2	109	123	137	150	164	178	191	205
5 3	113	127	141	155	169	183	198	212
5 4	117	131	146	160	175	189	204	218
5 5	120	135	150	165	180	195	210	225
5 6	124	139	155	170	186	201	217	232
5 7	128	144	160	176	192	208	223	239
5 8	132	148	164	181	197	214	230	247
5 9	135	152	169	186	203	220	237	254
5 10	139	157	174	192	209	227	244	261
5 11	143	161	179	197	215	233	251	269
6 0	147	166	184	203	221	240	258	277
6 1	152	171	189	208	227	246	265	284
6 2	156	175	195	214	234	253	273	292
6 3	160	180	200	220	240	260	280	300
6 4	164	185	205	226	246	267	288	308

Data based on the *1979 Build and Blood Pressure Study*

This is an average for all 30- to 39-year-old insured men. The average weight-versus-height index for this group is .0355 pounds per inch of height squared (which is the same as 25.0 kg per meter of height squared).

INCREASED MALE MORTALITY DUE TO ABOVE AVERAGE WEIGHT
For men 40 to 49 years old

Risk factor:	less	less	normal	+11%	+20%	+33%	+50%	+71%

	WEIGHT (in pounds)							
height (in feet and inches)	below average		average	above average				
	−20%	−10%		+10%	+20%	+30%	+40%	+50%
5 2	111	125	139	153	167	181	194	208
5 3	115	129	143	158	172	186	201	215
5 4	118	133	148	163	178	192	207	222
5 5	122	137	153	168	183	198	214	229
5 6	126	142	157	173	189	205	220	236
5 7	130	146	162	178	195	211	227	243
5 8	134	150	167	184	200	217	234	251
5 9	138	155	172	189	206	224	241	258
5 10	142	159	177	195	212	230	248	266
5 11	146	164	182	200	219	237	255	273
6 0	150	169	187	206	225	243	262	281
6 1	154	173	193	212	231	250	270	289
6 2	158	178	198	218	237	257	277	297
6 3	163	183	203	224	244	264	285	305
6 4	167	188	209	230	250	271	292	313

Data based on the *1979 Build and Blood Pressure Study*

This is an average for all 40- to 49-year-old insured men. The average weight-versus-height index for this group is .0361 pounds per inch of height squared (which is the same as 25.4 kg per meter of height squared).

INCREASED MALE MORTALITY DUE TO ABOVE AVERAGE WEIGHT

For men 50 to 62 years old

Risk factor:	less	less	normal	+11%	+20%	+33%	+50%	+71%
				WEIGHT (in pounds)				
height (in feet and inches)	below average		average	above average				
	−20%	−10%		+10%	+20%	+30%	+40%	+50%
5 2	112	125	139	153	167	181	195	209
5 3	115	130	144	158	173	187	202	216
5 4	119	134	149	163	178	193	208	223
5 5	123	138	153	169	184	199	215	230
5 6	126	142	158	174	190	205	221	237
5 7	130	147	163	179	195	212	228	244
5 8	134	151	168	184	201	218	235	252
5 9	138	155	173	190	207	224	242	259
5 10	142	160	178	195	213	231	249	267
5 11	146	165	183	201	219	238	256	274
6 0	150	169	188	207	226	244	263	282
6 1	155	174	193	213	232	251	271	290
6 2	159	179	199	218	238	258	278	298
6 3	163	184	204	224	245	265	286	306
6 4	168	189	209	230	251	272	293	314

Data based on the *1979 Build and Blood Pressure Study*

This is an average for all 50- to 62-year-old insured men. The average weight-versus-height index for this group is .0363 pounds per inch of height squared (which is the same as 25.5 kg per meter of height squared).

INCREASED FEMALE MORTALITY DUE TO ABOVE AVERAGE WEIGHT
For women 30 to 39 years old

Risk factor:	less	less	normal	+6%	+10%	+25%	+36%

height (in feet and inches)	WEIGHT (in pounds)						
	below average		average	above average			
	−20%	−10%		+10%	+20%	+30%	+40%
4 10	87	98	109	119	130	141	152
4 11	90	101	112	124	135	146	157
5 0	93	105	116	128	139	151	163
5 1	96	108	120	132	144	156	168
5 2	99	112	124	137	149	161	174
5 3	103	115	128	141	154	167	179
5 4	106	119	132	145	159	172	185
5 5	109	123	136	150	164	177	191
5 6	113	127	141	155	169	183	197
5 7	116	130	145	159	174	188	203
5 8	119	134	149	164	179	194	209
5 9	123	138	154	169	184	200	215
5 10	127	142	158	174	190	206	221
5 11	130	146	163	179	195	212	228
6 0	134	151	167	184	201	218	234

Data based on the *1979 Build and Blood Pressure Study*

This is an average for all 30- to 39-year-old insured women. The average weight-versus-height index for this group is .0323 pounds per inch of height squared (which is the same as 22.7 kg per meter of height squared).

INCREASED FEMALE MORTALITY DUE TO ABOVE AVERAGE WEIGHT
For women 40 to 49 years old

Risk factor:	less	less	normal	+6%	+10%	+25%	+36%

| height (in feet and inches) | WEIGHT (in pounds) | | | | | | |
| | below average | | average | above average | | | |
	−20%	−10%		+10%	+20%	+30%	+40%
4 10	90	102	113	124	136	147	158
4 11	93	105	117	129	140	152	164
5 0	97	109	121	133	145	157	169
5 1	100	112	125	137	150	162	175
5 2	103	116	129	142	155	168	181
5 3	107	120	133	147	160	173	187
5 4	110	124	137	151	165	179	192
5 5	113	128	142	156	170	184	199
5 6	117	132	146	161	175	190	205
5 7	121	136	151	166	181	196	211
5 8	124	140	155	171	186	202	217
5 9	128	144	160	176	192	208	224
5 10	132	148	164	181	197	214	230
5 11	135	152	169	186	203	220	237
6 0	139	157	174	191	209	226	244

Data based on the *1979 Build and Blood Pressure Study*

This is an average for all 40- to 49-year-old insured women. The average weight-versus-height index for this group is .0336 pounds per inch of height squared (which is the same as 23.6 kg per meter of height squared).

INCREASED FEMALE MORTALITY DUE TO ABOVE AVERAGE WEIGHT
For women 50 to 62 years old

Risk factor:	less	less	normal	+6%	+10%	+25%	+36%

| height (in feet and inches) | WEIGHT (in pounds) | | | | | | |
| | below average | | average | above average | | | |
	−20%	−10%		+10%	+20%	+30%	+40%
4 10	93	105	116	128	140	151	163
4 11	96	108	120	132	144	156	168
5 0	100	112	124	137	149	162	174
5 1	103	116	129	141	154	167	180
5 2	106	120	133	146	159	173	186
5 3	110	123	137	151	165	178	192
5 4	113	127	142	156	170	184	198
5 5	117	131	146	161	175	190	204
5 6	120	135	151	166	181	196	211
5 7	124	140	155	171	186	202	217
5 8	128	144	160	176	192	208	224
5 9	132	148	165	181	197	214	230
5 10	135	152	169	186	203	220	237
5 11	139	157	174	192	209	226	244
6 0	143	161	179	197	215	233	251

Data based on the *1979 Build and Blood Pressure Study*

This is an average for all 50- to 62-year-old insured women. The average weight-versus-height index for this group is .0346 pounds per inch of height squared (which is the same as 24.3 kg per meter of height squared).

tween height, weight, and risk of dying. Use the table that corresponds to your gender and age; then look up your height and weight. If you are between 21 and 29 years old, use the 30- to 39-year-old table; it is very close.

This first set of six tables does not distinguish between people with different frame sizes. If you have a large frame, you can be a few pounds heavier than these figures, with the same degree of risk. If you have a small frame, you will have to be a few pounds less than these figures for the same risk. (If you want to find out exactly how much weight variation is caused by frame size difference, take a look at the fourth set of tables.) If your table says that you have a seriously elevated risk of dying, you should be under the care of a doctor even if you feel healthy. Most likely, you won't have that much excess fat.

Only one of the six tables applies to you. Ignore the other five tables which are irrelevant to you. The table that applies to your gender and age group will give you a rough idea about your increased risk of dying due to excess fat. Of course, specific medical problems such as cardiovascular disease can make your risk much higher than is suggested by your table. *If your physician orders you to lose fat, heed his or her advice, no matter what your table says.*

Technical note for health professionals: The first set of 6 charts is based on a concept called the weight-versus-height index. You can calculate your weight-versus-height index (WH index) as follows:

$$\text{WH index} = \frac{\text{weight (in pounds)}}{\text{height} \times \text{height (in inches)}}$$

For example, if you are male, 33 years old, 72 inches tall, and weigh 184 pounds, your

$$\text{WH index} = \frac{184}{72 \times 72} = \frac{184}{5184} = .0355 \text{ pounds per inch squared.}$$

A WH index of .0355 is average for an insured male who is 30 to 35 years old, so this means that you have an average weight for your height.

We have identified the WH index that is used for each table. We have given the WH index in both English pound and inch units, and in the metric system. If you measure mass in kilograms and height in meters, use the metric WH index value.

Some of the insurance companies want to encourage you to be considerably leaner than these averages because they would like you to live as long as possible. Metropolitan Life Insurance Company has published tables of "desirable" heights versus weights for people with small, medium, and large bones for their height. This is referred to as small, medium, or large frame size.

The next pair of tables below (one for men, another for women) tells you how to measure yourself to find whether you have a small, medium, or large frame.

To make an approximation of your frame size . . . extend your arm and bend the forearm upward at a 90° angle. Keep fingers straight and turn the inside of your wrist toward your body. If you have a caliper, use it to measure the space between the two prominent bones on *either side* of your elbow. Without a caliper, place thumb and index finger of your other hand on these two bones. Measure the space between your fingers against a ruler or tape measure. Compare it with these tables that list elbow measurements for *medium-frame* men and women. *Measurements lower than those listed indicate you have a small frame. Higher measurements indicate a large frame.*

MEN	ELBOW BREADTH
5'1"–5'2"	2½"–2⅞"
5'3"–5'6"	2⅝"–2⅞"
5'7"–5'10"	2¾"–3"
5'11"–6'2"	2¾"–3⅛"
6'3"	2⅞"–3¼"

WOMEN	
4'9"–4'10"	2¼"–2½"
4'11"–5'2"	2¼"–2½"
5'3"–5'6"	2⅜"–2⅝"
5'7"–5'10"	2⅜"–2⅝"
5'11"	2½"–2¾"

Courtesy of Metropolitan Life Insurance Company. Adapted from *1983 Metropolitan Height and Weight Tables.*

Note: We have subtracted 1 inch from the heights on the original tables, which were for people wearing shoes. The tables are now for barefoot heights.

The next pair of tables on page 209 (one for men and one for women) is adapted from the 1959 Metropolitan Life Insurance Company tables of "desirable" weights, which are significantly less than average. A few scientists have criticized the 1959 tables for demanding that one be leaner than is really required to achieve good health. (Simopoulos, 1984; Andres, 1980; Thomas, 1977) We think that for most people the tables are healthy goals which will provide a better than average body shape. We do agree with those scientists, however; it is not *necessary* to be this lean to be in *normal* good health. Nevertheless we also think that most people will be stacking the health odds in their favor if they use these leaner than average figures as a goal.

The original tables have been adapted for use when nude by subtracting 1 inch from the height to correct for shoe height, and a clothing weight of 3 pounds has been subtracted for women and a weight of 5 pounds for men.

The next pair of tables on page 210 (again, one table for men and one for women) is adapted from the 1983 Metropolitan Life Insurance Company tables, which are based on mortality data from the 1979 Build Study. They represent the range of weights that are usually medically acceptable and consistent with normal good health. *If your weight is above or below this range, we strongly suggest that you see a physician.* A few scientists have criticized the 1983 tables for not suggesting that one be lean enough for *optimum* health, which though healthier than normal, requires more effort than normal health. In general we agree with these comments; however, remember that your genes have something to say about the matter too. A thin Pima Indian is not as likely to be healthy as one that these tables would consider too heavy. If you are interested in optimum health, see our *Life Extension: A Practical Scientific Approach* and *The Life Extension Companion* for further data.

Note that the changes made since the 1959 tables are greatest for women. The risk of excess fat is usually less for women than for men.

The original tables have been adapted for use when nude by subtracting 1 inch from the height to correct for shoe height, and a clothing weight of 3 pounds has been subtracted for women and 5 pounds for men.

In the final analysis the choice of your target, whether expressed as

DESIRABLE WEIGHTS FOR MEN AGED 25 AND OVER

HEIGHT		SMALL	MEDIUM	LARGE
FEET	INCHES	FRAME	FRAME	FRAME
5	1	107–115	113–124	121–136
5	2	110–118	116–128	124–139
5	3	113–121	119–131	127–143
5	4	116–124	122–134	131–147
5	5	119–128	125–138	133–151
5	6	123–132	129–142	137–156
5	7	127–136	133–147	142–161
5	8	131–140	137–151	146–165
5	9	135–145	141–155	150–169
5	10	139–149	145–160	154–174
5	11	143–153	149–165	159–179
6	0	147–157	153–170	163–184
6	1	151–162	157–175	168–189
6	2	155–166	162–180	173–194
6	3	159–170	167–185	177–199

Courtesy of the Metropolitan Life Insurance Company.

DESIRABLE WEIGHTS FOR WOMEN AGED 25 AND OVER

HEIGHT		SMALL	MEDIUM	LARGE
FEET	INCHES	FRAME	FRAME	FRAME
4	9	89–95	93–104	101–116
4	10	91–98	95–107	103–119
4	11	93–101	98–110	106–122
5	0	96–104	101–113	109–125
5	1	99–107	104–116	112–128
5	2	102–110	107–119	115–131
5	3	105–113	110–123	118–135
5	4	108–116	113–127	122–139
5	5	111–120	117–132	126–143
5	6	115–124	121–136	130–147
5	7	119–128	125–140	134–151
5	8	123–132	129–144	138–155
5	9	127–137	133–148	142–160
5	10	131–141	137–152	146–165
5	11	135–145	141–156	150–170

Courtesy of the Metropolitan Life Insurance Company.

DESIRABLE WEIGHTS FOR MEN OVER 25 YEARS OF AGE

HEIGHT FEET	INCHES	SMALL FRAME	MEDIUM FRAME	LARGE FRAME
5	1	123–129	126–136	133–145
5	2	125–131	128–138	135–148
5	3	127–133	130–140	137–151
5	4	129–135	132–143	139–155
5	5	131–137	134–146	141–159
5	6	133–140	137–149	144–163
5	7	135–143	140–152	147–163
5	8	137–146	143–155	150–171
5	9	139–149	146–158	153–175
5	10	141–152	149–161	156–179
5	11	144–155	152–165	159–183
6	0	147–159	155–169	163–187
6	1	150–163	159–173	167–192
6	2	153–167	162–177	171–197
6	3	157–171	166–182	176–202

Courtesy of the Metropolitan Life Insurance Company.

DESIRABLE WEIGHTS FOR WOMEN OVER 25 YEARS OF AGE

HEIGHT FEET	INCHES	SMALL FRAME	MEDIUM FRAME	LARGE FRAME
4	9	99–108	106–118	115–128
4	10	100–110	108–120	117–131
4	11	101–112	110–123	119–134
5	0	103–115	112–126	122–137
5	1	105–118	115–129	125–140
5	2	108–121	118–132	128–144
5	3	111–124	121–135	131–148
5	4	114–127	124–138	134–152
5	5	117–130	127–141	137–156
5	6	120–133	130–144	140–160
5	7	123–136	133–147	143–164
5	8	126–139	136–150	146–167
5	9	129–142	139–153	149–170
5	10	132–145	142–156	152–173
5	11	135–148	145–159	155–176

Courtesy of the Metropolitan Life Insurance Company.

body fat percentage or weight, is yours and your physician's if you have a weight-related medical problem. Most likely, though, you are not overweight enough to significantly increase your medical risk; if so, the choice is yours and yours alone. You must make this choice now before going on to the next step in designing your own personal fat loss program because your choice of techniques will depend on the distance between what you are now and what you want to be. Pick your target and go for it!

Durk has chosen a goal for himself of 10–12 percent body fat, which is in the male Olympic track and field athlete range. When his body fat percentage drops lower than 10 percent, he becomes excessively sensitive to cold and has to be very careful about eating regularly. Durk's body fat percentage as of May 21, 1981, was 13 percent. As of August 23, 1985, it was 11.2 percent. Sandy's chosen body fat goal is 15–17 percent, well within the female Olympic athlete range. On May 21, 1981, Sandy's body fat percentage was 16.4 percent. As of August 23, 1985, it was 16.8 percent. As of the latter date both Sandy and Durk are 42 years old.

LIST YOUR PHYSIOLOGICAL LIMITATIONS.

All the nutrients and even the foods used in our program may have annoying or even dangerous side effects, depending upon your own individual physiological state. Do you have heart disease, high blood pressure, hypothyroidism, ulcer, Parkinson's disease, schizophrenia, pigmented malignant melanoma (a type of cancer), diabetes, allergies to any of the substances or foods used in our techniques, or use MAO-inhibitor antidepressant drugs? All of these and more can influence your choice of techniques. *Even if you are in perfect health, be sure to check the Safety Appendix before using any nutrient, drug, or food as a fat loss aid.*

Your own genetic factors determine many physiological limitations and can be very important in determining your body weight and fat distribution. Do you have fat parents, brothers, or sisters? *Keep your genetic propensities firmly in mind when deciding on your fat loss goal.* If your *body* wants to have 35 percent body fat, you will have to drag it kicking and screaming all the way if *you* want to have 15 percent body fat. If you are in good health, you may be able to do it, but it is not going to be simple or fast, even though it will probably not require the conventional unpleasantness of extreme caloric restriction, constant hunger, and lengthy heavy exercise. In this case, 25 percent body fat might be a more reasonable and equally healthy goal.

Do you see your personal physician regularly and get a physical exam and clinical lab tests at least once a year? If you don't, we recommend that you do. Get a comprehensive checkup as described in "How You Can Use Our Program" before starting your fat loss program; your obesity may be due to a disease, or you may have a disease like hypertension or a cardiac arrhythmia that prevents you from safely using certain nutrient supplements and drugs such as phenylalanine, tyrosine, ephedrine, or phenylpropanolamine. A doctor's supervision is a must if you want to lose more than 10 percent of your body weight.

LIST YOUR PERSONAL PREFERENCES

Which of the techniques that we discussed did you find most personally appealing to you? There is no need to substitute unpleasant techniques for the unpleasantness of going hungry! If you find a technique unpleasant, you may be able to follow it for a short while, but in the long run you will lose interest. Our program is a long-term one designed to maintain a high ratio of muscle to fat on your body. This is not a temporary program, as most diets are. Remember, though, that you will have to use more of our techniques, or use them more vigorously, to lose all that fat than you will require to maintain your new leaner body once you have achieved your goal.

REVIEW OF FAT LOSS AND SUSTAINED FAT CONTROL METHODS

We have described 17 methods for modifying your fat-prone metabolism so that you can lose fat without ever being hungry, let alone being hungry for the remainder of your life. Some of the nutrient supplements can be used to affect more than one of these mechanisms. We have arranged both the book and this list primarily by mechanisms rather than by substances (nutrients or drugs) to emphasize why and how these techniques work. Some of the nutrient fat loss aids, such as GH releasers, only work when taken at certain times and under certain conditions, unlike most of the drugs with which you are familiar. That is why you must keep the mechanisms in mind when you use these techniques; this is not just a health food store shopping list. As we said at the start of the book, you will have to do a little hard thinking to replace a lot of hard work. The hard thinking is understanding why you are doing what you are doing so that you can do it safely and effectively. The hard work that you have escaped is a life filled with an hour or more of time-consuming exercise every day and denying yourself food when you are hungry.

Cutting down on your eating by willpower is not *part of our program and is generally ultimately ineffective.* For most people, this gives a big 0 in the long-term results department. Very few people are willing to tolerate voluntary hunger for the rest of their lives. Going hungry when there is lots of food around is very unnatural! Nearly all the people who lose weight by this technique put it right back on, and almost everything that goes back on is fat. The results of a typical diet without exercise are 25 percent lean muscle mass lost and 75 percent fat lost. This is an undesirable result because it is normally difficult for adults to regain lost muscle mass. If you have the willpower to eat a single very nutritious but boring food, we doubt that you would get fat eating as much as you wanted of the Ralston Purina High Protein Monkey Chow.

1. *Take growth hormone releasers.* The nutrient amino acid growth hormone releasers arginine and ornithine can increase your growth hormone level back up to that of a normal healthy person in his or her late teens, or of a young adult. The B vitamin niacin and the nutrient amino acid methionine can release GH. The amino acid

tryptophan can also release GH, especially when taken at bedtime. The prescription drug L-Dopa can also be a very effective GH releaser (propranolol is also required in the very obese), but it should only be used with a doctor's supervision. We have described other GH releasers and nutrients which facilitate GH release caused by other stimuli. You can generally regain your youthful ability to eat lots of food without putting on body fat. Even people who were chronically plump in their teens have had spectacular benefits from this technique. The growth hormone released by your pituitary will help maintain existing muscle mass without exercise and will enable you to put on muscle very rapidly with just 5 minutes per day of optional peak output exercise. Growth hormone also instructs your body *not* to manufacture fat for energy storage and to burn fats for energy. See Chapter 5, "Growth Hormone Releasers and Your Muscle-to-Fat Ratio." This method requires that you take these amino acid supplements at one or two specified times during the day.

2. *Eat carbohydrate foods (sugars and starches) that have a low glycemic index.* Carbohydrates, as a result of digestion, increase blood levels of glucose, a sugar your body's cells use for energy. Unfortunately these increased blood sugar levels also result in the release of insulin. Insulin, unlike growth hormone, causes your body to increase its fat stores by manufacturing and storing fat from any excess calories that you eat, even protein. Insulin also blocks some of the effects of growth hormone. To be lean and to have a high ratio of muscle to fat in your body, it is necessary to keep the ratio of growth hormone to insulin relatively high. Watching the glycemic indices of your food is very important even if you are not using GH releasers, both due to the fat synthesis and storage-enhancing abilities of insulin, and due to the carbohydrate craving caused by insulin-induced reactive hypoglycemia. You can help keep insulin down to reasonable but not too low levels by eating sugars and other carbohydrates that have a low glycemic index. But don't worry, that includes a lot of delicious goodies, including the fruit sugar fructose and ice cream! See Chapter 8, "Sweets—How to Have a Sweet Tooth Without Putting On Fat."

3. *Control your carbohydrate craving by substituting fructose (fruit sugar) for sucrose whenever you can in your usual diet.* Fructose has a low glycemic index and in published scientific studies helped people

follow low-calorie diets without hunger, fatigue, or anxiety. Fructose snacks before meals helped people eat less and still be satisfied. Reactive hypoglycemia and the intense carbohydrate craving accompanying it is much less likely to happen with fructose than with sucrose (common sugar). See Chapter 8, "Sweets—How to Have a Sweet Tooth Without Putting On Fat." Fructose has an added bonus; it is also a thermogenic agent; it helps your body burn excess calories for heat.

4. *Control your carbohydrate craving with the nutrient amino acid tryptophan.* Your brain levels of serotonin (made from tryptophan) control whether you crave carbohydrates or not. You may be able to turn off a carbohydrate craving with tryptophan supplements, as has been done by some people in published scientific experiments. See Chapter 8, "Sweets—How to Have a Sweet Tooth Without Putting On Fat."

5. *Control your carbohydrate cravings with niacin supplements.* Niacin can be effective in controlling reactive hypoglycemia. It helps keep your blood sugar levels above the hypoglycemic range longer with less intake of sugar or other carbohydrates, thereby curbing your appetite for more sugars and carbohydrates. Again, see Chapter 8.

6. *Control your carbohydrate cravings with supplements of the essential mineral nutrient chromium.* Either GTF (glucose tolerance factor) chromium or trivalent chromium chloride may improve your blood sugar and insulin regulation, thereby helping you avoid the carbohydrate cravings caused by symptoms resembling hypoglycemia. According to scientists at the USDA, chromium deficiency is widespread in America, and adequate supplies of chromium are absolutely necessary for proper blood sugar and insulin regulation. See Chapter 8.

7. *Curb your appetite without willpower by eating protein or fructose snacks before meals.* Studies show that these snacks allow you to eat less while eating as much as you want. In fact we include a formula for an appetite-reducing snack food which incorporates both fructose and hydrolyzed protein as well as other nutrients. See Chapter 9, "Appetite Control Without Willpower: Nutrients That Curb Appetite!"

8. *Reduce your appetite with supplements of the natural nutrient*

amino acid L-phenylalanine. L-phenylalanine has been shown in rat, monkey, and human studies to reduce appetite effectively at reasonable doses. L-phenylalanine causes a release of CCK, cholecystokinin, a polypeptide hormone that signals your brain that you are full and should stop eating. Phenylalanine and the nutrient amino acid tyrosine are usually effective antidepressants for anergic depressions. See Chapter 9.

9. *Increase your intake of fiber.* Fiber is low in the diets of most people living in western societies. Increasing your fiber intake speeds food through your digestive tract as much as 3 times faster. This may help you lose weight by reducing your absorption of calories. The fiber, which cannot be digested, makes you feel temporarily full on fewer calories. Fiber enables people to eat fewer calories without hunger. Fiber also slows the absorption of nutrients in your gut and can lower the effective glycemic index of carbohydrates taken with it. Fiber has been found in epidemiological studies to reduce the incidence of colon cancer, a major killer. See Chapter 9.

10. *Take choline and vitamin B-5 supplements.* These nutrients are made into acetylcholine in your brain and body. The acetylcholine is responsible for the contractions that move food along in your digestive tract. Increasing your supply of acetylcholine will help food move quickly through your system. See Chapter 9. Acetylcholine is also involved in the modulation of satiation and in the GH release caused by arginine and ornithine. Choline plus B-5 will also increase your muscle tone and help hold in that sagging belly, even without exercise.

11. *Take supplements of niacin and possibly L-carnitine (NOT D- or DL-carnitine) to directly modify your fat metabolism.* Niacin reduces fat synthesis so much that our recommended dose will reduce the fat in your bloodstream by more than most diets. These nutrients can also increase the burning of stored fats for energy and may help reduce fat stores. Niacin markedly reduces serum cholesterol, triglycerides, and VLDL (very low density lipoproteins), thereby causing a major improvement in your cardiovascular risk factor. Some studies indicate that L-carnitine is also effective in reducing serum lipids. See Chapter 11, "Fat Metabolism: How You Can Change It."

12. *Correct functional hypothyroidism.* Check with your doctor.

Functional hypothyroidism is fairly common, especially in those over forty. Your overweightness may be related to this. It is important to correct functional hypothyroidism so that you have a normal basal metabolic rate and sleeping body core temperature. Thyroid hormone is also essential for proper nervous system and immune system function. We are not suggesting increasing effective thyroid hormone activity to abnormally high levels; this is hazardous and will cause a loss of lean body mass. See Chapter 12, "Thermogenesis: The Cool Way to Lose Fat."

13. *Take substances that increase thermogenesis (brown fat tissue metabolism that produces heat by burning up excess calories).* Fructose has thermogenic effects. Thermogenic drugs include theophylline and ephedrine, which most healthy people may (optionally) use to increase their body's brown fat tissue metabolic rate. See Chapter 12.

14. *Increase thermogenesis by exposing yourself to cooler temperatures.* Turning down your thermostat just a few degrees can really help. See Chapter 12.

15. *Wear thermogenic clothing.* Thermogenic clothing can be as simple as wearing shorts around your home, or as complex as a jogging suit or three-piece business suit designed by a team of space age scientists. Thermogenic clothing can help you burn as many calories per day as running for an hour or more. Properly designed thermogenic shorts and pants can increase a male's production of the natural anabolic sex hormone testosterone, sometimes with an attendant increase in libido.

16. *Change your behavior so that you are just as satisfied with smaller amounts of food.* Use smaller dishes and control your portions. Pay more attention to your food so that you get your CCK satiation hormone released in your brain before you overeat. This is not the same thing as caloric restriction; we do not suggest that you leave the table hungry. Use biofeedback by tape-measuring and weighing yourself and looking at yourself nude in a mirror regularly to help reset your brain's weight control center. See Chapter 13, "Changing Your Behavior: How to Act Slim."

17. *Optional. Peak output exercise is capable of rapid muscle building and maintenance and good cardiovascular conditioning.* Used with a diet reduced in calories by appetite modification (or by diffi-

cult-to-sustain self-denial) vigorous exercise prevents most loss of muscle mass. You can use growth hormone releasers to increase the effectiveness of your exercise, so that with even 5 minutes a day of peak output exercise, you can get a dramatic increase in your muscle mass and equally dramatic reductions of your fat stores. See Chapter 14, "Peak Output Exercise: The Astronauts' Fast Exercise Method."

There are dozens of other useful techniques described in this book; the list above merely reviews the high points. You may be amazed at how much better you feel as well as look when you have your blood sugar, insulin, growth hormone, and fat cells under proper control.

You must be under a doctor's supervision during a weight loss program in which you plan to lose more than 10 percent of your body weight. Get a checkup from your doctor before starting our program. Then, get a checkup two months after starting and a checkup every year after that. We strongly recommend that you have these checkups even if your weight loss goal is less than 10 percent; prevention of illness is usually a lot easier than curing it, and you may be ill without knowing it.

Most people do not have a personal physician. This is very unfortunate. It is not advisable simply to choose a physician out of the telephone book when a problem arises. Your new doctor will not have access to your past medical records and will be unable to interpret your present condition in that light. A glucose tolerance test result that gradually rises over the years, but is still within the normal range, would alert a doctor who had been following this over the years to the possible development of adult-onset diabetes. If you see a different physician every time, your new doctor would not know your history and would have no way to make this judgment until you had become a diabetic.

We believe that the stresses of dieting, especially those related to free radical pathology, are sufficient to require more than the RDA's of several important vitamins and minerals. *We suggest that you take a properly formulated anti-free radical high potency vitamin-mineral supplement with each meal and at bedtime.* See the Safety Appendix for our suggested formulation and dosages.

For more on how to achieve optimum health, how to control free radical pathology, and the effects of vitamins and minerals and their deficiencies, see our *Life Extension: A Practical Scientific Approach,* and *The Life Extension Companion.*

16

Measuring Your Own Progress

It is very important to keep track of your progress in losing body fat by using the correct instruments and taking measurements regularly. Of course it is possible to lose body fat without keeping any records. However, the changes that take place will occur gradually, especially if you are following our suggestion to lose only 1 to 2 pounds of fat a week. Changes may not be easy to see in the short term. Keeping track of these gradual changes will provide two major benefits:

1. You will have the psychological satisfaction and motivation that results from seeing your success.

2. You will have an objective demonstration of your progress. A copy of these measurements can be given to your doctor to be kept with your medical records.

The tools that you will need are:

    a. a tape measure
    b. a skin-fold caliper
    c. a precise scale
    d. a camera (optional)

(For sources of skin-fold calipers and scales, see our Suppliers' Appendix.)

With a tape measure, you can keep track of your most fatty body measurements, usually the waistline or hips. Record this on the form that we have provided for you in Appendix 1, "Your Own Case History." Body fat is not distributed evenly and most people have a problem area that builds up fat more than the rest of their body. These problem areas are the last to disappear on any weight loss program, including ours. Remember, these fat depots are supposed to protect you against famine in the wild, like back in the bad old days.

If you are using peak output exercise, you should also use your tape to measure the diameter of the muscle groups involved (bicep, calf, chest, neck, etc.). Record these data too. If you don't, you may wonder if your eyes are fooling you when you think that your muscles look bigger after a total of only *one hour* of peak output exercise spread out over a three-week period.

Even without peak output exercise your muscles may appear to become larger, especially if you are a man. This is primarily due to improved muscular definition. Your subcutaneous fat layer surrounds your muscles, softening their angularity and concealing them. Reduce the thickness of that subcutaneous fat layer (which is measured by your skin-fold caliper), and your muscles look much more impressive, even if they aren't really any larger. Bodybuilders are very well aware that great muscular definition is more impressive than gross bulk alone, and they go to real extremes (such as lowering body fat levels to 3 to 4 percent) to get it.

It is very easy to use a skin-fold caliper, once you know how. The skin-fold measurements must be made in the proper places, and the caliper must be oriented properly during these measurements. Here is a set of drawings that show you where to make the measurements, and how to hold the caliper and orient the skin fold while making them. This is a tool that is widely used by professional athletes who must know their body composition in order to function optimally. You can now join their ranks!

After you have taken the two skin-fold measurements as indicated in the drawings, record the data. Make each skin-fold measurement 3 times so that you have an idea of how much random error you have in your measurements. Each measurement should be made independently; don't look at the last measurement when you make a new one, or this knowledge may affect your measurement. If your measurements are repeatable within 1 percentage point of body fat, you are doing a very good job in making the measurement. If you make three repeated sets of measurements at the same time and find that they vary by 3 percent or more, you will have to be more careful in making your measurements.

The biggest problem is in making the measurement in exactly the

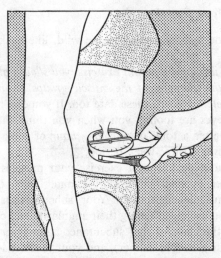

Women: The over-the-hip skin-fold measurement is taken as a vertical skin-fold over the iliac crest (the protruding top edge of the hipbone).

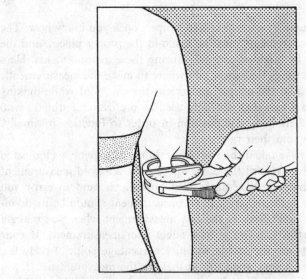

Women: The back of the arm skin-fold measurement is taken with the arm dangling and relaxed. It is a vertical skin-fold on the back of the arm half-way between the level of the spine of the shoulder blade and the bony projection at the elbow, with the elbow fully extended.

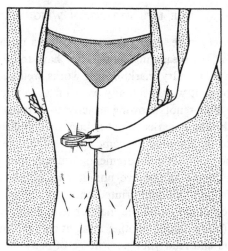

Men: The thigh skin-fold measurement is taken as a vertical skin-fold in the midline of the thigh (on the front side of the body), halfway between the groin ligament and the top of the kneecap.

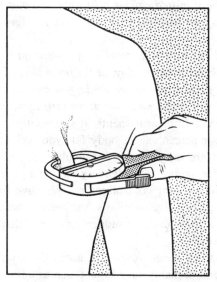

Men: The skin-fold measurement just below the shoulder blade is taken as a skin-fold running downward and to the side in the natural fold of the skin just below the shoulder blade.

same place every time. We make 2 tiny marks on our skins with indelible ink at the measuring spots. They have to be reinked about once a week. A laundry marking pen works well because it won't wash off, though it will eventually wear off as you grow new skin. Don't worry about not knowing exactly to a fraction of an inch where to make the 2 marks. What is important is that you measure your skin-fold thickness at the same spots every time.

From these skin-fold measurements you can find your body fat percentage with one of the two nomograms (a special ready-made graph used for calculations) printed on pages 225 and 226. You locate these measurements on the male or female nomogram. Draw a straight line (using a ruler or other straight surface) between the two measurements and read your percentage of body fat on the middle line. An example of a skin-fold computation is shown in Figure 3 on page 227. This woman has 28 percent body fat.

You should measure your body fat percentage once a week and record both the skin-fold caliper measurements and your nomogram calculated body fat percentage in Appendix 1, "Your Own Case History."

You should measure your total body weight on a precise scale or doctor's-style balance once a day, at the same time of day. We suggest that you take your weight before the largest meal of the day. If possible, weigh yourself nude, and look at yourself nude in a good mirror. Record these weight measurements. If you multiply your total body weight by your percentage of body fat, you will know how many pounds of fat are on your body. Calculate and record this figure every day. By weighing yourself every day, you provide biofeedback for your brain's weight control center. We have found that if we neglect to weigh ourselves regularly, our weights tend to creep up by a few pounds a week, until we suddenly discover that we weigh 10 or 15 pounds more.

Be sure that you weigh yourself at about the same time each day; your weight will probably vary by as much as a few pounds depending on the time of day. For most people, their maximum weight occurs right after their biggest meal of the day and their minimum weight when they wake up in the morning. While sleeping, you have

FIG.1

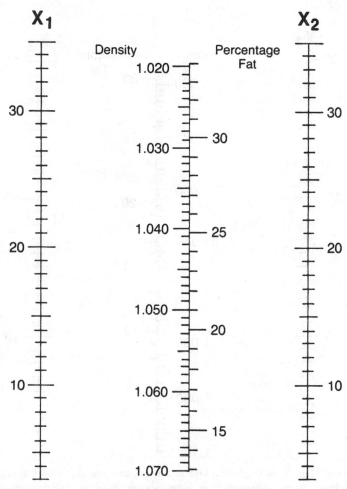

Young Women. X_1 = hip skin-fold thickness (mm) and X_2 = back of arm skin-fold thickness (mm). Adapted from Sloan and de V. Weir, "Nomograms for Prediction of Body Density and Total Body Fat from Skin-fold Measurements," *J. Appl. Physiol.* 28(2):221–22 (1970).

FIG. 2

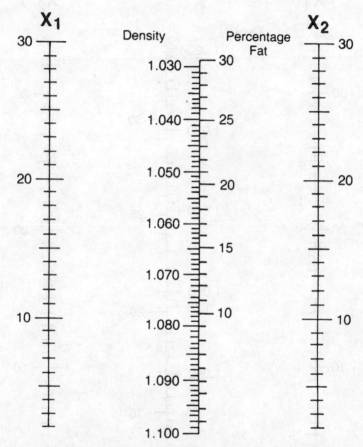

Young Men. X_1 = thigh skin-fold thickness (mm) and X_2 = back skin-fold thickness (mm). Adapted from Sloan and de V. Weir, "Nomograms for Prediction of Body Density and Total Body Fat from Skin-fold Measurements," *J. Appl. Physiol.* 28(2):221–22 (1970).

FIG. 3

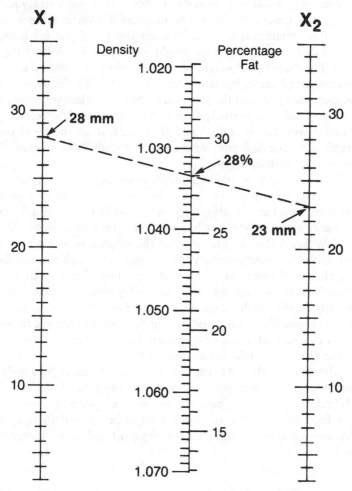

Example of a body fat percentage determination. This woman has a 23-mm back of the arm skin-fold thickness and a 28-mm hip skin-fold thickness. She has 28 percent body fat.

burned a considerable amount of food and some body fat to carbon dioxide and water vapor, which you exhale.

Your weight will vary from day to day even if you weigh yourself at the same time of day. Do not be surprised if it varies by a pound or two; this variation is natural. How do you tell if you are losing a pound or two a week if your weight varies that much from day to day? You record your weight on a graph and plot a trend line. This sounds complicated, but it is really very easy. Here is an example. Suppose that you start the program on Monday when you weigh 125 pounds. Each day you weigh yourself at the same time, record it in "Your Own Case History," and then mark it on the trend curve graph. On Tuesday you weighed 124 pounds, you weighed 125 pounds on Wednesday, etc.

Even though you gain weight on some days and lose some on others, the trend of the line is clearly downward by about 2 pounds per week. You can see this clearly on a trend line graph, but it would be hard to see it if you just had a list of dates and weights.

Now take a ruler and lay it along the graph points that you plotted. Move the ruler around so that it passes through the middle of the cluster of points and draw a straight line. This is your weight trend line. It averages out your day-to-day variations, and lets you see where you are heading in the long run and how fast you are getting there. If you don't plot a trend line, you will become unnecessarily discouraged by minor temporary increases in your weight. You might also lose weight too fast without realizing it.

Always remember, though, that you want to reduce your body fat percentage. Your weight is only part of the picture. If you are using GH releasers and doing peak output exercise, your weight may actually increase while you are losing a lot of fat. *Your daily tape measurements and weekly skin-fold measurements tell the most important story.*

Weight

Weight	Mon	Tue	Wed	Thr	Fri	Sat	Sun	Mon	Tue	Wed	Thr
130											
129											
128											
127											
126											
125	X		X								
124		X		X		X	X				
123					X			X			
122									X	X	
121											X
120											

Day

TAKING PHOTOS TO RECORD YOUR BODY APPEARANCE

Improving the appearance of your body is probably one of your major reasons for seeking to lose fat. You can optionally take photographs that record the gradual changes taking place as your body sheds excess fat. You don't just get thinner; your shape changes too. You can have your own "before" and "after" photos to marvel over (and include in your case history records). When taking these photographs, keep in mind:

1. Use the same lighting, lighting angle, body posture, and clothing in each photograph so they can be directly compared to each

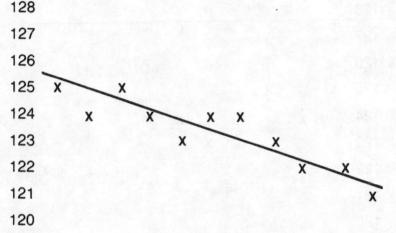

Draw a straight line through the middle of the cluster of points. This is your weight trend line. It averages out the random day-to-day variations in your weight and lets you see your long-term progress more clearly.

other. The less clothing the better. Don't expect to see any changes if you are wearing a three-piece suit in the photos; three-piece suits are designed to hide fat, and they are just as good at hiding leanness.

2. You can have a sort of "time-lapse" photography of your body changes by taking photos at frequent and equal time increments, such as once a week. If you are careful to pose the same way every time, you can even bind the stack of time-lapse photos together at the bottom and flip through them at a rate of a few photos per second, giving you your own crude time-lapse fat loss movie!

3. Make sure the angles you have chosen to photograph yourself

include a good view of the fattiest deposits on your body. Remember, nobody has to see these photos except yourself!

4. Frontal lighting tends to conceal changes in body shape, which occur as you lose fat and build muscle. Lighting that is more directly overhead tends to accentuate these changes and make them easier to see and evaluate.

Now it is time for you to become involved in Appendix 1, "Your Own Case History."

APPENDIX 1

Your Own Case History

Your own case history is important to you, so why not include your records of it in this book? The measurements—skin-fold caliper, scale, and tape measure—are all easy to do and take little time. You can follow your progress, even if it is slow and gradual. If you miss a measurement, don't worry, just continue on with the succeeding measurements. Be sure to use the same scale for all weight measurements, since scales can vary by a significant amount. The following record forms are for recording skin-fold measurements, percentage of body fat, weight, and tape measurements of fat problem areas. If you are doing peak output exercise, especially if you are using GH releasers too, you may want to tape-measure the muscles that you are exercising. Be sure to date all measurements.

Your medical records are another very important part of your own case history. When you go to your doctor for a comprehensive checkup before starting your program, ask him for copies of all the lab test results. When you are tested again in your next physical exam, ask for copies of that too. You will probably be delighted by the reductions in serum total cholesterol, LDL, VLDL, triglycerides (fats), and overall cardiovascular risk. You won't have to wait a year to see these results, especially if you are using our suggested dose of niacin. With niacin the changes will show up in your lipid panel test (serum fatty materials such as cholesterol, HDL, LDL, VLDL, triglycerides, etc.) after only a few weeks of regular use. GH releasers and your high potency anti-free radical vitamin and mineral supplement will also generally improve your lipid panel, though perhaps not as rapidly and dramatically as the niacin.

YOUR PERSONAL GROWTH HORMONE RELEASER SCHEDULE
Weekdays

TIME OF MEALS	TIME TO TAKE GH RELEASERS	TIME TO EXERCISE

YOUR PERSONAL GROWTH HORMONE RELEASER SCHEDULE
Weekends

TIME OF MEALS	TIME TO TAKE GH RELEASERS	TIME TO EXERCISE

DATE	SKIN-FOLD MEASUREMENTS		% BODY FAT	POUNDS BODY FAT (% body fat × weight)
	X_1	X_2		

For women: X_1 is hip (over the top edge of the pelvic bone) skin-fold thickness. X_2 is back of arm skin-fold thickness.

For men: X_1 is thigh (front, halfway between kneecap and crotch) skin-fold thickness. X_2 is back (below shoulder blade) skin-fold thickness.

TOTAL BODY WEIGHT

DATE	TIME OF DAY	TOTAL BODY WEIGHT

TAPE MEASUREMENT OF BODY PROBLEM AREA

MY PROBLEM AREA NO. 1 IS _____

DATE	TIME OF DAY	TAPE MEASUREMENT

MY PROBLEM AREA NO. 2 IS _____

DATE	TIME OF DAY	TAPE MEASUREMENT

TAPE MEASUREMENT OF EXERCISED MUSCLES

MY EXERCISED MUSCLE NO. 1 IS _____

DATE	TIME OF DAY	TAPE MEASUREMENT

MY EXERCISED MUSCLE NO. 2 IS _____

DATE	TIME OF DAY	TAPE MEASUREMENT

MY EXERCISED MUSCLE NO. 3 IS _____

DATE	TIME OF DAY	TAPE MEASUREMENT

MY EXERCISED MUSCLE NO. 4 IS _____

DATE	TIME OF DAY	TAPE MEASUREMENT

APPENDIX 2

How to Join Our Research Program

There is still a lot to be learned about fat control and life extension, and *YOU* can be a part of our ongoing research program investigating them. As a participant you will not be provided with nutrients, medical tests, or advice. We will be using information about your own case history, particularly clinical laboratory test results, that you send us. These data will be made available to research scientists, except that your identity will never be released without your explicit written permission. Remember, these procedures for fat control are experimental. The information about your case will help us and other scientists evaluate the techniques and improve them. If you would like to be a research subject, fill out the following questionnaire and send it to the address below.

If you do not have a personal physician and you are looking for one to perform our suggested physical exam and clinical laboratory tests, to supervise your own personal fat loss program, and to help you stay well, please write to us at the address given below. If we know of a physician in your area who is interested in working with you, we will send you his or her address and business phone number *IF you include a stamped, self-addressed envelope.* If we do not know of a doctor in your area, we will keep your request and return envelope on file and send you the data as soon as we can.

A note to physicians: We are seeking physicians interested in working with our experimental research subjects and with people who are attempting to enhance their health through improved nutrition. There are many people across the country without a personal physician who would welcome clinical testing and medical supervision, especially from a physician with an interest in nutrition and preventive medicine. Literally thousands of people have asked us, "Where can I find a doctor who will not think it strange that I want clinical laboratory tests when I am well and who will warn me if something appears amiss. I want a doctor who recognizes the importance of good nutrition, who is willing to work with well people to help keep them that way and to enhance health, not just save them after they become ill." Although we doubt that many physicians would be reluctant to administer these standard low-risk clinical laboratory tests, many people avoid health professionals except when ill because of their mistaken belief that most doctors will laugh at their interest in nutrition and prevention. These people would feel much more comfortable and confident knowing that a particular physician welcomed them as healthy clients, not just as sick patients.

If you are a physician who is interested in participating in such clinical research, or if you would simply like us to pass your name on to people in your area who are seeking a doctor, please write to us at the address below.

RESEARCH PROGRAM
P.O. Box 853
Redondo Beach, CA 90277

Important: *We are scientists, not physicians. We can not answer medical questions sent to us by our readers. Please see your personal physician. If you do not have one, you should find one at this time. You can also find a great deal of additional information by using the National Library of Medicine's computer literature searches. See Appendix 3, "Further Sources of Information" in this book. For more details see our chapter on this subject in* The Life Extension Companion.

HEALTH BACKGROUND INFORMATION

A copy of the information in this questionnaire will be made available to research scientists as part of their studies. Your name and address will be deleted and replaced by a code number.

Many questions can be answered either yes (Y) or no (N).

Name _____ Age _____ Sex _____

Height _____ Weight _____

Address _____

_____

Phone (home) _____ (work) _____

Family Information

Is your mother alive? _____ If so, what is her age? _____ If not, what did she die of and at what age? _____

_____

Is your father alive? _____ If so, what is his age? _____ If not, what did he die of and at what age? _____

_____

Is your grandmother (on your mother's side) alive? _____ If so, what is her age? _____ If not, what did she die of and at what age? _____

Is your grandfather (on your mother's side) alive? _____ If so, what is his age? _____ If not, what did he die of and at what age? _____

Is your grandmother (on your father's side) alive? _____ If so, what is her age? _____ If not, what did she die of and at what age? _____

Is your grandfather (on your father's side) alive? _____ If so, what is his age? _____ If not, what did he die of and at what age? _____

Are your parents and/or close relatives fat? yes _____ no _____

If yes, please describe on an additional sheet of paper: their relation to you, the nature of their problem, including age of onset, any medical consequences, and the outcome of their prior fat loss attempts.

Dietary Information

Do you eat a high-fat diet (examples: butter, fatty meats, oils)? _____ If yes, how much of what per week? _____

_____

Do you eat a lot of polyunsaturated fats such as safflower oil and corn oil? _____ If yes, how much of what per week? _____

Do you eat a high-carbohydrate (starch foods and sugars, such as rice, pasta, breads, cakes, etc.) diet? _____ If yes, how much of what per week? __

Do you eat a high-protein diet (examples: meat, fish, cheese)? _____ If yes, how much of what per week? _____

_____

Do you generally eat a portion of green leafy vegetables at least once daily? _____ More often? _____ What approximate quantity in ounces each day? _____

Do you generally eat a portion of yellow or orange vegetables at least once daily? _____ More often? _____ What approximate quantity in ounces each day? _____

Do you often enjoy sugar-containing foods (such as candy, cakes, soft drinks)? _____ How much of what per week? _____

Are you now trying to reduce your weight by limiting your caloric intake? _____ How and by how much? _____

Do you eat a lot of fiber-containing foods such as whole grains? _____ If yes, how much of what per week? _____

Do you drink milk? _____ How much daily and what type (e.g., skim, nonfat, low-fat, whole, etc.) _____
Do you eat a vegetarian diet? _____ If yes, do you eat eggs? _____, milk _____, or cheese _____?

Nutrient Supplement Information

Do you take a magnesium supplement? _____ If so, what type, how much, and how often? _____

List the nutrients (vitamins, minerals, amino acids, etc.) that you take daily. Please supply quantities taken and about how long you have been using them. If they are taken in divided doses throughout the day, please specify. If you take a multivitamin/mineral product, please list all the contents or list the distributor, manufacturer, and manufacturer's address so that we can ascertain the exact contents of your formula. If possible, just send us the product labels instead of writing it down. Thank you! _____

_____
_____
_____
_____
_____
_____
_____

Prescription and Recreational Drug Information

List the prescription and recreational drugs you take, how much, and how often you take them. Remember that coffee, tea, alcohol, and tobacco are recreational drugs too.

_____
_____
_____
_____
_____
_____

History of Major Illnesses

What major illnesses have you had, and when did you have them?

_____
_____
_____
_____

Are you frequently ill? _____ If yes, how often and with what? _____

_____

Are you now ill or suffering medical symptoms? _____ If so, describe the illness and list the symptoms. _____

_____

_____

_____

Life-style Factors

Do you smoke? _____ If so, what? Pipe? _____ Cigar? _____
Cigarettes? _____ How many per day? _____ How long have you
been smoking? _____
Answer the following with *N* for not at all, *L* for a little, *M* for moderately,
or *H* for heavily: To what extent do you drink beer? _____ wine?
_____ mixed drinks? _____ straight hard liquor? _____ If moder-
ately to heavy, how much of what? _____
Do you drink generally with meals? _____ generally on an empty stom-
ach? _____ Do you generally maintain a suntan? _____
Do you use a sun block? How often and what type? _____
Do you keep out of the sun? _____
Do you have a type A personality (hard-driving, "workaholic")?

_____

Are you under a lot of stress? _____ If yes, please describe it.

_____

_____

Do you exercise (check one) not at all? _____, a little? _____, moderately? _____, a great deal? _____. Describe the exercise.

_____

_____

_____

Do you take birth control pills? _____ If yes, what type and for how
long? _____
How many hours do you usually sleep per night? _____ Do you diet
often? _____

_____

What diets and weight loss programs have you tried, and what were the
results?

_____

_____

_____

_____

_____

_____

_____

_____

_____

What is your current weight? _____

What is your prior weight history? _____

_____

_____

_____

What is your present percentage of body fat (if known)? _____ If known, was it measured by skin-fold caliper, underwater weighing, electrical-impedance device, or ultrasonics? _____

Where, when, and by whom was it measured? _____

What are your tape measurements? _____

_____

_____

Additional Comments

(Attach further remarks, if desired.)_____

_____

_____

_____

_____

_____

If you have kept records (fat-fold caliper, scale, tape measure) of your weight loss program, please be sure to include these with the questionnaire.

Please also obtain a copy of your medical records from your physician and include them too.

WHAT IS YOUR BIGGEST AND MOST SERIOUS LONG-TERM HEALTH CONCERN? _____

_____

_____

_____

_____

WHAT IS YOUR MOST FREQUENT AND ANNOYING NONSERIOUS HEALTH PROBLEM? _____

_____

_____

_____

ARE YOU INTERESTED IN A MEDICALLY SUPERVISED FAT LOSS PROGRAM USING THESE TECHNIQUES? _____

ARE YOU INTERESTED IN A MEDICALLY SUPERVISED HEALTH-ENHANCEMENT AND PREVENTIVE MEDICINE PROGRAM? _____

WHAT WOULD YOU LIKE US TO DO NEXT? _____

_____

_____

_____

WHAT DO YOU WANT? This could include health-related books, services, products, etc. _____

_____

_____

_____

WHAT DO YOU DISLIKE? Again, we are interested in health-related books, services, products, etc. _____

_____

APPENDIX 3

Further Sources of Information

This book is based on the work of hundreds of scientists. If you would like to find out more about some of the topics discussed here, you can consult one or more of the information sources listed below. We hope you will do that. We prefer that readers actively investigate our information, rather than simply taking our word for it.

We have arranged the 386 different references by chapter or appendix so that you can more readily find research related to a particular subject by looking at the titles of the various papers. Nearly all of these references are published reports of original scientific research, published reviews of such work, or standard biomedical references.

INFORMATION SOURCES FOR LAYPERSONS

Books

Beller, Anne Scott, *Fat and Thin, a Natural History of Obesity,* New York: Farrar Straus Giroux (1977).

Brecher, E. M. *Licit and Illicit Drugs,* Boston: Little, Brown (1972).

Goldman, Bob with Patricia Bush, Ph.D., and Dr. Ronald Klatz, *Death in the Locker Room,* South Bend, Ind.: Icarus Press (1984). (About abuse of anabolic steroids.)

Morehouse and Gross, *Total Fitness in 30 Minutes a Week,* New York: Simon and Schuster (1975).

Pearson, Durk and Sandy Shaw, *Life Extension: A Practical Scientific Approach,* New York: Warner Books (1982).

Pearson, Durk and Sandy Shaw, *The Life Extension Companion,* New York: Warner Books (1984).

Pinckney, Pinckney, *The Encyclopedia of Medical Tests,* New York: Pocket Books (1978).

USDA, *Nutritive Value of American Foods in Common Units,* Agriculture Handbook No. 456, Agricultural Research Service, United States Dept. of Agriculture (1975).

USDA, *Composition of Foods, Dairy and Egg Products,* Agricultural Handbook No. 8-1, United States Dept. of Agriculture, Agricultural Research Service (1976).

USDA, *Composition of Foods, Nut and Seed Products,* Agricultural Handbook No. 8-12, United States Dept. of Agriculture, Human Nutrition Information Service (1984).

USDA, *Composition of Foods, Poultry Products,* Agricultural Handbook No. 8-5, United States Dept. of Agriculture, Science and Education Administration (1979).

Wurtman, Judith J., Ph.D., *The Carbohydrate Craver's Diet,* New York: Ballantine (1983).

Magazines

Rodin, Judith, "Taming the Hunger Hormone," *American Health,* Jan.-Feb. 1984.

Wurtman, Richard J., "Nutrients that Modify Brain Function," *Sci. Amer.,* Apr. (1982).

INFORMATION SOURCES FOR SCIENTISTS AND PHYSICIANS

Books

Armbrecht, Prendergast, Coe, editors, *Nutritional Intervention in the Aging Process,* New York: Springer-Verlag (1984).

Beers Jr., Roland F. and Edward Bassett, editors, *Nutritional Factors: Modulating Effects on Metabolic Processes,* New York: Raven Press, (1981).

Beeson, McDermott, Wyngaarden, editors, *Cecil Textbook of Medicine,* 15th ed., Philadelphia: Saunders (1979).

Blackburn, Grant, and Young, editors, *Amino Acids, Metabolism and Medical Applications,* Littleton, Mass.: John Wright-PSG Inc. (1983).

Brecher, E. M. *Licit and Illicit Drugs,* Boston: Little, Brown (1972).

Brown, Mitchell, Young, *Chemical Diagnosis of Disease,* New York: Elsevier p. 280 (1979).

Conn Jr., DeFelice, and Kuo, editors, *Health and Obesity,* New York: Raven Press (1983).

Garattini and Samanin, editors, *Anorectic Agents, Mechanisms of Action and Tolerance,* New York: Raven Press (1981).

Gilman, Goodman, Gilman, editors, *Goodman and Gilman's The Pharmacological Basis of Therapeutics,* 6th ed., New York: Macmillan (1980).

Greenwood, M. R. C., editor, "Behavioral and Self-Help Treatments," *Obesity,* New York: Churchill Livingstone (1983).

Jeanes, Allene and John Hodge, editors, *Physiological Effects of Food Carbohydrates,* ACS Symposium Series 15, ACS (1975).

Meites, Joseph, editor, *Neuroendocrinology of Aging,* New York: Plenum Press (1983).

Morehouse and Gross, *Total Fitness in 30 Minutes a Week,* New York: Simon and Schuster (1975).

Novin, Wyrwicka, and Bray, editors, *Hunger: Basic Mechanisms and Clinical Implications,* New York: Raven Press (1976).

Pearson, Durk and Sandy Shaw, *Life Extension: A Practical Scientific Approach,* New York: Warner Books (1982).

Pecile and Muller, editors, *Growth and Growth Hormone,* New York: Excerpta Medica Foundation (1972).

Phillips and Baetz, editors, *Diet and Resistance to Disease,* New York: Plenum Press (1981).

Present Knowledge in Nutrition, pp. 571–86, Washington, D.C.: The Nutrition Foundation, Inc. (1984).

Seiden and Dykstra, *Psychopharmacology, a Biochemical and Behavioral Approach,* New York: Van Nostrand Reinhold (1977).

Silverstone, T., editor, *Drugs and Appetite,* New York: Academic Press (1982).

Sipple and McNutt, editors, *Sugars in Nutrition,* New York: Academic Press (1974).

Stunkard and Stellar, editors, *Eating and Its Disorders,* New York: Raven Press (1984).

USDA, *Nutritive Value of American Foods in Common Units,* Agriculture Handbook No. 456, Agricultural Research Service, United States Dept. of Agriculture (1975).

USDA, *Composition of Foods, Dairy and Egg Products,* Agricultural Handbook No. 8-1, United States Dept. of Agriculture, Agricultural Research Service (1976).

USDA, *Composition of Foods, Nut and Seed Products,* Agricultural Handbook No. 8-12, United States Dept. of Agriculture, Human Nutrition Information Service (1984).

USDA, *Composition of Foods, Poultry Products,* Agricultural Handbook No. 8-5, United States Dept. of Agriculture, Science and Education Administration (1979).

Wurtman and Wurtman, editors, *Nutrition and the Brain,* New York: Raven Press (1979 and following). A continuing multivolume series.

NATIONAL LIBRARY OF MEDICINE COMPUTER LITERATURE SEARCHES (MEDLARS)

The National Library of Medicine contains the entire output of over 3000 of the world's most important biomedical publications, including current work in cancer, cardiovascular disease, and of course obesity. If it's a known medical condition, MEDLARS has data on it. The MEDLARS database is available, not only to scientists and physicians, but also to laypersons. A typical search will cost $35–$50 and may provide hundreds of references, with many of these accompanied by a brief summary of what is contained in the complete paper. If you want a complete copy of the paper, you will need to go to a nearby university medical library.

Listed below are the regional MEDLARS centers, allowing you to find the one closest to you. The actual search can be done entirely by mail. Just write or phone your local MEDLARS center for the search form. There are even services which sell complete papers, but these are expensive and unless you are located in the boondocks, you will probably find it more cost-effective to make copies of the papers yourself.

If you are of average intelligence, you can do your own literature research by searching the MEDLARS database for the scientific work of interest to you. For complete information on how to access the MEDLARS database, including an example of a filled-out search form and the resulting search data, see our *Life Extension: A Practical Scientific Approach* (Warner Books 1982) and *The Life Extension Companion* (Warner Books, 1984).

Medlars Regional Centers

GREATER NORTHEASTERN
REGIONAL MEDICAL LI-
BRARY PROGRAM
The New York Academy of Med-
icine
2 East 103rd Street
New York, NY 10029
Phone: 212-876-8763
States served: CT, DE, MA, ME,
NH, NJ, NY, PA, RI, VT
(plus Puerto Rico)

SOUTHEASTERN/ATLANTIC
REGIONAL MEDICAL LI-
BRARY SERVICES
(STARS)
University of Maryland
Health Sciences Library
111 South Greene Street
Baltimore, MD 21201
Phone 301-528-7637
States served: AL, FL, GA, MD,
MS, NC, SC, TN, VA, WV,
and the District of Columbia

REGION 3: REGIONAL MED-
ICAL LIBRARY
University of Illinois at Chicago
Library of the Health Sciences
Health Sciences Center
P.O. Box 7509
Chicago, IL 60680
Phone 312-996-2464
States served: IA, IL, IN, KY, MI,
MN, ND, OH, SD, WI

MIDCONTINENTAL RE-
GIONAL MEDICAL LI-
BRARY PROGRAM
(MCRML)

University of Nebraska
Medical Center Library
42nd and Dewey Avenue
Omaha, NE 68105
Phone 402-559-4326
States served: CO, KS, MO, NE,
UT, WY

SOUTH CENTRAL RE-
GIONAL MEDICAL LI-
BRARY PROGRAM
(TALON)
University of Texas
Health Science Center at Dallas
5323 Harry Hines Blvd.
Dallas, TX 75235
Phone: 214-688-2085
States served: AR, LA, NM, OK,
TX

PACIFIC NORTHWEST RE-
GIONAL HEALTH SCI-
ENCES LIBRARY SER-
VICE (PNRHSLS)
Health Sciences Library
University of Washington
Seattle, WA 98195
Phone: 206-543-8262
States served: AK, ID, MT, OR,
WA

PACIFIC SOUTHWEST RE-
GIONAL MEDICAL LI-
BRARY SERVICE
(PSRMLS)
UCLA Biomedical Library
Center for the Health Sciences
Los Angeles, CA 90024
Phone: 213-825-1200
States served: AZ, CA, HI, NV

SCIENTIFIC LITERATURE REFERENCES

1: Why You Can Benefit from Our New Natural High-tech Approach

Bray, "The Myth of Diet in the Management of Obesity," *Am. J. Clin. Nutr.* 23(9):1141–1148 (1970).

Bray, "Diet and Exercise as Treatment for Obesity," in Conn, Jr., DeFelice, and Kuo, *Health and Obesity,* New York: Raven Press (1983).

Fisher and Lachance, "Nutrition Evaluation of Published Weight-Reducing Diets," *J. Amer. Diet. Assoc.* 85:450–454 (1985).

Itallie, "Diets for Weight Reduction: Mechanisms of Action and Physiological Effects," *Int. J. Obesity* 2:113–122 (1978).

Rosenblatt, Stencel, "Weight Control: A National Obsession," published by Congressional Quarterly, Inc., Nov. 19, 1982.

Wooley and Wooley, "Should Obesity Be Treated at All," in *Eating and Its Disorders,* edited by Stunkard and Stellar, New York: Raven Press (1984).

2: Why Nature Makes You Fat

Andres, "Effect of Obesity on Total Mortality," *Int. J. Obesity* 4 (1980).

Assimacopoulos-Jeannet, Jeanrenaud, "The Hormonal and Metabolic Basis of Experimental Obesity," in Albrink, editor, *Clinics in Endocrinology and Metabolism,* Vol. 5, pp. 337–365, Philadelphia: Sanders (1976).

Bazzarre, Johanson, Huseman, Varma, Blizzard, "Human Growth Hormone Changes with Age," *Proc. 3rd Int. Symp. on Growth Hormone,* Milan, North Holland, Amsterdam (1975).

Beller, Anne Scott, *Fat and Thin, a Natural History of Obesity,* New York: Farrar Straus Giroux (1977).

Bray, "Diet and Exercise as Treatment for Obesity," in Conn Jr., DeFelice, and Kuo, *Health and Obesity,* New York: Raven Press (1983).

Cahill Jr., "Disorders of Carbohydrate Metabolism," in Beeson, McDermott, Wyngaarden, editors, *Cecil Textbook of Medicine,* 15th ed., Philadelphia: Saunders, pp. 1969–1989 (1979).

Christy, "Anterior Pituitary Function in Normal Subjects and in Patients with Systemic Diseases," in Beeson, McDermott, Wyngaarden, editors, *Cecil Textbook of Medicine,* 15th ed., Philadelphia: Saunders, pp. 2085–2091 (1979).

Coleman, "Obesity Genes: Beneficial Effects in Heterozygous Mice," *Science* 203:663–665 (1979).

Larner, "Insulin and Oral Hypoglycemic Drugs," in Gilman, Goodman, Gilman, *Goodman and Gilman's The Pharmacological Basis of Therapeutics,* 6th ed., pp. 1497–1523, New York: Macmillan (1980).

Murad, Haynes, "Adenohypophyseal Hormones and Related Substances," in Gilman, Goodman, Gilman, *Goodman and Gilman's The Pharmacological Basis of Therapeutics,* 6th ed., pp. 1369–1396, New York: Macmillan (1980).

"Muscle Loss Occurs in Women with Aging Just as It Does in Men," p. 13 of Special Report on Aging 1980, United States Dept. of Health and Human Services, NIH, NIA. (No GH stimulation by exercise in persons over 30 found in Baltimore Longitudinal Study of Aging.)

Ratzmann and Gottschling, "Abnormal Growth Hormone Response in Obesity with Normal Carbohydrate Tolerance and Normal Thyroid Function," *Endokrinologie* Band 72 Heft 2: 149–154 (1978).

Rosenblatt, Stencel, "Weight Control: A National Obsession," published by Congressional Quarterly, Inc., Nov. 19, 1982.

Wooley and Wooley, "Should Obesity Be Treated at All?" in Stunkard and Stellar, editors, *Eating and Its Disorders,* New York: Raven Press (1984).

Zadik, Chalew, McCarter Jr., Meistas, Kowarski, "The Influence of Age on the 24-Hour Integrated Concentration of Growth Hormone in Normal Individuals," *J. Clin. Endocrin. Metab.* 60(3):513–516 (1985).

3: Fat Loss Versus Weight Loss

Bazzarre, Johanson, Huseman, Varma, Blizzard, "Human Growth Hormone Changes with Age," *Proc. 3rd Int. Symp. on Growth Hormone,* Milan, North Holland, Amsterdam (1975).

Brownell and Wadden, "Behavioral and Self-Help Treatments," in *Obesity* (edited by M. R. C. Greenwood), New York: Churchill Livingstone (1983).

Bray, "Diet and Exercise as Treatment for Obesity," in Conn Jr., DeFelice, Kuo, editors, *Health and Obesity,* New York: Raven Press (1983).

Fisher and Lachance, "Nutrition Evaluation of Published Weight-Reducing Diets," *J. Amer. Diet. Assoc.* 85:450–454 (1985).

Itallie, "Diets for Weight Reduction: Mechanisms of Action and Physiological Effects," *Int. J. Obesity* 2:113–22 (1978).

"Muscle Loss Occurs in Women with Aging Just as It Does in Men," p. 13 of Special Report on Aging 1980, U.S. Dept. of Health and Human Services, NIH, NIA. (No GH stimulation by exercise in persons over 30 found in Baltimore Longitudinal Study of Aging.)

Phillips and Baetz, editors, *Diet and Resistance to Disease,* New York: Plenum Press (1981).

Sours, Frattali, Brand, Feldman, Forbes, Swanson, Paris, "Sudden Death Associated with Very Low Calorie Weight Reduction Regimens," *Am. J. Clin. Nutr.* 34:453–461 (1981).

Wurtman, J., P. Moses, and R. J. Wurtman, "Prior Carbohydrate Consumption Affects the Amount of Carbohydrate that Rats Choose to Eat," *J. Nutr.* (1983).

Zadik, Chalew, McCarter Jr., Meistas, Kowarski, "The Influence of Age on the 24-Hour Integrated Concentration of Growth Hormone in Normal Individuals," *J. Clin. Endocrin. Metab.* 60(3):513–516 (1985).

4: How You Can Use Our Program

Drop, Sabbe, Visser, "The Effect of Puberty and Short Term Oral Administration of Testosterone Undecanoate on HGH Patients," *Clin. Endocr.* 16:375–381 (1982).

Fisher and Lachance, "Nutrition Evaluation of Published Weight-Reducing Diets," *J. Amer. Diet. Assoc.* 85:450–454 (1985).

Fleck and Hagerman, "Athletes' Body-fat Charts Show Interesting Modern Trends," *The Olympian,* July 1981.

Illig, Prader, "Effect of Testosterone on HGH Secretion in Patients with Anorchia and Delayed Puberty," *J. Clin. Endocrin. Metab.* 30:615–618 (1970).

Job, Donnadieu, Garnier, Evain-Brion, Roger, Chaussain, "Ornithine Stimulation Test, Correlation to Subsequent Response to HGH Therapy," *Evaluation of Growth Hormone Secretion: Pediat. Adolesc. Endocr.,* Karger, 12:86–102 (1983).

Kaplan, Grumbach, "The Ontogenesis of Hypothalamic-Hypophysiotrophic Releasing Factor Regulation of HGH Secretion," in Pecile and Muller, editors, *Growth and Growth Hormone,* New York: Excerpta Medica Foundation, pp. 382–388 (1972).

Phillips and Baetz, editors, *Diet and Resistance to Disease,* New York: Plenum Press (1981).

Prader, Ferrandez, Zachmann, Illig, "The Effect of HGH Treatment on

Growth, Bone Age, and Skinfold Thickness in 44 Children with Growth Hormone Deficiency," in Pecile and Muller, editors, *Growth and Growth Hormone,* New York: Excerpta Medica Foundation, pp. 452–457 (1972).

Tanner, "Human Growth Hormone," *Nature* 237:433–39 (1972).

Tanner, Whitehouse, Hughes, Vince, *Arch. Dis. in Childh.* 46:745 (1971).

Tanner, Whitehouse, "The Pattern of Growth in Children with Growth Hormone Deficiency Before, During, and After Treatment," in Pecile and Muller, editors, *Growth and Growth Hormone,* New York: Excerpta Medica Foundation, pp. 429–451 (1972).

Zachmann, Prader, "Anabolic and Androgenic Effect of Testosterone in Sexually Immature Boys and Its Dependency on Growth Hormone," *J. Clin. Endocr.* 30:85–95 (1970).

5: *Growth Hormone Releasers and Your Muscle-to-Fat Ratio, or Sandy's Lucky Break: A Broken Foot Leads to a Breakthrough*

Assimacopoulos-Jeannet, Jeanrenaud, "The Hormonal and Metabolic Basis of Experimental Obesity," in Albrink, editor, *Clinics in Endocrinology and Metabolism,* Vol. 5, pp. 337–365, Philadelphia: Saunders (1976).

Barbarino, De Marinis, Troncone, "Growth Hormone Response to Propranolol and L-Dopa in Obese Subjects," *Metabolism* 27(3):275–278 (1978).

Barbul, et al., "Arginine: A Thymotropic and Wound-Healing Promoting Agent," *Surgical Forum* 28:101–103 (1977).

Barbul, Rettura, Levenson, Seifter, "Thymotropic Actions of Arginine (ARG), Ornithine (ORN), and Growth Hormone (GH)," *Fed. Proc. Abstr.* 37(3): No. 282 (Federation of American Societies for Experimental Biology, 62nd annual meeting, Atlantic City, N.J.), April 9–14, 1978.

Bazzarre, Johanson, Huseman, Varma, Blizzard, "Human Growth Hormone Changes with Age," *Proc. 3rd Int. Symp. on Growth Hormone,* Milan, North Holland, Amsterdam (1975).

Beard, "The Effects of Parenteral Injection of Synthetic Amino Acids Upon the Appearance, Growth, and Disappearance of Emge Sarcoma in Rats," *Arch. Biochem.* 1:177–186 (1943).

Bohannon, Karam, Forsham, "Endocrine Responses to Sugar Ingestion in Man," *J. Am. Diet. Assoc.* 76:555–560 (1980).

Boyd, Lebowitz, Pfeiffer, "Stimulation of Human Growth Hormone Secretion by L-Dopa," *New Engl. J. Med.* 283:1425–1429 (1970).

Bray, "Diet and Exercise as Treatment for Obesity," in Conn Jr., DeFelice, and Kuo, editors, *Health and Obesity,* New York: Raven Press (1983).

Brown, Gajdusek, Gibbs Jr., and Asher, "Potential Epidemic of Creutzfeldt-Jakob Disease from Human Growth Hormone Therapy," *New Engl. J. Med.* 313:728–731 (1985).

Bruni, Meites, "Effects of Cholinergic Drugs on Growth Hormone Release," *Life Sci.* 23:1351–1358 (1978).

Buckler, Bold, Taberner, London, "Modification of Hormonal Responses to Arginine by Alpha-Adrenergic Blockade," *Br. Med. J.* iii:153–154 (1969).

Casanueva, Betti, Cella, Muller, Mantegazza, "Effect of Agonists and Antagonists of Cholinergic Neurotransmission on Growth Hormone Release in the Dog," *Acta Endocrinologica* 103:15–20 (1983).

Casanueva, Betti, Frigerio, Cocchi, Mantegazza, Muller, "Growth Hormone-Releasing Effect of an Enkephalin Analog in the Dog: Evidence for Cholinergic Mediation," *Endocrinology* 106:1239–1245 (1980).

Casanueva, Villanueva, Cabranes, Cabezas-Cerrato, Fernandez-Cruz, "Cholinergic Mediation of Growth Hormone Secretion Elicited by Arginine, Clonidine, and Physical Exercise in Man," *J. Clin. Endocrin. Metab.* 59(3):526–530 (1984).

Cahill Jr., "Disorders of Carbohydrate Metabolism," in Beeson, McDermott, Wyngaarden, editors, *Cecil Textbook of Medicine,* 15th ed., Philadelphia: Saunders, pp. 1969–1989 (1979).

Catt, "Growth Hormone," *The Lancet,* pp. 933–939, May 2, 1970.

Christy, "Anterior Pituitary Function in Normal Subjects and in Patients with Systemic Diseases," in Beeson, McDermott, Wyngaarden, editors, *Cecil Textbook of Medicine,* 15th ed., Philadelphia: Saunders, pp. 2085–2091 (1979).

Christy, "Assessment of Anterior Pituitary Function," in Beeson, McDermott, Wyngaarden, editors, *Cecil Textbook of Medicine,* 15th ed., Philadelphia: Saunders, pp. 2091–2094 (1979).

D'Alessandro, Bellastella, Esposito, Gasbarro, "Levodopa and L-Arginine to Test GH Release in Obesity," *New Engl. J. Med.* 290:575 (1974).

Delitala, Frulio, Pacifico, Maioli, "Participation of Cholinergic Muscarinic Receptors in Glucagon- and Arginine-Mediated Growth Hormone Secretion in Man," *J. Clin. Endocrin. Metab.* 55:1231–1233 (1982).

Drop, Sabbe, Visser, "The Effect of Puberty and Short Term Oral Administration of Testosterone Undecanoate on HGH Patients," *Clin. Endocr.* 16:375–381 (1982).

El-Khodary, Ball, Oweiss, Canary, "Insulin Secretion and Body Composition in Obesity," *Metabolism* 21:641–655 (1972).

Freinkel, "Hypoglycemic Disorders," in Beeson, McDermott, Wyngaarden, editors, *Cecil Textbook of Medicine,* 15th ed. Philadelphia: Saunders, pp. 1989–1997 (1979).

Frohman, Bernardis, Burek, Maran, Dhariwal, "Hypothalamic Control of Growth Hormone Secretion in the Rat," in Pecile and Muller, editors, *Growth and Growth Hormone,* New York: Excerpta Medica Foundation, pp. 271–282 (1972).

Gerich, Lorenzi, Bier, Tsalikian, Schneider, Karam, Forsham, "Effects of Physiologic Levels of Glucagon and Growth Hormone on Human Carbohydrate and Lipid Metabolism," *J. Clin. Invest.* 57:875–884 (1976).

Gibbs Jr., Joy, Heffner, Franko, Miyazaki, Asher, Parisi, Brown, Gajdusek, "Clinical and Pathological Features and Laboratory Confirmation of Creutzfeldt-Jakob Disease in a Recipient of Pituitary-Derived Human Growth Hormone," *New Engl. J. Med.* 313:734–738 (1985).

Gill-Ad, Topper, Laron, "Oral Clonidine as a Growth Hormone Stimulation Test," *The Lancet,* pp. 278–280 (1979).

Handwerger, Grandis, Barry, Crenshaw, "Stimulation by Ornithine of Ovine Placental Lactogen Secretion," *J. Endocr.* 88:283–288 (1981).

Hanson, "Serum Growth Hormone Response to Exercise in Non-Obese and Obese Normal Subjects," *Scand. J. Clin. Lab. Invest.* 31(2):175–178 (1973).

Holvey, editor, "Pituitary—Anterior Lobe Disorders: Diagnosis," *The Merck Manual of Diagnosis and Therapy,* 12th ed., pp. 1138–1139 (1972).

Illig, Prader, "Effect of Testosterone on HGH Secretion in Patients with Anorchia and Delayed Puberty," *J. Clin. Endocrin. Metab.* 30:615–618 (1970).

Imura, Kato, Ikeda, Morimoto, Yawata, "Effect of Adrenergic-Blocking or -Stimulating Agents on Plasma Growth Hormone, Immunoreactive Insulin, and Blood Free Fatty Acid Levels in Man," *J. Clin. Invest.* 50:1069–1079 (1971).

Irie, Sakuma, Shizume, Nakao, "The Effect of Nicotinic Acid Administration on Plasma Growth Hormone Concentrations," *Proc. Soc. Exptl. Biol. Med.* 126:708 (1967).

Irie, Tsushima, Sakuma, "Effect of Nicotinic Acid Administration on Plasma HGH, FFA, and Glucose in Obese Subjects and in Hypopituitary Patients," *Metabolism* 19:972–979 (1970).

Isidori, Monaco, Cappa, "A Study of Growth Hormone Release in Man

After Oral Administration of Amino Acids," *Curr. Med. Res. Opin.* 7(7):475–481 (1981).

Jacoby, Greenstein, Sassin, Weitzman, "The Effect of Monoamine Precursors on the Release of Growth Hormone in the Rhesus Monkey," *Neuroendocrin.* 14:95–102 (1974).

Jenkins et al., "Glycemic Index of Foods: A Physiological Basis for Carbohydrate Exchange," *Am. J. Clin. Nutr.* 34:362–366 (1981).

Job, Donnadieu, Garnier, Evain-Brion, Roger, Chaussain, "Ornithine Stimulation Test, Correlation to Subsequent Response to HGH Therapy," *Evaluation of Growth Hormone Secretion: Pediat. Adolesc. Endocr.,* Karger, 12:86–102 (1983).

Johnson, et al., "Hormonal Responses to Exercise in Racing Cyclists," *Proc. Physiological Soc.,* pp. 23P–24P, April 1974.

Josefsberg, Kauli, Keret, Brown, Bialik, Greenberg, Laron, "Tests for HGH Secretion in Childhood," *Evaluation of Growth Hormone Secretion: Pediat. Adolesc. Endocr.,* Karger, 12:66–74 (1983).

Kaplan, Grumbach, "The Ontogenesis of Hypothalamic-Hypophysiotropic Releasing Factor Regulation of HGH Secretion," in Pecile and Muller, editors, *Growth and Growth Hormone,* New York: Excerpta Medica Foundation, pp. 382–388 (1972).

Kenny, "Provocative Tests for Growth Hormone Deficiency," in Pecile and Muller, editors, *Growth and Growth Hormone,* New York: Excerpta Medica, pp. 415–420 (1972).

Knopf, Conn, Fajans, Floyd, Guntsche, Rull, "Plasma Growth Hormone Response to Intravenous Administration of Amino Acids," *J. Clin. Endocr.* 25:1140–1144 (1965).

Koch, Berg, De Armond, Gravina, "Creutzfeldt-Jakob Disease in a Young Adult with Ideopathic Hypopituitarism: Possible Relation to the Administration of Cadaveric Human Growth Hormone," *New Engl. J. Med.* 313:731–733 (1985).

Lal, Martin, De La Vega, Friesen, "Comparison of the Effect of Apomorphine and L-Dopa on Serum Growth Hormone Levels in Man," *Clin. Endocr.* 4:277–285 (1975).

Lal, Tolis, Martin, Brown, Guyda, "Effect of Clonidine on Growth Hormone, Prolactin, Luteinizing Hormone, Follicle-Stimulating Hormone, and Thyroid-Stimulating Hormone in the Serum of Normal Men," *J. Clin. Endocrin. Metab.* 41:827–832 (1975).

Larner, "Insulin and Oral Hypoglycemic Drugs," in Gilman, Goodman, Gilman, *Goodman and Gilman's The Pharmacological Basis of Therapeutics,* 6th ed., pp. 1497–1523, New York: Macmillan (1980).

Laron, Karp, Pretzelan, Kauli, Keret, Doron, "The Syndrome of Familial

Dwarfism and High Plasma Immunoreactive Human Growth Hormone (IR-HGH)," in Pecile and Muller, editors, *Growth and Growth Hormone*, New York: Excerpta Medica Foundation, pp. 458–482 (1972).

Leppaluoto, Rapeli, Varis, Ranta, "Secretion of Anterior Pituitary Hormones in Man: Effects of Ethyl Alcohol," *Acta Physiol. Scand.* 95:400–406 (1975).

Leveston, Cryer, "Endogenous Cholinergic Modulation of Growth-Hormone Secretion in Normal and Acromegalic Humans," *Metab.* 29:703–706 (1980).

Levy, Montanez, Feaver, Murphy, Dunn, "Effect of Arginine on Tumor Growth in Rats," *Cancer Res.* 14:198–200 (1954).

Lotter, Woods, "Injections of Insulin and Changes of Body Weight," *Physiol. Behav.* 18:293–297 (1977).

MacKay, Calloway, Barnes, "Hyperalimentation in Normal Animals Produced by Protamine Insulin," *Nutr.* 20:59–66 (1940).

Manchester, "The Interrelationship of the in Vitro Actions of Growth Hormone to Those in Vivo and to Effects of Insulin," in Pecile and Muller, editors, *Growth and Growth Hormone*, New York: Excerpta Medica Foundation, pp. 150–154 (1972).

Martin, "Functions of Central Nervous System Neurotransmitters in Regulation of Growth Hormone Secretion," *Fed. Proc.* 39(11):2902–2906 (1980).

Martin, "Neuroendocrine Regulation of Growth Hormone Secretion," *Evaluation of Growth Hormone Secretion: Pediat. Adolesc. Endocr.*, Karger, 12:1–26 (1983).

Massara, Strumia, "Increase in Plasma Growth Hormone Concentration in Man After Infusion of Adrenaline-Propranolol," *J. Endocr.* 47:95–100 (1970).

Massara, Camanni, "Effect of Various Adrenergic Receptor Stimulating and Blocking Agents on Human Growth Hormone Secretion," *J. Endocr.* 54:195–206 (1972).

Meites, "Role of Biogenic Amines in the Control of Prolactin and Growth Hormone Secretion," *Psychopharm. Bull.*, pp. 120–121 (Oct. 1976).

Merimee, et al., "Arginine-Initiated Release of Human Growth Hormone," *New Engl. J. Med.* 183(26):1425–1429 (1969).

Milner, Stepanovich, "Effect of Dietary Arginine on Ehrlich Ascites Tumor Cells," *Fed. Proc. Abstr.* 37(3): Abstract No. 773 (Federation of American Societies for Experimental Biology, 62nd annual meeting, Atlantic City, N.J.), April 9–14, 1978.

Milner, Stepanovich, "Inhibitory Effect of Dietary Arginine on Growth of Ehrlich Ascites Tumor Cells in Mice," *J. Nutr.* 109:489–491 (1979).

Mims, Stein, Bethune, "The Effect of a Single Dose of L-Dopa on Pituitary Hormones in Acromegaly, Obesity, and Normal Subjects," *J. Clin. Endocrin. Metab.* 37:34–39 (1973).

Moretti, Fabbri, Gnessi, Bonifacio, Fraioli, Isidori, "Pyridoxine (B₆) Suppresses the Rise in Prolactin and Increases the Rise in Growth Hormone Induced by Exercise," *New Engl. J. Med.* 307(7):444–445 (1982).

Murad, Haynes, "Adenohypophyseal Hormones and Related Substances," in Gilman, Goodman, Gilman, *Goodman and Gilman's The Pharmacological Basis of Therapeutics,* 6th ed., pp. 1369–1396, New York: Macmillan (1980).

"Muscle Loss Occurs in Women with Aging Just as It Does in Men," p. 13 of Special Report on Aging 1980, United States Dept. of Health and Human Services, NIH, NIA. (No GH stimulation by exercise in persons over 30 found in Baltimore Longitudinal Study of Aging.)

Pecile, Muller, Felici, Netti, "Nervous System Participation in Growth Hormone Release from Anterior Pituitary Gland," in Pecile and Muller, editors, *Growth and Growth Hormone,* New York: Excerpta Medica Foundation, pp. 261–270 (1972).

Pimstone, "Human Growth Hormone in Protein-Calorie Malnutrition," in Pecile and Muller, *Growth and Growth Hormone,* New York: Excerpta Medica Foundation, pp. 389–401 (1972).

Podolsky, Burrows, Zimmerman, Pattavina, "Effect of Chronic Potassium Depletion on Growth Hormone Release in Man," in Pecile and Muller, editors, *Growth and Growth Hormone,* New York: Excerpta Medica Foundation, pp. 402–407 (1972).

Prader, Ferrandez, Zachmann, Illig, "The Effect of HGH Treatment on Growth, Bone Age, and Skinfold Thickness in 44 Children with Growth Hormone Deficiency," in Pecile and Muller, editors, *Growth and Growth Hormone,* New York: Excerpta Medica Foundation, pp. 452–457 (1972).

Prinz et al., "Growth Hormone Levels During Sleep in Elderly Males," presented at the 29th annual Gerontological Society Conference, Oct. 13, 1976.

Prudden, Nishihara, Ocampo, "Studies on Growth Hormone. III: The Effect on Wound Tensile Strength of Marked Postoperative Anabolism Induced with Growth Hormone," *Surg. Obstet. Gynecol.* 107:481 (1958).

Quabbe, Helge, Kubicki, "Nocturnal Growth Hormone Secretion: Correlation with Sleeping EEG in Adults and Pattern in Children and Adolescents with Non-Pituitary Dwarfism, Overgrowth, and Obesity," *Acta Endocrinologica* 67:767–783 (1971).

Ratzmann and Gottschling, "Abnormal Growth Hormone Response in Obesity with Normal Carbohydrate Tolerance and Normal Thyroid Function," *Endokrinologie* Band 72 Heft 2: 149–154 (1978).

Rettura, Barbul, Seifter, "Ornithine Inhibits Two Murine Tumors" *Fed. Proc. Abstr.* 37(3): Abstract No. 779 (Federation of American Societies for Experimental Biology, 62nd annual meeting, Atlantic City, N.J.), April 9–14, 1978.

Rettura, Levinson, Seifter, "Anti-Tumor and Anti-Stress Actions of L-Ornithine," *Fed. Proc. Abstr.* (72nd annual meeting Amer. Soc. Biol. Chem., St. Louis, Mo., May 31–June 4, 1981), 40(6): Abstract No. 840 (1981).

Rodin, "Taming the Hunger Hormone," *American Health,* Jan.-Feb. 1984.

Rodin and Spitzer, "The Effects of Type of Sugar Ingested on Subsequent Eating Behavior," 4th International Congress on Obesity, The Sheraton Centre, New York, N.Y., Oct. 5–8, 1983.

Salvadorini, Saba, Forli, Tusini, Galeone, "Effect of Cytidine Diphosphate Choline on Growth Hormone Secretion in Patients with Brain or Pituitary Lesions," *Endocrinol. Japon.* 27:265–271 (1980).

Samuels, Shapiro, "Thyroid Hormone Stimulates De Novo Growth Hormone Synthesis in Cultured GH1 Cells," *Proc. Nat. Acad. Sci. USA* 73:3369–3373 (1976).

Seifter, Rettura, Barbul, Levenson, "Arginine: An Essential Amino Acid for Injured Rats," *Surgery,* pp. 224–230, August 1978.

Sonntag, Forman, Miki, Trapp, Gottschall, Meites, "L-Dopa Restores Amplitude of Growth Hormone Pulses in Old Male Rats to That Observed in Young Male Rats," *Neuroendocrin.* 34:163–168 (1982).

Sorkin, Pierpaoli, Fabris, Bianchi, "Relation of Growth Hormone to Thymus and the Immune Response," in Pecile and Muller, editors, *Growth and Growth Hormone,* New York: Excerpta Medica, pp. 132–142 (1972).

Spitz, Gonen, Rabinowitz, "Growth Hormone Release in Man Revisited: Spontaneous vs. Stimulus-Initiated Tides," in Pecile and Muller, editors, *Growth and Growth Hormone,* New York: Excerpta Medica Foundation (1972).

Strauch, Pandos, Bricaire, "Fructose Induced Growth Hormone Release," *J. Clin. Endocrin. Metab.* 32(4):582–584 (1971).

Takeda, Tominaga, Tei, Kitamura, Taga, Murase, Taguchi, Miwatani, "Inhibitory Effect of L-Arginine on Growth of Rat Mammary Tumors Induced by 7,12-Dimethylbenz(a)anthracene," *Cancer Res.* 35:2390–2393 (1975).

Tanner, "Human Growth Hormone," *Nature* 237:433–439 (1972).

Tanner, Whitehouse, Hughes, Vince, *Arch. Dis. in Childh.* 46:745 (1971).

Tanner, Whitehouse, "The Pattern of Growth in Children with Growth Hormone Deficiency Before, During, and After Treatment," in Pecile and Muller, editors, *Growth and Growth Hormone,* New York: Excerpta Medica Foundation, pp. 429–451 (1972).

Weisburger, Yamamoto, Glass, Frankel, "Prevention by Arginine Glutamate of the Carcinogenicity of Acetamide in Rats," *Toxicol. Appl. Pharmacol.* 14:163–175 (1969).

Woolf and Lee, "Effect of the Serotonin Precursor, Tryptophan, on Pituitary Hormone Secretion," *J. Clin. Endocrin. Metab.* 45:123 (1977).

Zachmann, Prader, "Anabolic and Androgenic Effect of Testosterone in Sexually Immature Boys and Its Dependency on Growth Hormone," *J. Clin. Endocr.* 30:85–95 (1970).

Zadik, Chalew, McCarter Jr., Meistas, Kowarski, "The Influence of Age on the 24-Hour Integrated Concentration of Growth Hormone in Normal Individuals," *J. Clin. Endocrin. Metab.* 60(3):513–516 (1985).

7: Not All Calories Are Created Equal—Eat to Lose!

Coulston, Hollenbeck, Liu, Williams, Starich, Mazzaferri, Reaven, "Effect of Source of Dietary Carbohydrate on Plasma Glucose, Insulin, and Gastric Inhibitory Polypeptide Responses to Test Meals in Subjects with Noninsulin-Dependent Diabetes Mellitus," *Am. J. Clin. Nutr.* 40:965–970 (1984).

Jenkins, Wolever, Jenkins, Josse, Wong, "The Glycaemic Response to Carbohydrate Foods," *The Lancet,* pp. 388–391 (Aug. 18, 1984).

Jenkins, David J. A. et al., "Glycemic Index of Foods: A Physiological Basis for Carbohydrate Exchange," *Am. J. Clin. Nutr.* 34:362–366 (1981).

8: Sweets: How to Have a Sweet Tooth Without Putting On Fat

Akgun and Ertel, "Plasma Glucose and Insulin After Fructose and High-Fructose Corn Syrup Meals in Subjects with Non-Insulin-Dependent Diabetes Mellitus," *Diabetes Care* 4(4):464–467 (1981).

Anderson, Polansky, Bryden, Roginski, Patterson, Reamer, "Effect of Exercise (Running) on Serum Glucose, Insulin, Glucagon, and Chromium Excretion," *Diabetes* 31:212–216 (1982).

Berthoud, "Cephalic Phase Insulin Response as a Predictor of Body Weight Gain and Obesity Induced by a Palatable Cafeteria Diet," *J. Obesity and Weight Regulation* 4:120–128 (1985).

Bohannon, Karam, Forsham, "Advantage of Fructose Ingestion (FTT) over Sucrose (STT) and Glucose (GTT) in Humans," *Diabetes* 27(suppl. 2):438 (1978).

Bohannon, Karam, Forsham, "Endocrine Responses to Sugar Ingestion in Man," *J. Amer. Diet. Assoc.* 76(6):555–560 (1980).

Brunzell, "Use of Fructose, Xylitol, or Sorbitol as a Sweetener in Diabetes Mellitus," *Diabetes Care* 1(4):223–230 (1978).

Cerasi, Li, Luft, "Some Metabolic Changes Induced by Acute Administration of HGH and Its Reduced-Alkylated Derivative in Man," in Pecile and Muller, editors, *Growth and Growth Hormone*, New York: Excerpta Medica Foundation, pp. 363–370 (1972).

Colford, "Sugar Assn. Sour on Coke," *Advertising Age*, pp. 12, 19, August (1985).

Coronary Drug Project, "Clofibrate and Niacin in Coronary Heart Disease," *J. Am. Med. Assoc.* 231:360–381 (1975).

Crapo, Kolterman, "The Metabolic Effect of 2-Week Fructose Feeding in Normal Subjects," *Amer. J. Clin. Nutr.* 39:525–534 (1984).

Crapo, Scarlett, Kolterman, "Comparison of the Metabolic Responses to Fructose and Sucrose Sweetened Foods," *Amer. J. Clin. Nutr.* 36:256–261 (1982).

Doisy, Streeten, Freiberg, Schneider in Prasad, editor, *Trace Elements in Human Health and Disease*, pp. 79–104, New York: Academic Press, (1976).

Evans, Roginski, Mertz, "Interaction of the Glucose Tolerance Factor (GTF) with Insulin," *Biochem. Biophys. Res. Comm.* 50:718–722 (1973).

Glinsmann, Feldman, Mertz, "Plasma Chromium After Glucose Administration," *Science* 152:1243–1245 (1966).

Glinsmann, Mertz, "Effect of Trivalent Chromium on Glucose Tolerance," *Metab. Clin. Exp.* 15:510–520 (1966).

"Glycemic Effects of Carbohydrates," *J. Amer. Diet. Assoc.* 84(12):1487–1488 (1984).

Gurson, Saner, "Effect of Chromium on Glucose Utilization in Marasmic Protein-Calorie Malnutrition," *Am. J. Clin. Nutr.* 24:1313–1319 (1971).

Gurson, Saner, "The Effect of Glucose Loading on Urinary Excretion of Chromium in Normal Adults in Individuals from Diabetic Families and in Diabetics," *Am. J. Clin. Nutr.* 31:1158–1161 (1978).

Hayashi, Larner, Sato, "Hormonal Growth Control of Cells in Culture," *In Vitro* 14:23–30 (1978).

Hopkins, Price, "Effectiveness of Chromium (III) in Improving the Impaired Glucose Tolerance of Middle-Aged Americans," *Western Hemisphere Nutr. Congr. II*, pp. 40–41 (1968).

Hopkins, Ransome-Kuti, Majaj, "Improvement of Impaired Carbohydrate Metabolism in Malnourished Infants," *Am. J. Clin. Nutr.* 21:203–211 (1968).

Jenkins, David J. A. et al., "Glycemic Index of Foods: A Physiological Basis for Carbohydrate Exchange," *Am. J. Clin. Nutr.* 34:362–366 (1981).

Katzen and Mahler, *Diabetes, Obesity, and Vascular Disease*, Parts 1 and 2, New York: Halsted Press/John Wiley (1978).

Levine, Streeten, Doisy, "Effect of Oral Chromium Supplementation on the Glucose Tolerance of Elderly Human Subjects," *Metab. Clin. Exp.* 17:114–125 (1968).

Liu, Abernathy, "Chromium and Insulin in Young Subjects with Normal Glucose Tolerance," *Am. J. Clin. Nutr.* 35:661–667 (1982).

Liu, Coulston, Hollenbeck, Reaven, "The Effect of Sucrose Content in High and Low Carbohydrate Diets on Plasma Glucose, Insulin, and Lipid Responses in Hypertriglyceridemic Humans," *J. Clin. Endocrin. Metab.* 59(4):636–642 (1984).

Liu, Morris, "Relative Chromium Response as an Indicator of Chromium Status," *Am. J. Clin. Nutr.* 31:972–976 (1978).

Makinen, "Sugars and the Formation of Dental Plaque," in *Sugars in Nutrition* (Sipple and McNutt, editors), New York: Academic Press (1974).

Mertz, "Chromium Occurrence and Function in Biological Systems," in *Physiol. Rev.* 49:163–203 (1969).

Offenbacher, Pi-Sunyer, "Beneficial Effects of Chromium-Rich Yeast on Glucose Tolerance and Blood Lipids in Elderly Subjects," *Diabetes* 29:919–925 (1980).

Pi-Sunyer, Offenbacher, "Chromium," in *Present Knowledge in Nutrition*, pp. 571–586, Washington, D.C.: The Nutrition Foundation, Inc. (1984).

Polansky, Anderson, Bryden, Glinsmann, "Chromium (Cr) and Brewer's Yeast Supplementation of Human Subjects: Effect on Glucose Tolerance, Serum Glucose, Insulin and Lipid Parameters," *Fed. Proc.* 41:391 (1982).

Porikos, Booth, Van Itallie, "Effect of Covert Nutritive Dilution on the Spontaneous Food Intake of Obese Individuals: a Pilot Study," *Am. J. Clin. Nutr.* 30(10):1638–44 (Oct. 1977).

Riales, Albrink, "Effect of Chromium Chloride Supplementation on Glucose

Tolerance and Serum Lipids Including High-Density Lipoprotein of Adult Men," *Am. J. Clin. Nutr.* 34:2670–2678 (1981).

Rizzino, Rizzino, Sato, "Defined Media and the Determination of Nutritional and Hormonal Requirements of Mammalian Cells in Culture," *Nutr. Rev.* 37:369–378 (1979).

Rodin, "Taming the Hunger Hormone," *American Health,* Jan.-Feb. 1984.

Rodin and Spitzer, "The Effects of Type of Sugar Ingested on Subsequent Eating Behavior," 4th International Congress on Obesity, The Sheraton Centre, New York, N.Y., Oct. 5–8, 1983.

Samundsen, "Has Aspartame an Aftertaste?" *J. Food Sci.* 50:1510, 1512 (1985).

Shansky, "Vitamin B-3 in the Alleviation of Hypoglycemia," *Drug and Cosmetic Industry,* Oct. 1981.

Sprince, et al., "Protectants Against Acetaldehyde Toxicity: Sulfhydryl Compounds and Ascorbic Acid," *Fed. Proc.* 33(3), Part 1, March (1974).

Tipton, Cook, "Trace Elements in Human Tissues II: Adult Subjects from the U.S.," *Health Phys.* 9:103–145 (1963).

Tipton, Schroeder, Perry Jr., Cook, "Trace Elements in Human Tissues III: Subjects from Africa, the Near and Far East and Europe," *Health Phys.* 11:403–451 (1965).

Tuman, Doisy, in Hoekstra, Suttie, Ganther, Mertz, editors, *Trace Element Metabolism in Animals II,* pp. 768–788, Baltimore: University Park Press (1974).

Wurtman, Judith J., Ph.D., *The Carbohydrate Craver's Diet,* New York: Ballantine (1983).

Wurtman, Richard J., "Nutrients that Modify Brain Function," *Sci. Amer.,* Apr. (1982).

Wurtman, J. and R. Wurtman, "Suppression of Carbohydrate Consumption as Snacks and at Mealtime by DL-Fenfluramine or Tryptophan," in *Anorectic Agents: Mechanisms of Action and Tolerance* (edited by Garattini and Samanin), New York: Raven Press (1981).

Wurtman, Moses, Wurtman, "Prior Carbohydrate Consumption Affects the Amount of Carbohydrate that Rats Choose to Eat," *J. Nutr.* (1983).

9: *Appetite Control Without Willpower: Nutrients That Curb Appetite!*

Anderson, "Dietary Fiber in Diabetes," in Spiller, Kay, editors, *Medical Aspects of Dietary Fiber,* New York: Plenum Press, 1980.

Anderson, Chen, "Plant Fiber: Carbohydrate and Lipid Metabolism," *Am. J. Clin. Nutr.* 32:346–63 (1979).

Anderson, Chen, Sieling, "Hypolipidemic Effects of High-Carbohydrate High-Fiber Diets," *Metabolism* 29:551–58 (1980).

Anderson, Sieling, "High-Fiber Diets for Obese Diabetic Patients," *Obesity Bariat. Med.* 9:109 (1980).

Anderson, Ward, "High Carbohydrate High Fiber Diets for Insulin-Treated Men with Diabetes Mellitus," *Am. J. Clin. Nutr.* 32:2312–2321 (1979).

Booth, Chase, Campbell, "Relative Effectiveness of Protein in the Late Stages of Appetite Suppression in Man," *Physiol. Behav.* 5:1299–1302 (1970).

Borison et al., "Metabolism of an Antidepressant Amino Acid," poster session at Apr. 9–14, 1978, FASEB, Atlantic City, N.J. (Discusses L-phenylalanine and depression.)

Cahill, Aoki, Rossini, "Metabolism in Obesity and Anorexia Nervosa," in Wurtman and Wurtman, *Nutrition and the Brain,* Vol. 3, New York: Raven Press (1979).

Cohen, Cohen, Pickar, Murphy, "Naloxone Reduces Food Intake in Humans," *Psychosom. Med.* 47(2):132–138 (1985).

Dulloo, Miller, "Thermogenic Drugs for the Treatment of Obesity: Sympathetic Stimulants in Animal Models," *Br. J. Nutr.* 52:179–196 (1984).

Ehrenpreis, Balagot, Comaty, Myles, "Naloxone Reversible Analgesia in Mice Produced by D-Phenylalanine and Hydrocinnamic Acid, Inhibitors of Carboxypeptidase A," in *Advances in Pain Research and Therapy,* Vol. 3, by John J. Bonica et al., New York: Raven Press (1979).

Fernstrom and Faller, "Neutral Amino Acids in the Brain: Changes in Response to Food Ingestion," *Neurochem.* 30:1531–1538 (1978).

Fernstrom and Wurtman, "Brain Serotonin Content: Increase Following Ingestion of Carbohydrate Diet," *Science* 174:1023–1025 (1971).

Garattini and Samanin, editors, *Anorectic Agents, Mechanisms of Action and Tolerance,* New York: Raven Press (1981), p. 146. (Discusses cholinergic mechanisms of feeding regulation.)

Gelenberg et al., "Tyrosine for the Treatment of Depression," *Am. J. Psychiat.* 137(5):622-623 (1980).

Gibbs, Falasco, McHugh, "Cholecystokinin-Decreased Food Intake in Rhesus Monkeys," *Am. J. Physiol.* 230(1):15–18 (1976).

Gibbs, Young, Smith, "Cholecystokinin Decreases Food Intake in Rats," *J. Comp. Physiol. Psychol.* 84:488–495 (1973).

Glassman, Jackson, Walsh, Roose, "Cigarette Craving, Smoking Withdrawal, and Clonidine," *Science* 226:864–66 (1984).

J. Amer. Med. Assoc. 243(4):343 (Jan. 25, 1980). (Clonidine reduces heroin-withdrawal symptoms.)

Jenkins, Leeds, Newton, Cummings, "Effect of Pectin, Guar Gum, and Wheat Fiber on Serum Cholesterol," *The Lancet* 1:1116–1118 (1975).

Kiehm, Anderson, Ward, "Beneficial Effects of a High Carbohydrate High Fiber Diet on Hyperglycemic Diabetic Men," *Am. J. Clin. Nutr.* 29:895–899 (1976).

Kirby, Anderson, Sieling, Rees, Chen, Miller, Kay, "Oat-Bran Intake Selectively Lowers Serum Low-Density Lipoprotein Cholesterol Concentrations of Hypercholestremic Men," *Am. J. Clin. Nutr.* 34:824–829 (1981).

McCarthy, Dettmar, Lynn, Sanger, "Anorectic Actions of the Opiate Antagonist Naloxone," *Neuropharm.* 20:1347–1349 (1981).

Meyer, Grossman, "Release of Secretin and Cholecystokinin," in *Gastrointestinal Hormones* (Demling, editor), pp. 50–53, Stuttgart: Georg Thieme Verlag (1972).

Mickelsen, Makdani, Cotton, Titcomb, Colmey, Gatty, "Effects of a High Fiber Bread Diet on Weight Loss in College-Age Males," *Am. J. Clin. Nutr.* 32:1703–1709 (1979).

Morley, "Minireview—The Ascent of Cholecystokinin (CCK) from Gut to Brain," *Life Sci.* 30:479–493 (1982).

Morley, Levine, "Stress-Induced Eating Is Mediated Through Endogenous Opiates," *Science* 209:1259–1260 (1980).

Porte and Woods, "Regulation of Food Intake and Body Weight by Insulin," *Diabetologia,* 20:274–280 (1981).

Reddy, Watanabe, Mori, "Effect of Conventional and Unconventional Dietary Fibers in Colon Carcinogenesis," in Furda, *Unconventional Sources of Dietary Fiber,* Washington, D.C.: American Chemical Society (1983).

Rodin, "Taming the Hunger Hormone," *American Health,* Jan.-Feb. 1984.

Rodin and Spitzer, "The Effects of Type of Sugar Ingested on Subsequent Eating Behavior," 4th International Congress on Obesity, The Sheraton Centre, New York, N.Y., Oct. 5–8, 1983.

Scala, "The Physiological Effects of Dietary Fiber," in Jeanes and Hodge, *Physiological Effects of Food Carbohydrates,* Washington, D.C.: American Chemical Society (1975).

Seiden and Dykstra, "Acetylcholine and Behavior," in *Psychopharmacology, a Biochemical and Behavioral Approach,* New York: Van Nostrand Reinhold (1977), p. 230. (Discusses cholinergic mechanisms of feeding regulation.)

Shekelle et al., "Dietary Vitamin A and Risk of Cancer in the Western Electric Study," *The Lancet,* pp. 1185–1190, Nov. 28, 1981.

Smith and Sauder, "Food Cravings, Depression, and Premenstrual Problems," *Psychosom. Med.* XXXI(4):281–287 (1969).

Smith, Gibbs, "Cholecystokinin and Satiety: Theoretic and Therapeutic Implications," in *Hunger: Basic Mechanisms and Clinical Implications* (edited by Novin, Wyrwicka, and Bray), New York: Raven Press (1976).

Smith, Gibbs, Jerome, et al., "The Satiety Effects of Cholecystokinin: a Progress Report," *Peptides* 2:57–59 (1981).

Taylor, Mathew, Ho, Weinman, "Serotonin Levels and Platelet Uptake During Premenstrual Tension," in Ho, Schoolar, Usdin, editors, *Serotonin in Biological Psychiatry, Advances in Biochemical Psychopharmacology,* Vol. 34, New York: Raven Press (1982).

Wilkins, Jenkins, Steiner, "Efficacy of Clonidine in Treatment of Alcohol Withdrawal State," *Psychopharm.* 81:78–80 (1983).

Wurtman, Judith J., Ph.D., *The Carbohydrate Craver's Diet,* New York: Ballantine (1983).

Wurtman, J. and R. Wurtman, "Suppression of Carbohydrate Consumption as Snacks and at Mealtime by DL-Fenfluramine or Tryptophan," in *Anorectic Agents: Mechanisms of Action and Tolerance* (edited by Garattini and Samanin), New York: Raven Press (1981).

Wurtman, Richard J., "Nutrients that Modify Brain Function," *Sci. Amer.,* Apr. 1982.

Wurtman, Moses, Wurtman, "Prior Carbohydrate Consumption Affects the Amount of Carbohydrate that Rats Choose to Eat," *J. Nutr.,* 1983.

Vetter, "Fiber as a Food Ingredient." *Food Technology,* pp. 64–69, Jan. (1984).

10: Diet Pills: What You Need to Know

Barnes and Galton, *Hypothyroidism: The Unsuspected Illness,* New York: Crowell (1976).

Bray, Greenway, "Pharmacological Approaches to Treating the Obese Patient," in *Clinics in Endocrinology and Metabolism,* Vol. 5 No. 2, p. 455 (Albrink, ed.), Philadelphia: Saunders (1976).

Cahill, Aoki, Rossini, "Metabolism in Obesity and Anorexia Nervosa," in

Wurtman and Wurtman, *Nutrition and the Brain,* Vol. 3, New York: Raven Press (1979).

Carruba, Ricciardi, Muller, Mantegazza, "Anorectic Effect of Lisuride and Other Ergot Derivatives in the Rat," *Europ. J. Pharm.* 64(2/3):133–141 (1980).

Cohen, Cohen, Pickar, Murphy, "Naloxone Reduces Food Intake in Humans," *Psychosom. Med.* 47(2):132–138 (1985).

Garattini and Samanin, editors, *Anorectic Agents, Mechanisms of Action and Tolerance,* New York: Raven Press (1981).

Gibbs, Falasco, McHugh, "Cholecystokinin-Decreased Food Intake in Rhesus Monkeys," *Am. J. Physiol.* 230(1):15–18 (1976).

Gibbs, Young, Smith, "Cholecystokinin Decreases Food Intake in Rats," *J. Comp. Physiol. Psychol.* 84:488–495 (1973).

Gilman, Goodman, Gilman, *Goodman and Gilman's The Pharmacological Basis of Therapeutics,* 6th ed., New York: Macmillan (1980).

Harrower, Yap, Nairn, Walton, Strang, Craig, "Growth Hormone, Insulin, and Prolactin Secretion in Anorexia Nervosa and Obesity During Bromocriptine Treatment," *Brit. Med. J.* 2:156 (1977).

Henman, "Guarana (Paullinia Cupana Var. Sorbilis): Ecological and Social Perspectives of an Economic Plant of the Central Amazon Basin," *J. Ethnopharmacology* 6:311–338.

Himms-Hagen, "Nonshivering Thermogenesis, Brown Adipose Tissue, and Obesity," in Beers and Bassett, *Nutritional Factors: Modulating Effects on Metabolic Processes,* New York: Raven Press (1981).

Landsberg and Young, "Diet-Induced Changes in Sympathoadrenal Activity: Implications for Thermogenesis and Obesity," *Obesity and Metabolism* 1(1):5–33 (1981).

Leibowitz, "Identification of Catecholamine Receptor Mechanisms in the Perifornical Lateral Hypothalamus and Their Role in Mediating Amphetamine and L-Dopa Anorexia," in *Central Mechanisms of Anorectic Drugs* (Garattini and Samanin, editors), p. 39, New York: Raven Press (1978).

Margules, Moisset, Lewis, Shibuya, Pert, "Beta-Endorphin Is Associated with Overeating in Genetically Obese Mice (ob/ob) and Rats (fa/fa)," *Science* 202:988–991 (1978).

McCarthy, Dettmar, Lynn, Sanger, "Anorectic Actions of the Opiate Antagonist Naloxone," *Neuropharm.* 20:1347–1349 (1981).

Morley, "Minireview: The Ascent of Cholecystokinin (CCK) from Gut to Brain," *Life Sci.* 30:479–493 (1982).

Munro and Ford, "Drug Treatment of Obesity," in Silverstone, *Drugs and Appetite,* New York: Academic Press (1982).

Rall, "Central Nervous System Stimulants," in Gilman, Goodman, Gilman, *Goodman and Gilman's The Pharmacological Basis of Therapeutics,* 6th ed., New York: Macmillan, pp. 592–607 (1980).

Rothwell, Stock, Wyllie, "Sympathetic Mechanisms in Diet-Induced Thermogenesis: Modification by Ciclazindol and Anorectic Drugs," *Br. J. Pharmacol.* 74(3):539–46 (1981).

Schmitt, Luqman, McCool, Lenz, Ahmad, Nolan, Stephan, Sunder Danowski, "Unresponsiveness to Exogenous TSH in Obesity," *Int. J. Obesity* 1:185–190 (1977).

Silverstone and Kyriakides, "Clinical Pharmacology of Appetite," in Silverstone, editor, *Drugs and Appetite,* New York: Academic Press (1982).

Smith, Gibbs, Jerome, et al., "The Satiety Effects of Cholecystokinin: A Progress Report," *Peptides* 2:57–59 (1981).

Thomson, White, Echols, "The Effect of L-Dopa Therapy in Parkinson's Disease," *Arizona Med.* 27:5 (1970).

Vardi, Oberman, Rabey, Streifler, Ayelow, Herzberg, "Weight Loss in Patients Treated with Levodopa," *J. Neurol. Sci.* 30:33 (1976).

Wurtman, Wurtman, "Suppression of Carbohydrate Consumption as Snacks and at Mealtime by DL-Fenfluramine or Tryptophan," in *Anorectic Agents: Mechanisms of Action and Tolerance* (edited by Garattini and Samanin), New York: Raven Press (1981).

Yen, Allan, Pearson, Acton, Greenberg, "Prevention of Obesity in AVY/a Mice by Dehydroepiandrosterone," *Lipids* 12(5):409–413 (1977).

11: Fat Metabolism—How You Can Change It

Babayan, "Medium Chain Length Fatty Acid Esters and Their Medical and Nutritional Applications," *J. Amer. Oil Chem. Soc.,* pp. 49A–51A, Jan. 1981.

Becklake, "Respiratory Disease; Physical and Chemical Irritants: Radiation," in Beeson, McDermott, Wyngaarden, editors, *Cecil Textbook of Medicine,* 15th ed., Philadelphia: Saunders, pp. 1001–1002 (1979).

Bjorksten, "The Crosslinkage Theory of Aging," *J. Am. Geriatr. Soc.* 16:408–427 (1968).

Borum, "Carnitine," *Ann. Rev. Nutr.* 3:233–259 (1983).

Borum and Fisher, editors, "Health Effects of Dietary Carnitine," Nov. 1983, prepared for the Bureau of Foods, Food and Drug Administration, Dept. of Health and Human Services, Washington, D.C. 20204

(Life Sciences Research Office, Federation of American Societies for Experimental Biology, 9650 Rockville Pike, Bethesda, MD 20814).

Bukowiecki, Lupien, Follea, Jahjah, "Effects of Sucrose, Caffeine, and Cola Beverages on Obesity, Cold Resistance, and Adipose Tissue Cellularity," *Am. J. Physiol.* 244(4):R500–7 (Apr. 1983).

Carlson, Froberg, Nye, "Acute Effects of Nicotinic Acid on Plasma, Liver, Heart, and Muscle Lipids. Nicotinic Acid in the Rat II," *Acta Med. Scand.* 180:571–579 (1966).

Carlson, Nye, "Acute Effects of Nicotinic Acid in the Rat. Plasma and Liver Lipids and Blood Glucose. Nicotinic Acid in the Rat I," *Acta Med. Scand.* 179:453–460 (1966).

Carlson, Oro, "The Effect of Nicotinic Acid on the Plasma Free Fatty Acids," *Acta Med. Scand.* 172:641–645 (1962).

Charman et al., "Nicotinic Acid in the Treatment of Hypercholesterolemia," *J. Angiology,* Jan. (1973).

Coronary Drug Project, "Clofibrate and Niacin in Coronary Heart Disease," *J. Am. Med. Soc.* 231:360–381 (1975).

Deyl, et al., "Aging of the Connective Tissue: Collagen Cross Linking in Animals of Different Species and Equal Age," *Exp. Geront.* 6:227–233 (1971).

Froberg, "Metabolism of Lipids in Blood and Tissues During Exercise," in *Biochemistry of Exercise, Medicine and Sport,* Karger, Vol. 3, pp. 100–113 (1969).

Harkins, Sarett, "Nutritional Evaluation of Medium-Chain Triglycerides in the Rat," *J. Amer. Oil Chem. Soc.* 45:26–30 (1968).

Hittner, et al., "Retrolental Fibroplasia and Vitamin E in the Preterm Infant —Comparison of Oral Versus Intramuscular Administration," *Pediatrics* 73:238–249 (1984).

Hittner, et al., "Prevention and Management of Retrolental Fibroplasia," *Hosp. Pract.* 19:85–94, 99 (1984).

Kaunitz, Slanetz, Johnson, Babayan, Barsky, "Nutritional Properties of Saturated Fatty Acids of Medium Chain-length," *J. Amer. Oil Chem. Soc.* 35:10–13 (1958).

Kirk, Chieffi, "Variation with Age in Elasticity of Skin and Subcutaneous Tissue in Human Individuals," *J. Derm.* 17:373–380 (1962).

Larner, "Insulin and Oral Hypoglycemic Drugs," in Gilman, Goodman, Gilman, *Goodman and Gilman's The Pharmacological Basis of Therapeutics,* 6th ed., pp. 1497–1523, Macmillan (1980).

Lassers, Wahlqvist, Kaijser, Carlson, "Effect of Nicotinic Acid on Myocardial Metabolism in Man at Rest and During Exercise," *J. Appl. Physiol.* 33:72–80 (1972).

Lavau and Hashim, "Effect of Medium-Chain Triglyceride on Lipogenesis and Body Fat in the Rat," *J. Nutr.* 108:613–620 (1978).

Maebashi, Sato, Kawamura, Imamura, Yoshinaga, "Lipid-Lowering Effect of Carnitine in Patients with Type-IV Hyperlipoproteinemia," *The Lancet,* pp. 805–807 (Oct. 14, 1978).

Miettinen et al., *Acta Med. Scand.* 186:247–253 (1969). (Study found a decrease in serum cholesterol of 25 percent and triglycerides of 30 percent in human subjects after 2 weeks on 3 grams of niacin per day.)

Pike, Brown, "Hepatocytes," in *Nutrition, an Integrated Approach,* New York: John Wiley, pp. 569–593 (1975).

Senior, Van Itallie, Isselbacher, Shwachman in Senior, Van Itallie, Greenberger, *Medium Chain Triglycerides,* pp. 247–260 (1968).

Shansky, "Vitamin B-3 in the Alleviation of Hypoglycemia," *Drug and Cosmetic Industry* (Oct. 1981).

Steinberg, "Tocopherols in Treatment of Primary Fibrositis, Including Dupuytren's Contracture, Periarthritis of the Shoulder, and Peyronie's Disease," *A.M.A. Arch. Surg.,* pp. 824–833 (c. 1950, no date or volume number on photocopy of paper).

Sundaram, et al., "Alpha-Tocopherol and Serum Lipoproteins," *Lipids,* 16(4):223–227 (1981). (Vitamin E treatment of fibrocystic breast disease.)

Tanzer, "Cross-Linking of Collagen," *Science* 180:561–566 (1973).

Verzar, "The Aging of Collagen," *Sci. Amer.,* Apr. (1963).

12: Thermogenesis—The Cool Way to Lose Fat

Arch, Ainsworth, "Reduction of Obesity in Mice with a Novel Type of Thermogenic Beta-Adrenergic Agonist," *Int. J. Obesity* 7:85–95 (1983).

Astrup, Lundsgaard, Madsen, Christensen, "Enhanced Thermogenic Responsiveness During Chronic Ephedrine Treatment in Man," *Am. J. Clin. Nutr.* 42:83–94 (1985).

Bagchi, Brown, Urdanivia, Sundick, "Induction of Autoimmune Thyroiditis in Chickens by Dietary Iodine," *Science* 230:325–327 (1985).

Bartness, Ruby, Wade, "Dietary Obesity in Exercising or Cold-Exposed Syrian Hamsters," *Physiol. Behav.* 32:85–90 (1984).

Bean, Spies, "A Study of Nicotinic Acid and Related Pyridine and Pyrazine Compounds on the Temperature of the Skin of Human Beings," *Am. Heart J.* 20:62–75 (1940).

Borum, "Carnitine," *Ann. Rev. Nutr.* 3:233–259 (1983).

Borum and Fisher, editors, "Health Effects of Dietary Carnitine," Nov. 1983, prepared for Bureau of Foods, Food and Drug Administration, Dept. of Health and Human Services, Washington, D.C. 20204 (Life Sciences Research Office, Federation of American Societies for Experimental Biology, 9650 Rockville Pike, Bethesda, MD 20814).

Boyd, Lebowitz, Pfeiffer, "Stimulation of Human Growth Hormone Secretion by L-Dopa," *New Engl. J. Med.* 283:1425–1429 (1970).

Brecher, E. M. *Licit and Illicit Drugs,* Boston: Little, Brown (1972).

Bukowiecki, Lupien, Follea, Jahjah, "Effects of Sucrose, Caffeine, and Cola Beverages on Obesity, Cold Resistance, and Adipose Tissue Cellularity," *Am. J. Physiol.* 244(4):R500–7 (Apr. 1983).

Carlson, Hsieh, *Control of Energy Exchange,* New York: Macmillan (1970).

"Chemical Clue to Obesity Found," *Science News,* p. 295, Nov. 8, 1980.

Danforth Jr., Daniels, Katzeff, Ravussin, Garrow, "Thermogenic Responsiveness in Pima Indians," *Clinical Research* 29:663a (1981).

Danforth Jr., Horton, Sims, "Nutritionally-Induced Alterations in Thyroid Hormone Metabolism," in Beers and Bassett, *Nutritional Factors: Modulating Effects on Metabolic Processes,* New York: Raven Press (1981).

Danforth Jr., Sims, Horton, Goldman, "Correlation of Serum Triiodothyronine Concentrations (T3) with Dietary Composition, Gain in Weight, and Thermogenesis in Man," *Diabetes* 24:406 (1975).

Dauncey, "Influence of Mild Cold on 24 H Energy Expenditure, Resting Metabolism and Diet-Induced Thermogenesis," *Br. J. Nutr.* 45:257–267 (1981).

Dulloo, Miller, "Thermogenic Drugs for the Treatment of Obesity: Sympathetic Stimulants in Animal Models," *Br. J. Nutr.* 52:179–196 (1984).

Elliot, "Blame It All on Brown Fat Now," *J. Amer. Med. Assoc.* 243:1983–1984 (1980).

Finer, Swan, Mitchell, "Hypothalamic Function and Energy Output in Obesity," *J. Obesity Weight Regulation* 4:(2)87–97 (1985).

Himms-Hagen, "Nonshivering Thermogenesis, Brown Adipose Tissue, and Obesity," in Beers and Bassett, *Nutritional Factors: Modulating Effects on Metabolic Processes,* New York: Raven Press (1981).

Himms-Hagen, "Thermogenesis in Brown Adipose Tissue as an Energy Buffer," *New Engl. J. Med.* 311:1549–1558 (1984).

Hirata, Nagasaka, "Enhancement of Calorigenic Response to Cold and to Norepinephrine in Physically Trained Rats," *Jpn. J. Physiol.* 31:657–665 (1981).

Jung, Shetty, James, Barrand, Callingham, "Reduced Thermogenesis in Obesity," *Nature* 279:322–323 (1979).

Landsberg, Young, "Diet-Induced Changes in Sympathoadrenal Activity:

Implications for Thermogenesis and Obesity," *Obesity and Metabolism* 1:5–33 (1981).

Lassers, Wahlqvist, Kaijser, Carlson, "Effect of Nicotinic Acid on Myocardial Metabolism in Man at Rest and During Exercise," *J. Appl. Physiol.* 33:72–80 (1972).

LeBlanc, Dussault, Lupien, Richard, "Effect of Diet and Exercise on Norepinephrine-Induced Thermogenesis in Male and Female Rats," *J. Appl. Physiol.: Respirat. Environ. Exercise Physiol.* 52(3):556–561 (1982).

McMinn, "A Third Variable in Obesity: The Effects of Brown Adipose Tissue on Thermogenesis," *Obesity and Metabolism* 1:209–222 (1981).

Minh, "Assays on Physical Hygiene and Sport," *M. Medicina* (1980).

Morgan, Goldberg, "Brown Adipose Tissue," *Obesity and Metabolism* 1:198–208 (1981).

"Obesity Linked to Metabolism in Brown Fat," *Chem. Eng. News,* pp. 25–26, Feb. 16, 1981.

Perkins, Rothwell, Stock, Stone, "Activation of Brown Adipose Tissue Thermogenesis by the Ventromedial Hypothalamus," *Nature* 289:401–402 (1981).

Rose, Williams, *Br. J. Nutr.* 24:1091–1107 (1970).

Rothwell, Stock, "Effects of Age on Diet-Induced Thermogenesis and Brown Adipose Tissue Metabolism in the Rat," *Int. J. Obesity* 7:583–589 (1983).

Rothwell, Stock, Wyllie, "Sympathetic Mechanisms in Diet-Induced Thermogenesis: Modification by Ciclazindol and Anorectic Drugs," *Br. J. Pharmacol.* 74(3):539–546 (1981).

Simonson, Tappy, Felber, "Thermogenic Effect of Fructose and Glucose in Man," *Diabetes* 34:74A: No. 295 (1985).

Stock, Rothwell, "Diet-Induced Thermogenesis and Brown Fat in Animals," *Int. J. Obesity* 7:501–504 (1983).

Stock, Rothwell, "Diet-Induced Thermogenesis: A Role for Brown Adipose Tissue," in Beers and Bassett, *Nutritional Factors: Modulating Effects on Metabolic Processes,* New York: Raven Press (1981).

Strong, Goldman, "A Linearized, Time Dependent Model of the Heat Transfer and Thermoregulatory Responses Occurring Upon Immersion in Cold Water," Report No. T7/82, Natick, Mass.: U.S. Army Research Institute of Environmental Medicine (1982).

Trayhurn, Douglas, McGuckin, "Brown Adipose Tissue Thermogenesis Is 'Suppressed' During Lactation in Mice," *Nature* 298:59–60 (1982).

Wellman, Marmon, "Synergism Between Caffeine and dl-Phenylpropanolamine on Brown Adipose Tissue Thermogenesis in the Adult Rat," *Pharmacol. Biochem. Behav.* 22(5):781–785 (1985).

Yakovlev, *Athlete Nutrition M.* (1967) (as published in "Nutrition and Sport" by the International Federation of Bodybuilders).

13: Changing Your Behavior—How to Act Slim

Blackburn, Greenberg, "Multidisciplinary Approach to Adult Obesity Therapy," *Int. J. Obesity* 2:133–142 (1978).

Bray, "The Myth of Diet in the Management of Obesity," *Am. J. Clin. Nutr.* 23(9):1141–1148 (1970).

Bray, "Diet and Exercise as Treatment for Obesity," in Conn Jr., DeFelice, and Kuo, *Health and Obesity*, New York: Raven Press (1983).

Brownell and Wadden, "Behavioral and Self-Help Treatments," in *Obesity* (edited by M. R. C. Greenwood), New York: Churchill Livingstone (1983).

Clausen, Silfen, Coombs, Ayers, Altschul, "Relationship of Dietary Regimens to Success, Efficiency, and Cost of Weight Loss," *J. Am. Diet. Assoc.* 77:249–257 (1980).

Greenwood, M. R. C., editor, *Obesity*, New York: Churchill Livingstone (1983).

Johnson, Stalonas, Christ, Pock, "The Development and Evaluation of a Behavioral Weight-Reduction Program," *Int. J. Obesity* 3:229–238 (1979).

Laughlin, Fisher, and Sherrard, "Blood Pressure Reductions During Self-Recording of Home Blood Pressure," *Amer. Heart J.* 98(5):629–634 (Nov. 1979).

Steffee, "The Medical Syndrome of Obesity," *Primary Care* 9(3):581–593 (1982).

Stuart, Guire, "Some Correlates of the Maintenance of Weight Lost Through Behavior Modification," *Int. J. Obesity* 2:225–235 (1978).

Stunkard, Penick, "Behavior Modification in the Treatment of Obesity," *Arch. Gen. Psychiatry* 36:801–806 (1979).

Stunkard, Wadden, "Behavior Therapy and Obesity" in Conn Jr., DeFelice, and Kuo, editors, *Health and Obesity*, New York: Raven Press (1983).

Volkmar, Stunkard, Woolston, Bailey, "High Attrition Rates in Commercial Weight Reduction Programs," *Arch. Intern. Med.* 141:426–428 (1981).

14: Peak Output Exercise—The Astronauts' Fast Exercise Method

Astrand, "Quantification of Exercise Capability and Evaluation of Physical Capacity in Man," in Sonnenblick and Lesch, editors, *Exercise and Heart Disease,* Grune & Stratton, pp. 87–103 (1977).

Davies, Quintanilka, Brooks, Packer, "Free Radicals and Tissue Damage Produced by Exercise," *Biochem. Biophys. Res. Commun.* 107(4):1198–1205 (1982).

Dillard, Litov, Savin, Dumelin, Tappel, "Effects of Exercise, Vitamin E, and Ozone on Pulmonary Function and Lipid Peroxidation," *J. Appl. Physiol.: Respirat. Environ. Exercise Physiol.* 45(6):927–932 (1978).

Flamm, Demopoulos, Seligman, Tomasula, DeCrescito, Ransohoff, "Ethanol Potentiation of Central Nervous System Trauma," *J. Neurosurg.* 46:328–335 (March 1977).

Grande, Taylor, "Adaptive Changes in the Heart, Vessels, and Patterns of Control Under Chronically High Loads," in *Handbook of Physiology, Circulation,* Vol. 3, p. 2615, Bethesda, Md.: American Physiological Society (1965).

Gyore, Frenkl, Meszaros, "Human Exercise and Enzyme Induction," *Mammalian Biochemistry* 95:445 (1981).

Higuchi, Cartier, Chen, Holloszy, "Superoxide Dismutase and Catalase in Skeletal Muscle: Adaptive Response to Exercise," *J. Geront.* 40:281–286 (1985).

Holloszy, "Adaptations of Muscular Tissue to Training," in Sonnenblick and Lesch, editors, *Exercise and Heart Disease,* New York: Grune & Stratton, pp. 25–38 (1977).

Luck and Engel, "Arrythmia and Social Drinking," *Ann. Int. Med.* 98(2):253–254 (1983).

Master, Rosenfeld, "Two-Step Exercise Test: Current Status After Twenty-five Years," *Mod. Conc. Cardiovasc. Dis.* 36:19–24 (1967).

Morehouse, Dr. Laurence A. and Leonard Gross, *Total Fitness in 30 Minutes a Week,* hardback, New York: Simon and Schuster (1975); paperback reprint, New York: Pocket Books (1975). (A popular book.)

Morehouse, Dr. Laurence A. and Leonard Gross, *Maximum Performance,* New York: Pocket Books (1977). (Also a popular book.)

Murad, Haynes, "Adenohypophyseal Hormones and Related Substances," in Gilman, Goodman, Gilman, *Goodman and Gilman's The Pharmacological Basis of Therapeutics,* 6th ed., pp. 1369–1396, New York: Macmillan (1980).

"Muscle Loss Occurs in Women with Aging Just as It Does in Men," p. 13

of Special Report on Aging 1980, U.S. Dept. of Health and Human Services, NIH, NIA. (No GH stimulation by exercise in persons over 30 found in Baltimore Longitudinal Study of Aging.)

Nagle, Balke, Naughton, "Graduational Step Tests for Assessing Work Capacity," *J. Appl. Physiol.* 20:745–748 (1965).

Ollivier, Boschat, Bercovici, "Physical Training and Blood Lipids: A Study in 270 Healthy Subjects," *Chemical Abstracts* 95:22225r (1981).

Oscai, Mole, Brei, "Cardiac Growth and Respiratory Enzyme Levels in Male Rats Subjected to a Running Program," *Am. J. Physiol.* 220:1944–1948 (1971).

Oscai, Mole, Holloszy, "Effects of Exercise on Cardiac Weight and Mitochondria in Male and Female Rats," *Am. J. Physiol.* 220:1944–1948 (1971).

Packer, "Vitamin E, Physical Exercise, and Tissue Damage in Animals," *Med. Biol.* 62:105–109 (1984).

Sitaram, Weingartner, Caine, Gillin, "Choline: Selective Enhancement of Serial Learning and Encoding of Low Imagery Words in Man," *Life Sci.* 22:1555–60 (1978).

Sitaram, Weingartner, Gillin, "Human Serial Learning: Enhancement with Arecholine and Choline and Impairment with Scopolamine Correlate with Performance on Placebo," *Science* 201:274–276 (1978).

Song and Rubin, "Ethanol Produces Muscle Damage in Human Volunteers," *Science* 175:327–328 (1972).

Williams, Wood, Haskell, Vranizan, "The Effects of Running Mileage and Duration on Plasma Lipoprotein Levels," *J. Amer. Med. Assoc.* 247:2674–2679 (1982).

15: Designing Your Own Personal Program

Andres, "Effect of Obesity on Total Mortality," *Int. J. Obesity* 4:381–386 (1980).

"Increased Female Mortality and Increased Male Mortality," charts adapted from the 1979 *Build and Blood Pressure Study,* Society of Actuaries and the Association of Life Insurance Medical Directors of America.

Simopoulos, Itallie, "Body Weight, Health, and Longevity," *Ann. Int. Med.* 100:285–295 (1984).

Thomas, William V., "Obesity and Health," booklet published by Congressional Quarterly, Inc., June 17, 1977.

Appendixes

APPENDIX 5: SAFETY APPENDIX

Akerblom, Siltanen, Kallio, "Does Dietary Fructose Affect the Control of Diabetes in Children?" *Acta Med. Scand.* Suppl. 542:197–202 (1972).

Akgun, Ertel, "A Comparison of Carbohydrate Metabolism after Sucrose, Sorbitol, and Fructose Meals in Normal and Diabetic Subjects," *Diabetes Care* 3:582 (1980).

Anderson, Story, Zettwoch, Sieling, "Long-Term Safety of Fructose Intake for Diabetic Men," *Diabetes* 33(1):5A (May 1984).

Astrup, Lundsgaard, Madsen, Christensen, "Enhanced Thermogenic Responsiveness During Chronic Ephedrine Treatment in Man," *Am. J. Clin. Nutr.* 42:83–94 (1985).

Bagchi, Brown, Urdanivia, Sundick, "Induction of Autoimmune Thyroiditis in Chickens by Dietary Iodine," *Science* 230:325–327 (1985).

Barbul, et al., "Arginine: A Thymotropic and Wound-Healing Promoting Agent," *Surgical Forum* 28:101–103 (1977).

Barbul, Rettura, Levenson, Seifter, "Thymotropic Actions of Arginine (ARG), Ornithine (ORN), and Growth Hormone (GH)," *Fed. Proc. Abstr.* 37(3): No. 282 (Federation of American Societies for Experimental Biology, 62nd annual meeting, Atlantic City, N.J.), April 9–14, 1978.

Bar-On, Stein, "Effect of Glucose and Fructose Administration on Lipid Metabolism in the Rat," *J. Nutr.* 94:95 (1968).

Bean, "Some Aspects of Pharmacological Use and Abuse of Water-Soluble Vitamins," in Hathcock, Coons, editors, *Nutrition and Drug Interactions,* New York: Academic Press, pp. 667–685 (1978).

Beard, "The Effects of Parenteral Injection of Synthetic Amino Acids upon the Appearance, Growth, and Disappearance of Emge Sarcoma in Rats," *Arch. Biochem.* 1:177–186 (1943).

Bergstrom, Hultman, Roch-Norland, "Lactic Acid Accumulation in Connection with Fructose Infusion," *Acta Med. Scand.* 184:359–64 (1968).

Bohannon, Karam, Forsham, "Advantages of Fructose Ingestion (FTT) over Sucrose (STT) and Glucose (GTT) in Humans," *Diabetes* 27 (Suppl. 2):438 (1978).

Bohannon, Karam, Forsham, "Endocrine Responses to Sugar Ingestion in Man," *J. Am. Diet. Assoc.* 76(6):555–560 (1980).

Brecher, E. M., *Licit and Illicit Drugs,* Boston: Little, Brown (1972).

Brown, Mitchell, Young, editors, *Chemical Diagnosis of Disease*, New York: Elsevier, p. 280 (1979).

Brunzell, "Use of Fructose, Xylitol, or Sorbitol as a Sweetener in Diabetes Mellitus," *Diabetes Care* 1:223 (1978).

Campbell, Bolli, Cryer, Gerich, "Pathogenesis of the Dawn Phenomenon in Patients with Insulin-Dependent Diabetes Mellitus," *New Engl. J. Med.* 312(23):1473–1479 (1985).

Charman et al., "Nicotinic Acid in the Treatment of Hypercholesterolemia," *J. Angiology*, Jan. 1973.

Chevalier, Wiley, Leveille, "The Age-Dependent Response of Serum Triglycerides to Dietary Fructose," *Proc. Soc. Exptl. Biol. Med.* 139:220 (1972).

Christy, "Assessment of Anterior Pituitary Function," in Beeson, McDermott, Wyngaarden, editors, *Cecil Textbook of Medicine*, 15th ed., Philadelphia: Saunders, pp. 2091–2094 (1979).

Coltart, Crossley, "Influence of Dietary Sucrose on Glucose and Fructose Tolerance and Triglyceride Synthesis in the Baboon," *Clin. Sci.* 38:427 (1970).

Coronary Drug Project, "Clofibrate and Niacin in Coronary Heart Disease," *J. Am. Med. Assoc.* 231:360–381 (1975).

Crapo, Kolterman, "The Metabolic Effects of 2-Week Fructose Feeding in Normal Subjects," *Am. J. Clin. Nutr.* 39:525–534 (1984).

Crapo, Kolterman, Olefsky, "Effects of Oral Fructose in Normal, Diabetic, and Impaired Glucose Tolerance Subjects," *Diabetes Care* 3:575 (1980).

Crapo, Reaven, Olefsky, "Plasma Glucose and Insulin Responses to Orally Administered Simple and Complex Carbohydrates," *Diabetes* 25:741 (1976).

Dobmeyer et al., *New Engl. J. Med.* 308(14):814–816 (1983).

Droge, Mannel, Falk, Lehmann, Schmidt, Hacker-Shahin, Janicke, "Suppression of Cytotoxic T Lymphocyte Activation by L-Ornithine," *J. Immunol.* 134(5):3379–3383 (1985).

Dulloo, Miller, "Thermogenic Drugs for the Treatment of Obesity: Sympathetic Stimulants in Animal Models," *Br. J. Nutr.* 52:179–196 (1984).

Fields, Renato, Ferrentti, Smith Jr., Reiser, "Effect of Copper Deficiency on Metabolism and Mortality in Rats Fed Sucrose or Starch Diets," *J. Nutr.* 113:1335–1345 (1983).

Fields, Smith Jr., Holbrook, Reiser, "Tissue Distribution of ^{67}Cu in Copper Deficient Rats Fed Fructose or Starch," *Fed. Proc.* 44:753 (1985).

Garb, Solomon, *Laboratory Tests in Common Use*, New York: Springer Publishing (1971).

Gilbert, "Caffeine as a Drug of Abuse," in Gibbins, Israel, Kalant, Popham,

Schmidt, Smart, editors, *Research Advances in Alcohol and Drug Problems,* Vol. 3, pp. 49–176, New York: John Wiley (1976).

Gotto, Bierman, Conner, Ford, Frantz, Glueck, Grundy, Little, "Recommendations for Treatment of Hyperlipidemia in Adults," American Heart Association Special Report No. 72-204-A (1984).

Gougerot-Pocidalo, Jacquet, Pocidalo, "Demonstration of the Depressive Effect of Normobaric Oxygen on the Mouse Lymphoid System," *C. R. Seances Acad. Sci.* Series 3, 294(18):925–7 (1982).

Greden, Fontaine, Lubetsky, Chamberlain, "Anxiety and Depression Associated with Caffeinism Among Psychiatric Inpatients," *Am. J. Psychiat.* 135:963–966 (1978).

Hathcock, "Quantitative Evaluation of Vitamin Safety," an accredited continuing medical education topic of the month from *Pharmacy Times,* pp. 104–113 (1985).

Hill, "Effect of Fructose on Rat Lipids," *Lipids* 5:621 (1970).

Holbrook, Fields, Smith Jr., Reiser, "Intraperitonial (IP) Injection of ^{67}Cu to Cu Deficient Rats Fed Fructose or Starch Diets: Tissue Distribution and Excretion," *Fed. Proc.* 44:754 (1985).

Holbrook, Smith Jr., Reiser, "Effects of Fructose or Starch Feeding on Mineral Balances in Humans Consuming a Low Copper Diet," *J. Am. Coll. Nutr.* 4:353 (1985).

Holvey, editor, "Pituitary—Anterior Lobe Disorders: Diagnosis," in *The Merck Manual of Diagnosis and Therapy,* Rahway, N.J.: Merck Sharp and Dohme, 12th ed., pp. 1138–1139 (1972).

Huttunen, Karro, Makinen, Scheinin, "Effects of Sucrose, Fructose, and Xylitol in Glucose, Lipid, and Urate Metabolism," *Acta Odontol. Scand.* Suppl. 70:239–45 (1975).

Job, Donnadieu, Garnier, Evain-Brion, Roger, Chaussain, "Ornithine Stimulation Test," *Pediat. Adolesc. Endocr.* 12:86–102 (Basel, Karger: 1983).

Johnson, Stuart, Bowman, "Bioavailability of Copper from Various Foods in the Presence of Different Carbohydrates," *Fed. Proc.* 44:756 (1985).

Kritchevsky, Tepper, "Influence of Dietary Carbohydrate on Lipid Metabolism in Rats," *Med. Exptl.* 19:329 (1969).

Levy, "Drugs Used in the Treatment of Hyperlipoproteinemias," in Gilman, Goodman, Gilman, *The Pharmacological Basis of Therapeutics,* pp. 834–847, New York: Macmillan (1980).

Levy, Montanez, Feaver, Murphy, Dunn, "Effect of Arginine on Tumor Growth in Rats," *Cancer Res.* 14:198–200 (1954).

Manso, Jover, Mayor, Velasco, Romero, "Effects of Galactose, Glucose and Fructose on Carbohydrate-Lipid Metabolism," *J. Med.* 10:479 (1979).

Maruhama, MacDonald, "Some Changes in the Triglyceride Metabolism of Rats on High Fructose or Glucose Diets," *Metabolism* 21:835 (1972).

Matsukura, Taminato, Kitano, Seino, Hamada, Uchihashi, Nakajima, Hirata, "The Effects of Environmental Tobacco Smoke on Urinary Cotinine Excretion in Nonsmokers," *New Engl. J. Med.* 311:828–832 (1984).

McCully, "Homocysteinemia and Arteriosclerosis," *Amer. Heart J.* 83:571–573 (1972).

Merimee, et al., "Arginine-Initiated Release of Human Growth Hormone," *New Engl. J. Med.* 183(26):1425–1429 (1969).

Miettinen et al., *Acta Med. Scand.* 186:247–253 (1969). (Study found a decrease in serum cholesterol of 25 percent and triglycerides of 30 percent in human subjects after two weeks on 3 grams of niacin per day.)

Miller, Drucker, Owens, Craig, Woodward, "Metabolism of Intravenous Fructose and Glucose in Normal and Diabetic Subjects," *J. Clin. Invest.* 31:115–25 (1952).

Miller, Hayes, "Vitamin Excess and Toxicity," in Hathcock, ed. *Nutritional Toxicology,* Vol. 1, New York: Academic Press, pp. 81–133 (1982).

Milner, Stepanovich, "Effect of Dietary Arginine on Ehrlich Ascites Tumor Cells," *Fed. Proc. Abstr.* 37(3): Abstract No. 773 (Federation of American Societies for Experimental Biology, 62nd annual meeting, Atlantic City, N.J.), April 9–14, 1978.

Milner, Stepanovich, "Inhibitory Effect of Dietary Arginine on Growth of Ehrlich Ascites Tumor Cells in Mice," *J. Nutr.* 109:489–491 (1979).

Mohler, Polc, Cumin, Pieri, Kettler, "Nicotinamide Is a Brain Constituent with Benzodiazepine-Like Actions," *Nature* 278:563–565 (1979).

Mosher, "Nicotinic Acid Side Effects and Toxicity: A Review," *Am. J. Psychiat.* 126(9):1290–1296.

Murad, Haynes, "Adenohypophyseal Hormones and Related Substances," in Gilman, Goodman, Gilman, *Goodman and Gilman's The Pharmacological Basis of Therapeutics,* 6th ed., pp. 1369–1396, New York: Macmillan (1980).

Nestel, Carroll, Havenstein, "Plasma Triglyceride Response to Carbohydrates, Fats and Caloric Intake," *Metab.* 19:1 (1970).

Newbold, "Niacin and the Schizophrenic Patient," *Am. J. Psychiat.* 127(4):535–536 (1970). Includes Mosher's reply to the article.

Nikkila, "Influence of Dietary Fructose and Sucrose on Serum Triglycerides in Hypertriglyceridemia and Diabetes," in Sipple and McNuff, editors, *Sugars in Nutrition,* New York: Academic Press (1974).

Nikkila, Kekki, "Effects of Dietary Fructose and Sucrose on Plasma Triglyceride Metabolism in Patients with Endogenous Hypertriglyceridemia," *Acta Med. Scand.* Suppl. 542:221 (1972).

Nikkila, Ojala, "Acute Effects of Fructose and Glucose on the Concentration and Removal Rate of Plasma Triglyceride," *Life Sci.* 5:89–94 (1966).

Nikkila, Ojala, "Induction of Hypertriglyceridemia by Fructose in the Rat," *Life Sci.* 4:937 (1965).

Pelkonen, Aro, Nikkila, "Metabolic Effects of Dietary Fructose in Insulin-Dependent Diabetes of Adults," *Acta Med. Scand.* Suppl. 542:187–193 (1972).

Pereyo-Torrellas, "P-Aminobenzoic-Acid-Related Compounds and Systemic Lupus," *Arch. Dermatol.* 114:1097 (1978).

Perheentupa, Raivio, "Fructose-Induced Hyperuricemia," *The Lancet* 2:528–531 (1967).

Pinckney, Pinckney, *The Encyclopedia of Medical Tests,* New York: Pocket Books (1978).

Press, Tamborlane, Sherwin, "Importance of Raised Growth Hormone Levels in Mediating the Metabolic Derangements of Diabetes," *New Engl. J. Med.* 310:810–815 (1984).

Prudden, Nishihara, Ocampo, "Studies on Growth Hormone. III: The Effect on Wound Tensile Strength of Marked Postoperative Anabolism Induced with Growth Hormone," *Surg. Obstet. Gynecol.* 107:481 (1958).

"Pyridoxin-Responsive Homocystinuria," *Nutr. Rev.* 39:16–18 (1981).

Raivio, Becker, Meyer, Greene, Nuki, Seegmiller, "Stimulation of Human Purine Synthesis De Novo by Fructose Infusion," *Metab.* 24:861–869 (1975).

Rall, "Central Nervous System Stimulants: The Xanthines," in Gilman, Goodman, Gilman, *Goodman and Gilman's The Pharmacological Basis of Therapeutics,* 6th ed., New York: Macmillan, pp. 592–607 (1980).

Reddy, Watanabe, Mori, "Effect of Conventional and Unconventional Dietary Fibers in Colon Carcinogenesis," in Furda, editor, *Unconventional Sources of Dietary Fiber,* Washington, D.C.: American Chemical Society (1983).

Reiser, Smith Jr., Scholfield, Powell, Yang, Mertz, "Indices of Copper Status and Lipogenesis in Humans Consuming a Typical American Diet Containing Either Fructose or Starch," *Fed. Proc.* 44:751 (1985).

Rettura, Barbul, Seifter, "Ornithine Inhibits Two Murine Tumors," *Fed. Proc. Abstr.* 37(3): Abstract No. 779 (Federation of American Societies for Experimental Biology, 62nd annual meeting, Atlantic City, N.J.), April 9–14, 1978.

Rettura, Levinson, Seifter, "Anti-Tumor and Anti-Stress Actions of L-Orni-thine," *Fed. Proc. Abstr.* (72nd Annual Meeting American Soc. Biol. Chem., St. Louis, May 31–June 4, 1981) 40(6): Abstract No. 840 (1981).

Schmidt, Lin, Gwynne, Jacobs, "Fasting Early Morning Rise in Peripheral Insulin: Evidence of the Dawn Phenomenon in Nondiabetes," *Diabetes Care* 7(1):32–35 (1984).

Seifter, Rettura, Barbul, Levenson, "Arginine: An Essential Amino Acid for Injured Rats," *Surgery,* pp. 224–230, August 1978.

Shekelle et al., "Dietary Vitamin A and Risk of Cancer in the Western Electric Study," *The Lancet,* pp. 1185–1190 (Nov. 28, 1981).

Simko, "Increase in Serum Lipids on Feeding Sucrose: The Role of Fructose and Glucose," *Am. J. Clin. Nutr.* 33:2217 (1980).

Smith Jr., Fields, Holbrook, Reiser, "Retention and Excretion of ^{67}Cu of Copper Deficient Rats Fed Fructose or Starch Diets," *Fed. Proc.* 44:752 (1985).

Sved, Fernstrom, Wurtman, "Tyrosine Administration Reduces Blood Pressure and Enhances Brain Norepinephrine Release in Spontaneously Hypertensive Rats," *Proc. Natl. Acad. Sci. USA* 76(7):3511–3514 (July 1979).

Takeda, Tominaga, Tei, Kitamura, Taga, Murase, Taguchi, Miwatani, "Inhibitory Effect of L-Arginine on Growth of Rat Mammary Tumors Induced by 7,12-Dimethylbenz(a)anthracene," *Cancer Res.* 35:2390–93 (1975).

Tanner, "Human Growth Hormone," *Nature,* 237:433–439 (1972).

Tews, Bradford, Harper, "Induction of Lysine Imbalance in Rats: Relationships Between Tissue Amino Acids and Diet," *J. Nutr.* 111:968–978 (1981).

Thenen, Mayer, "Effects of Fructose and Other Dietary Carbohydrates on Plasma Glucose, Insulin, and Lipids in Genetically Obese (Ob/Ob) Mice," *Proc. Soc. Exptl. Biol. Med.* 153:464 (1976).

Turner, Bierman, Brunzell, Chait, "Effect of Dietary Fructose on Triglyceride Transport and Glucoregulatory Hormones in Hypertriglyceridemic Men," *Am. J. Clin. Nutr.* 32:1043–1050 (1979).

Waterman, "Nutrient Toxicities in Animals and Man: Niacin," in Rechcígel, Jr., editor, *Handbook Series in Nutrition and Food, Section E: Nutritional Disorders,* Vol. 1, Cleveland: CRC Press, pp. 29–42 (1978).

Weisburger, Yamamoto, Glass, Frankel, "Prevention by Arginine Glutamate of the Carcinogenicity of Acetamide in Rats," *Toxicol. Appl. Pharmacol.* 14:163–175 (1969).

Wiseman, "Active Transport of Amino Acids by Sacs of Everted Small

Intestine of the Golden Hamster (Mesocricetus auratus)," *J. Physiol.* 133:626–630 (1956).

APPENDIX 6: SUPERMARKET SHOPPING GUIDE

"Extended Glycemic Index of Foods" and "Nutritive Values of Common Foods," both in *Nutritive Value of American Foods in Common Units,* Agriculture Handbook No. 456, Agricultural Research Service, United States Dept. of Agriculture (1975). (Does not include glycemic indices; see below.)

Glycemic indices chart adapted from: Brunzell, "Use of Fructose, Xylitol, or Sorbitol as a Sweetener in Diabetes Mellitus," *Diabetes Care* 1(4):223–230 (1978).

Jenkins, Wolever, Jenkins, Josse, Wong, "The Glycaemic Response to Carbohydrate Foods," *The Lancet,* pp. 388–391 (Aug. 18, 1984).

Jenkins, Wolever, Taylor, Barker, Fielden, Baldwin, Bowling, Newman, Jenkins, Goff, "Glycemic Index of Foods: a Physiological Basis for Carbohydrate Exchange," *Amer. J. Clin. Nutr.* 34:362–366 (1981).

"ARGININE AND LYSINE CONTENT OF FOODS"

Composition of Foods, Dairy and Egg Products, Agricultural Handbook No. 8-1, United States Dept. of Agriculture, Agricultural Research Service (1976).

Composition of Foods, Nut and Seed Products, Agricultural Handbook No. 8-12, United States Dept. of Agriculture, Human Nutrition Information Service (1984).

Composition of Foods, Poultry Products, Agricultural Handbook No. 8-5, United States Dept. of Agriculture, Science and Education Administration (1979).

APPENDIX 4

Suppliers' Appendix

We had intended to include a listing of several suppliers who offer the equipment and nutrients that we discuss in this book. Due to the very limited time allowed by this book's publication schedule to evaluate the products and prepare this list, we have decided to make this vendor information available by mail to those who send in the postpaid card printed on the endpaper of this book. We did not want to recommend equipment or suppliers that we had not had plenty of time to evaluate, and we thought that you would rather send in a postpaid card than get immediate but possibly half-baked recommendations. Send in the card if you would like to receive information from sources for skin-fold calipers, blood pressure meters, pulse rate meters, electronic scales, gym equipment, thermogenic clothing, all of the nutritional supplements described in this book, standardized ephedrine-containing herbs, urine- and blood-glucose-measuring supplies, and medically supervised behavior change weight loss clinics of proven effectiveness. You will receive information from several different companies; competition and comparison shopping are your best assurances of reasonable prices.

You will also receive information on a new health enhancement newsletter which we will publish if there is sufficient interest. With the exception of immunology and public health, modern medicine once focused primarily on treating disease rather than preventing it. Health maintenance organizations were controversial years ago, but now they have become respectable and popular. It is easier to prevent most diseases than to cure them. The next logical concept after health maintenance is health enhancement. Our health enhancement newsletter is all about staying well and performing at your best, in spite of possible adverse life-style factors that you choose not to change, or genes that predispose you to problems such as cardiovascular disease or cancer. This will not be the endless recital of no-no's that you find in so many health newsletters. It will be full of positive affirmative information that you can use to maintain and improve the function of both your mind and body.

If the postpaid card has been removed, write to:

SUPPLIER INFORMATION
P.O. BOX 92996
WORLDWAY POSTAL CENTER
5800 West Century Blvd.
Los Angeles, CA 90009

Warning: Many nutrient supplement sales outfits have claimed in their advertisements that they were selling formulas approved or developed by us (they were almost always deceiving you), or they implied that we were associated with them (generally more lies). In our opinion some of these deceptive products have been dangerous to more than the purchaser's bank account. We have had to spend a fortune (of our own funds, which could have otherwise been used for research purposes) on legal fees having lawyers prepare cease-and-desist orders to try to halt this fraud. For every one we shut down, two more seem to spring up. This will undoubtedly continue to happen, especially now with respect to fat loss products and with respect to fat loss clinics. Any collection of idiots and rip-off artists can claim to be using our techniques, so be careful!

If an outfit claims or implies that they are associated with us, please write us at the above address, including a copy of the advertising in question. We will tell you whether we are in fact associated with them (unlikely) and then will most likely send the stuff to our lawyers for another cease-and-desist order. Thank you for your help in cleaning up an unsavory mess.

We have come to the conclusion that exhortations, complaints, and cease-and-desist orders will not do an adequate job of controlling the bad guys. What will really do the most good is to provide alternative products and services of our own. We are currently seeking experienced reputable entrepreneurs and venture capitalists to start just such a series of businesses based on our knowledge. For example, we would very much like to help establish a chain of medically supervised *fat loss clinics which would use, market, and collect further research data on these techniques, and offer an unconditional satisfaction-or-your-money-back guarantee!*

APPENDIX 5

Safety

INTRODUCTION—READ THIS FIRST

Mark Twain once said, "Be careful about reading health books. You might die of a misprint." Heed his warning, and ours as well. Some of the items discussed here, such as caffeine and theophylline, are not really nutrients even though they are natural constituents of food, and others are over-the-counter (nonprescription) drugs such as phenylpropanolamine and ephedrine, or prescription drugs such as L-Dopa. Most of the items in this appendix are nutrients, and some of them are essential for life; nevertheless, even these essential nutrients can be misused.

Do not assume that even natural nutrients are always safe for everyone in any dose under all circumstances. They are not. Nothing is perfectly safe! Too much of anything, even water or oxygen, is toxic.

Other health books may *seem* less complicated because they do not include any information on the possible complications and risks of the techniques and nutritional supplements that they advocate. We feel that where safety is concerned, ignorance is not bliss.

This Safety Appendix may seem long and detailed. That is because we have included all of the problems that we know of that may be encountered in the use of the nutrients and nonprescription drugs, even when the frequency of occurrence is very small. Many of these safety precautions apply only to people who have certain diseases or specific genetic defects, and only 1 person in 100,000 might have to be concerned with some of them. We have even included some warnings or cautions that are purely hypothetical; we have never heard or read of these problems happening, but we think that they *might* be possible under certain unusual circumstances. This attention to unlikely or rare conditions and circumstances does take up quite a bit of space. Since this book may be read by millions of people, it would be irresponsible for us to do less. Other precautions apply to everyone. If you read our caution about caffeine, you will probably be a bit surprised at some of its rare adverse effects. Information of this type is included, not to alarm you, but to serve as an essential guide to safe and effective use.

This appendix is meant to be used as a reference. Read the parts that deal with things that you want to take. If you do not intend to use ephedrine, for example, you don't have to bother reading those safety precautions.

Before you take anything, whether nutrient, natural food constituent, over-the-counter drug, or prescription drug, read the relevant precautions and warnings, as well as any on the product package. Before taking prescription drugs, you should also read the package insert or look the drug up in the Physicians' Desk Reference. You can find this invaluable reference in any public library, a doctor's or pharmacist's office, and most large book stores. We have *not* duplicated all the warnings and precautions for prescription drugs.

You should take safety seriously. It is generally possible to use the substances discussed in this book safely if you are an adult, are healthy (but not pregnant or lactating), are prudent, follow directions, and carefully read and heed all relevant precautions and warnings *before* starting.

Remember that many of these procedures for fat loss, altering appetite and carbohydrate and fat metabolism, rapidly building muscles, and improving cardiovascular fitness are experimental. Some of them have not been used by large numbers of medically monitored people for long periods of time. None of the nutrients have been approved by the FDA as fat loss aids. Since our first book was published four years ago, hundreds of thousands of people have been using nutrient supplements such as arginine, choline, ornithine, phenylalanine, tyrosine, tryptophan, vitamin B-1–vitamin C–cysteine combinations, and properly designed free-radical-scavenging nutrient supplements without reported serious adverse effects. However, you should remember that only a small percentage of these health food store patrons were medically tested and supervised, and that neither we nor anyone else knows of all possible adverse effects.

Our program and the substances that we discuss in this book must NOT be used by pregnant or lactating women, children, adolescents, people who are seriously ill, people who refuse to have an annual physical exam, and fools who ignore their physician's advice, or who think that if 1 gram of something is good, 2 grams is sure to be better.

Medical supervision is always desirable, and it is necessary if your desired fat loss is over 10 percent of your body weight.

A physician's advice is absolutely necessary if you are ill or hyperobese, particularly if you have cardiovascular, kidney, or liver disease, cancer, a psychosis, or diabetes or thyroid problems. Certain diseases, such as the latter two, can contribute to excessive weight gain.

Don't gamble with your health. Have your doctor give you a complete physical exam before you start, even if you are in apparent good health. Unfortunately, about half *of the people who have hypertension (high blood pressure), diabetes, or hypothyroidism are* not *aware that they are ill, so play safe and get a thorough checkup.* See Chapter 4, "How You Can Use Our Program," for the clinical laboratory tests that we think should be part of your checkup. Of course, your physician may order other tests as well.

Unless otherwise specified, the doses given are the maximum total amounts that one can normally take per day.

APPETITE-SPOILING FORMULA

You can use the following snack formula about 1 to 2 hours before lunch or dinner to decrease your subsequent appetite. This subsequent appetite decrease may more than make up for the snack calories in many people. This formula does not provoke a large insulin release and the subsequent reactive-hypoglycemia-induced carbohydrate craving and overeating that would be caused by most common sweet snacks. This formula may also be used as a small snack between meals. Since fructose is more slowly absorbed than sucrose, and since the fiber further slows its absorption, you may want to take this snack about an hour before you usually become hungry. Because of the tryptophan and carbohydrates in the formula, you may feel a little sleepy after eating it, as you may after eating a large lunch. This sedative effect is medically harmless, but be cautious when driving or when engaged in potentially dangerous tasks. Tryptophan does not cause the increase in reaction time and the loss of coordination that are common with other sedatives and tranquilizers. You may experience a niacin flush, if you are not accustomed to it (see the information on niacin below). These effects are harmless.

The hydrolyzed protein in this formula will interfere with amino acid GH releasers, and the fiber could excessively slow their absorption. See the "Carbohydrate-Craving Control Formula" later in this appendix for an appetite control formula that you can take around the time that you take GH releasers.

DOSE: Suggested contents per dose:

hydrolyzed protein	10 to 30 grams
tryptophan	250 to 500 milligrams
fruit juice extract	to taste
fructose	10 to 35 grams
fiber	10 to 30 grams

GTF chromium	25 to 50 micrograms
or	
trivalent chromium	25 to 50 micrograms
niacin	50 to 200 milligrams
vitamin C	250 milligrams to 1 gram
vitamin B-6	20 to 50 milligrams
optionally, caffeine	0 to 200 milligrams
optionally, MCT	0 to 20 grams
(medium-chain triglycerides, with antioxidants)	

The constituents of this and similar formulas are FDA-recognized only as nutrients, and neither these nutrients nor this formula have been approved as appetite-modifying aids.

ARGININE AND ORNITHINE

Arginine and ornithine are nutrient amino acids. Arginine is found in especially large quantities in foods such as dairy products and chicken and turkey meat. (That old wives' tale about the benefits of chicken soup has some truth in it, after all! Arginine can stimulate the immune system.) Arginine is a building block for proteins.

Our approach to GH releaser use is to try to replicate the levels of GH and the patterns of pulsatile release found in healthy athletic persons in their late teens to early twenties. Do not attempt to attain higher GH peaks, or to maintain the peak levels continuously.

A review on human growth hormone itself has said: "There are no known side effects, even from large doses. Very high doses in certain other species have a diabetogenic effect, but this does not occur in man or the rat." (Tanner, 1972) (Dr. Tanner's comments refer to healthy humans, not to those with diabetes mellitus—sugar/insulin diabetes—or the pituitary disease acromegaly.)

Warning: GH RELEASERS MUST NOT BE USED BY PERSONS WITH DIABETES MELLITUS OR BORDERLINE DIABETICS! You should have your physician test you for diabetes mellitus with a glucose tolerance test before using GH releasers. If you have diabetes mellitus or borderline diabetes, the released GH will make your illness worse. We strongly advise against the use of GH releasers by cancer patients or persons with pituitary disease, unless prescribed by their physician. Persons with ocular or brain herpes infections must not use supplemental arginine or ornithine.

Diabetes mellitus has a strong hereditary component; if any of your relatives have diabetes mellitus, your chances of having it or developing it are greatly increased. The most common symptoms include frequent urination, thirst, abnormally high fluid consumption, itching, dry skin, hunger, weakness, slow wound healing, and loss of weight. Unfortunately, you may be diabetic and not have any of these symptoms. About half of the people who have diabetes mellitus do not know it, and some do not have any of the above symptoms; hence a glucose tolerance test performed by your physician is necessary.

GH releasers do not cause cancer and have reduced the incidence of cancer in experimental animals. (Barbul, 1977; Barbul, 1978; Beard, 1943; Levy, 1954; Milner, 1978; Milner, 1979; Rettura, 1978; Rettura, 1981; Takeda, 1975; Weisburger, 1969) However, if you do have cancer, it would be most prudent not to take them, since the increased GH levels might arguably promote preexisting cancer growth more than they improved the function of your immune system. The decision to use GH releasers as an adjunct to immunotherapy under these circumstances must be left to your immunologist and personal physician.

Caution: We have had five anecdotal reports of arginine or ornithine reactivating latent herpes viruses. In three cases, the subjects repeated the experiment, with the same results. In all cases, the symptoms disappeared within a week after discontinuing the arginine or ornithine. This does not appear to be a common phenomenon. We know of many people who have latent herpes viruses who have had no reactivation problems; nevertheless, if you have ocular or brain herpes, you should *not* use these two nutrient amino acid supplements.

Caution: Excessive growth hormone levels can cause the skin to grow faster than it wears away, leading to thickening and roughening. This effect is reversible; if the GH levels are reduced to the normal teenage range, the excess skin will wear away in a month or two. It may not even be possible to obtain sufficiently high GH levels to cause this with any of the nutrient GH releasers that we have described. We have received no reports of it from gung-ho athletes and bodybuilders, some of whom greatly exceeded our recommended doses, even though we specifically asked them to watch for this possible side effect.

Warning: Extremely high levels of GH over an extended period of time may produce joint or larynx growth. These effects are irreversible. These effects occur at extremely high sustained GH levels in the disease acromegaly (characteristic of pituitary-disease giants). The amounts of GH involved in the latter disease are far above the amounts involved in our use of GH releasers. In our seven years of GH releaser experience, we have not observed any of these effects in any of our experimental subjects, at any dose, even at amounts up to seven times higher than our recommended maximums. We ourselves have used growth hormone releasers daily for the past seven years at doses that were usually twice our recommended maximums and have not experienced this problem. Even Durk's twenty-two-year-old MIT class ring still fits exactly the same as when he got it in 1964. We have never seen any evidence that these nutrient GH releasers can produce the extremely high sustained GH levels that are found in acromegaly; however, very frequent huge overdoses of injected human GH may do this, and there are experimental drugs that might be capable of doing this, too.

Caution: Taking arginine or ornithine in the doses required for growth hormone release may cause an increase in libido or irritability, particularly in males.

Arginine and ornithine may cause irritability in a few males, which may usually be relieved by tryptophan supplements of 250 milligrams (or 1/4 gram; 1000 milligrams = 1 gram) taken as required, preferably on an empty stomach, or 500 milligrams to 2 grams of tryptophan at bedtime. Do not take more than 2 grams per day of tryptophan supplements. A dose of 250 milligrams of tryptophan will rarely cause drowsiness during the day, but a 500-milligram dose may do so in some people. Vitamins B-6 (30 milligrams) and C (250 milligrams) are necessary cofactors for this use of tryptophan.

Caution: Arginine and ornithine may also cause a temporary nausea, weakness, and hypoglycemia-like symptoms, as can other GH releasers and GH itself. Arnold Schwarzenegger used to have a barf bucket next to his workout station when he was younger. He said that if he didn't work out hard enough to throw up, he wasn't working hard enough to really build his muscles. The nausea was apparently caused by the heavy-exercise-induced GH release in the young Arnold. When he grew older, this stopped happening, presumably because of his age-related reduction in GH release during exercise. Nausea is most likely in conjunction with a GH-releaser-supplemented long hard workout, or around dawn if the GH releasers are taken at bedtime. This is most likely to be a problem with gung-ho bodybuilders and athletes who eschew moderation. Most people do not experience GH-releaser-related nausea. *Nausea and weakness rarely occur if you increase your GH releaser dose slowly over a week or two, starting at about one quarter of our recommended doses.* If any unusual symptoms develop, discontinue use and see your physician.

Caution: We have had six anecdotal reports of arthritis being worsened by arginine or ornithine. In four cases, the experiment was repeated with the same results. In all six cases, the arthritis went back to its prior condition within a week after discontinuing the supplements. In two cases, a dosage reduction to one quarter of our suggested maximum was sufficient to eliminate the symptoms. This does not seem to be a common phenomenon.

Caution: We also had a report of ornithine reversibly worsening an existing psychosis, and one that arginine hydrochloride might cause diarrhea.

Caution: Arginine and ornithine compete with the essential amino acid lysine to cross your blood-brain barrier and enter your brain. You could conceivably induce a brain lysine deficiency if you frequently took large quantities of arginine or ornithine at the same time as your meals. (Tews, 1981) Therefore, don't regularly take these GH releaser supplements within 2 to 3 hours of a meal. You wouldn't want to do so anyway, because the amino acids from the protein in the meal would interfere with the blood-brain barrier transport of the GH releaser amino acids, and the insulin released by the meal would tend to block the effects of the GH. Do not take a protein or multi–amino acid supplement within 2 to 3 hours of GH releaser use, because of competition.

DOSE: We recommend that you begin by taking 2 grams of arginine or 1 gram of ornithine on an empty stomach at the times specified in Chapter 6, "Growth Hormone Releaser Dosage Schedules." You may slowly increase the total daily arginine supplement dosage to 6 to 12 grams (or ornithine to 3 to 6 grams) depending on your weight, over a period of 2 weeks. You may use up to twice as much if directed to do so by your physician. (These doses are for a weight range of 50 to 100 kilograms, or 110 to 220 pounds. Persons with higher body weights should not use more unless directed to do so by their physician.) A gram of ornithine will release about as much GH as 2 grams of arginine.

DOSE SCHEDULE: Use arginine or ornithine *only* at the times and under the conditions specified in the schedules in Chapter 6.

COFACTOR DOSE: *We strongly suggest that you also take 3 grams of choline and 1 gram of vitamin B-5 daily when you are using arginine or ornithine as GH releasers.* These nutrients will increase brain acetylcholine levels; brain acetylcholine is involved in GH release from arginine, ornithine, and sleep. See "Choline" in this appendix.

The amounts of arginine that we suggest taking on an empty stomach for GH release are about the same as could be obtained from selected foods. If you ate a high-protein diet with turkey and chicken as your major protein source, you could get as much as 8 to 10 grams of arginine per day. (Of course, this arginine contained in food would be much less effective as a GH releaser because of blood-brain barrier transport competition from other amino acids, due to the dose being divided and spread out over the entire day, and due to the insulin released by the meals.) The arginine dose used for GH release in most of the human experiments was 30 grams by intravenous injection. That dose was chosen to be more than enough to saturate the GH release mechanism for pituitary function diagnostic tests. In most people, the smaller doses that we suggest should still give a substantial GH release. Do NOT take 30 grams per day of arginine.

Caution: Don't try to have the highest GH levels in your athletic club; please do not take more GH releasers than our suggested doses. You want late-teens-to-early-twenties GH levels and release patterns, but no more. If your blood sugar regulation is normal as measured by a glucose tolerance test, and if you follow our instructions, you will have no more problems with hyperglycemia than a healthy teenager.

Arginine and ornithine are available in capsules and as powders. The capsules have two problems: they are more expensive, and the handful of capsules that you will have to take can give you a stomachache. The stomachache is caused by the mechanical effects of a lot of hard capsules. People are not birds, so we do not have gizzards to grind up hard lumps. The capsules will dissolve in about 20 to 30 minutes, but they can be distinctly uncomfortable until then.

All references to arginine and ornithine in this book are to L-arginine and L-ornithine, the natural isomers, and their acid addition salts. The synthetic D and DL forms are not widely available to laypersons and have not been evaluated for our purposes.

Arginine and ornithine are available in two chemical forms, as the amino acid free bases (these two amino acids are more basic than acidic), and as acid addition salts. "Arginine" and "ornithine" alone on a bottle refer to the free bases. Examples of the acid addition salts are the hydrochloric acid (HCl) addition salts arginine HCl and ornithine HCl. If you wish to take the less expensive powders, forget about the unneutralized free bases; they taste ghastly. In fact, arginine free base smells rather like dog vomit. The hydro-chloric acid addition salts don't smell or taste as bad, but your body can metabolize the basic arginine and ornithine to neutral metabolites, leaving your body with an excess of hydrochloric acid that might cause diarrhea and acid indigestion, or even acidosis in some sensitive individuals.

We are currently working on a multicomponent powder formulation to make the free bases much more palatable. This will have three advantages over free-base tablets or capsules: (1) lower cost; (2) faster absorption; (3) no mechanical stomach irritation from a dozen or more large tablets or hard gelatin capsules. In addition, it will not have a potential problem with excess acid.

We think that the use of arginine as a GH releaser may be biochemically more conservative than the use of ornithine because arginine is common in the normal human diet. Normal diets contain a negligible trace amount of ornithine. You make the ornithine that you need from arginine in your body, the normal human serum levels of ornithine being about half those of arginine.

The use of arginine (and, less frequently, ornithine) as GH-releasing agents to test pituitary function in humans is well accepted, and arginine has been proposed as a wound-healing accelerator in human surgery. (Holvey, 1972; Barbul, 1977; Barbul, 1978; Christy, 1979; Job, 1983; Merimee, 1969; Murad, 1980; Prudden, 1958; Seifter, 1978)

Arginine and ornithine are recognized by the FDA only as nutrients and have not been approved by the FDA as growth-hormone-releasing agents or as fat loss aids.

Important note to persons with impaired glucose tolerance: Caution: Hyperglycemia (excessive blood sugar) induced by high levels of released GH may be a problem for people with preexisting impaired glucose tolerance. Glucose tolerance is a measure of how effectively and rapidly you can metabolize a sudden big dose of glucose and keep your peak blood sugar level under control. Your personal physician should perform a glucose tolerance test on you before you use GH releasers. If the results of your test show that you are diabetic or a borderline diabetic, you must NOT use GH releasers. If your glucose tolerance is mildly impaired, but you are definitely not diabetic, you may be able to use GH releasers with caution, if you make sure that you do not become hyperglycemic. Hyperglycemia is harmful and must be avoided.

Arginine, ornithine, or any other substance that increases growth hormone release may contribute to the "dawn effect." In diabetics (Campbell, 1985) there is a decrease in glucose tolerance with resulting hyperglycemia that occurs around dawn. This is believed to be caused by the normal predawn increase in circulating growth hormone, which blocks some of the sugar-utilizing effects of insulin. GH-induced hyperglycemia does not occur in normal humans because of a compensatory release of insulin. (Schmidt, 1984; Press, 1984) Dawn-effect hyperglycemia might occur in some individuals with impaired glucose tolerance if they use a bedtime GH releaser. If this occurs, you may feel symptoms similar to hypoglycemia, such as weakness and nausea, because the high levels of GH are blocking the movement of blood sugar into your cells by insulin.

Many cases of impaired glucose tolerance can be improved by taking a nutrient supplement of 200 micrograms per day of trivalent chromium or of GTF chromium (also called glucose-tolerance-factor chromium). Some people, especially the elderly and those plagued by symptoms resembling hypoglycemia or by hyperglycemia, are apparently unable to convert dietary chromium into GTF chromium. In these cases, they should take the GTF chromium rather than an ordinary chromium supplement. Many people in the United States are thought to be chromium-deficient. See Chapter 8, "Sweets: How to Have a Sweet Tooth Without Putting On Fat," for further information on chromium and blood sugar control.

There are three rules to help prevent hyperglycemia when using GH releasers:

1. *Take 200 micrograms per day of GTF chromium if you are not allergic to yeast, or 200 micrograms per day of trivalent chromium if you are.*

2. *Caution: Do not eat a high-glycemic-index meal or snack within 3 hours before or 2 hours after taking GH releasers. This will also make your GH releasers much more effective, too.* If you have a mildly impaired glucose tolerance and use GH releasers, you may get enough GH released for you to become hyperglycemic if you eat a high-glycemic-index food at the same time. A large enough GH release can block insulin so much that your blood sugar might rise above normal despite the additional insulin that the elevated blood sugar releases. You wouldn't want to eat like this anyway, because the insulin release from a high-glycemic-index meal or snack would tend to block the effects of the GH, too.

3. *Substitute low-glycemic-index carbohydrates for high-glycemic-index carbohydrates in your diet. This, too, will substantially increase the effectiveness of your GH releasers.*

Caution: If you are definitely not diabetic or a borderline diabetic but have mildly impaired glucose tolerance, you must make sure *that you do not become hyperglycemic if you take GH releasers.* You can easily measure your blood sugar at 20-minute intervals for 4 hours after taking a GH releaser dose by using an inexpensive test strip available without a prescription from any large drugstore (or see the Suppliers' Appendix). Only one drop of blood from a pinprick is required. Further information is given in "Clinical Laboratory Tests" in this appendix. Of course, if there has been no hyperglycemia after a few experiments, it is not necessary to test yourself every time. You should retest yourself if you increase your dose, however. Do not attempt to use these home tests to diagnose whether or not you are a diabetic or borderline diabetic; that must be done by your physician.

Caution: If you are taking large amounts of vitamins C or B-1, or the amino acid cysteine, or some other free-radical-scavenging nutrients, these test strips can give alarmingly false values due to interference with the test's chemistry by the nutrients. See "Clinical Laboratory Tests" in this appendix for alternate blood and urine sugar tests that are not subject to this interference.

A technical note on ornithine for physicians, scientists, and other health professionals: At extremely high concentrations, ornithine (specifically the natural isomer L-ornithine) has been shown to inhibit the early phase of induction of cytotoxic T-cell lymphocyte responses. (Droge, 1985) This effect is specific to L-ornithine; this effect was not produced by the chemical analogs D-ornithine, L-lysine, or putrescine, or the possible L-ornithine precursors L-histidine, and L-alanine. According to the authors of this paper, there was no evidence of general toxicity to the responding white cell population in any of their experiments, at any ornithine concentration tested (up to 0.1 M). A variety of immune system functions were measured, and only this one particular aspect was inhibited. The very selective immunosuppressive effect was temporary and dependent on unphysiologically extremely high ornithine concentrations being present at the same time and place as the attempt at immunization.

The experiments were performed in mice, and with mouse lymphocytes in tissue culture. This effect was observed in vitro in mouse lymphocyte tissue cultures only at ornithine concentrations that are higher than could be attained if our maximum suggested oral dose were instantly and completely absorbed throughout the body without any homeostatic regulation of ornithine levels. This homeostatic regulation normally controls serum L-ornithine at levels that are about 20 times lower than required to produce this effect. The extremely high L-ornithine levels that are necessary for this effect were experimentally attained in vivo by L-ornithine injection into the foot pads of the mice performed at the same time and at the same site as the attempt at immunization against foreign tissue.

For example, scaling the mouse experimental dose given in the authors' Figure 1 to a human dose, about 100 grams of ornithine would have to be injected at the same time and in the same place as the immunizing antigen to produce a temporary localized 50 to 70 percent reduction in the activation of the cytotoxic T-lymphocytes. Moreover, the peak local concentration of L-ornithine when given by foot pad injection would be far higher than when administered orally, since L-ornithine (and L-arginine) are slowly absorbed from the gut (10 to 20 times slower than glycine or L-alanine). (Wiseman, 1956) Intravenous L-ornithine injections of 30 grams have been used in humans as a test to assess the release of pituitary GH; these levels might be high enough to produce some effect, but it should be kept in mind that dilution of the intravenously injected L-ornithine solution will occur much more rapidly than if the solution were injected into a mouse's foot pads.

In our opinion, the experiments that caused selective partial immunosuppression used doses and conditions that are remote from the L-ornithine dose and use conditions that we have suggested. These data do underline the fact that anything can be hazardous in excessive quantities, especially when taken by injection. As the famous sixteenth-century physician Paracelsus said, "Only the dose determines that a thing is not poison." Indeed, four days of pure oxygen at one atmosphere (five times its normal level) is far more immunosuppressive in mice, completely destroying the thymus, source of the T-cells, not just causing very selective temporary localized inhibition of one aspect of the immune response. (Gougerot-Pocidalo, 1982)

Some of the data in the Droge paper actually suggests that, at our suggested dose, T-cell immunostimulation rather than suppression may occur. Several other papers have clearly and unambiguously shown that T-cell immunostimulation and increased resistance to transplanted cancer cells and increased resistance to cancer induced in animals by common human carcinogens can be caused by doses of arginine or ornithine similar to those that we have suggested. (Barbul, 1977; Barbul, 1978; Beard, 1943; Levy, 1954; Milner, 1978; Milner, 1979; Rettura, 1978; Rettura, 1981; Takeda, 1975; Weisburger, 1969) We would like to see more research into the use of these two amino acids as adjuncts in the immunotherapy of human cancer.

B-1

See "Vitamin B-1–Vitamin C–Cysteine Formula" near the end of this appendix.

BETA-CAROTENE

The material that makes carrots orange, beta-carotene, is quite effective when taken orally for reducing your chances of sunburn, premature skin aging, skin cancer, and smoking-induced lung cancer. We suggest 20,000 to 30,000 I.U. per day, taken with the fattiest meal of the day to facilitate absorption of this water-insoluble, fat-soluble nutrient, and to minimize your chances of gastric upset. Do not be alarmed when your feces turn orange; it is the beta-carotene, not blood. Blood colors the feces black, not orange. At these doses, the skin on the soles of your feet and on the palms of your hands (especially calluses) may be tinted slightly orange. If you regularly take very large doses (much larger than we have recommended), your skin can gradually become as orange as a carrot. This happens slowly; you will not wake up and suddenly discover that you have turned orange overnight. The *Merck Manual of Diagnosis and Therapy* says that while this may alarm the patient, it is harmless. If you take very large quantities for an extended period of time, it will take as much as several weeks to get back to your normal skin color after you discontinue use.

CAFFEINE

Caffeine is one of the world's most popular and reasonably safe stimulants. It can increase the amount of work many people can do and stimulate a more rapid and clearer flow of thought. For example, in the proper dose, it can help most typists work faster and with fewer errors. If too much caffeine is used or if it is taken too rapidly, though, performance may be worsened. Caffeine's most famous and common side effects are "the jitters," excessive stimulation (a "wired" feeling), irritability, insomnia, restlessness, and anxiety. Sensitivity to the effects of caffeine varies widely, and tolerance to the brain stimulation effects develops fairly rapidly with regular use.

Note that coffee contains many substances other than just caffeine. It also contains oils that are sensitive to oxidation by exposure to the air. These oils can become rancid, especially when coffee is held in a pot all day. Rancid oils are known to increase cancer risks. Therefore, be sure to drink only fresh coffee (including freshly prepared instant coffee), if you choose to use it.

Caution: Tolerance and a limited degree of psychological dependence may develop with caffeine, and a severe withdrawal headache may occur. (Greden, 1978) *Caffeine can even become a drug of abuse in some individuals.* (Gilbert, 1976) *Caffeine increases the secretion of stomach acid, which can be blocked with the anti-ulcer drug cimetidine. Caffeine should not be used by heart patients, ulcer patients, the ulcer-prone, or those with active gastritis unless directed by their physician. It should not be used by persons with hypersensitivity or idiosyncrasy to caffeine and other methylxanthines (coffee, tea, theophylline, colas, cocoas, chocolates, etc.). Caffeine worsens the symptoms of panic or anxiety disorders, so if you suffer from these, it is probably best to avoid coffee, colas, tea, and possibly cocoa and chocolate, which all contain caffeine or closely related natural methylxanthine stimulants. Caffeine overdose may cause insomnia, anorexia, nausea, vomiting, irritability, headache, diarrhea, tachycardia (abnormally fast heartbeat), and cardiac arrhythmias.* (Rall, 1980) *A dose of 200 milligrams of caffeine (about 2 cups of coffee) has been reported to cause cardiac arrhythmias in 3 out of 7 normals and in 6 out of 12 heart patients! It also caused tachycardia in 3 of 12 heart patients.* (Dobmeyer, 1983)

CAPSULES VERSUS TABLETS VERSUS POWDERS

There can be substantial differences between the results obtained with the same active ingredients if they are administered in different dosage forms. Dr. Harry Demopoulos, a scientist and pathologist at New York University, performed a three-year study of people taking megadoses of various self-selected nutrient supplements. He found that about 85 percent of the reported adverse effects were due to allergies or other adverse reactions to the binders, fillers, and excipients in the tablets. In 85 percent of the cases, these symptoms vanished when tablets were replaced with hard gelatin capsules containing the pure nutrient supplement powders. That is one of the reasons why we strongly suggest that you avoid tablets and take gelatin capsules or the pure powders instead. Another reason is dissolution time variation; cheap tablets may take hours to dissolve, whereas gelatin capsules reliably dissolve in about 20 minutes, and soluble powders dissolve almost immediately. Dissolution can be a major problem with vitamin C and niacin tablets; an acidic tablet (such as ascorbic acid or nicotinic acid) that gets into your intestines before it dissolves will irritate them (it is supposed to be alkaline there, not acid) and can cause diarrhea.

Capsules cost more than tablets, but we think that they are worth every extra penny. A survey has shown that the majority of health professionals responding preferred capsules to tablets.

Mechanical irritation to your stomach can be a big problem if you take a handful of tablets. People are not turkeys; we do not have a gizzard to grind up hard lumps. Capsules can cause mechanical irritation, too, but they soften faster, so the discomfort is over sooner. Soft gelatin capsules cause even less mechanical trouble, but you have to be sure that the filler oil necessary for soft gelatin encapsulation of powders has been chosen to have a high stability (no safflower, corn, or other polyunsaturated oils!) and is protected from potentially hazardous rancidity by free-radical-scavenging antioxidants. Powders do not have these problems; their big problem is taste. Arginine, for example, tastes awful. We are working on an arginine powder formulation that is palatable enough to be mixed with fruit juice and swallowed without gagging. This is quite a challenge!

CARBOHYDRATE-CRAVING CONTROL FORMULA

This formula is specifically designed to help you control and satisfy your carbohydrate craving. It does not provoke the subsequent reactive hypoglycemia-induced carbohydrate craving that would be caused by most common sweet snacks. It does not include fiber, nor does it alter your appetite for fats or protein. This formula may be used as a small snack between meals. Since fructose is more slowly absorbed than sucrose, you may want to take this about 30 minutes to 1 hour before you usually crave carbohydrates. Because of the tryptophan and carbohydrates in the formula, you may feel a little sleepy after eating it, as you may after eating a large lunch. This sedative effect is medically harmless, but be cautious when driving or when engaged in potentially dangerous tasks. Tryptophan does not cause the increase in reaction time and the loss of coordination that is common with other sedatives and tranquilizers. The niacin may cause flushing, if you are not accustomed to it. (See niacin, below.) These effects are harmless. *This formula will not interfere with GH releaser use.*

DOSE: Suggested contents per dose:

GTF chromium	25 to 50 micrograms
or	
trivalent chromium chloride	25 to 50 micrograms
niacin	30 to 200 milligrams
tryptophan	250 to 500 milligrams
vitamin B-6	20 to 50 milligrams
vitamin C	200 to 500 milligrams
fructose	15 to 30 grams

The ingredients in this and similar formulas are FDA-recognized only as nutrients, and neither the nutrients nor the formula have been approved as aids for appetite modification or fat loss.

CCK OR CHOLECYSTOKININ

CCK (cholecystokinin) functions as a satiety signal: it makes you feel full and satisfied when you eat. We have previously mentioned that certain nutrients, such as L-phenylalanine and tryptophan, cause the release of CCK, and that behavioral techniques should be helpful in stimulating CCK release, too. What about taking CCK itself?

Some purveyors of nutrient supplements are now selling products labeled as CCK. Beware of such products. In our opinion, they are very unlikely to be CCK, and even if they are, an oral CCK product won't be effective. See our comments on CCK in Chapter 10.

CHOLINE

Choline is a nutrient.

DOSE: 3 grams of choline a day is a reasonable dose for most healthy adults. That is the dose MIT students took when they developed better memories and abilities to learn lists of words. Begin at 1 gram of choline and about 1/4 gram of vitamin B-5 a day, taken in the morning, or with your GH releasers. Over a period of several days, increase the dose to 3 grams of choline and 1 gram of vitamin B-5 a day.

Caution: Because choline can increase muscle tone, overdose can cause a muscle tension headache or stiff, tight muscles, especially in the neck and shoulders. If too much choline and too much B-5 are taken too fast, intestinal cramps (from the excess acetylcholine formed from the choline with the help of the B-5) can result. Choline plus vitamin B-5 will reduce your gut transit time, and a few people may experience diarrhea if they take too much too quickly. If any of these problems occur, skip taking your choline and B-5 for 1 or 2 days, then reduce your dose of choline and B-5 by half and then, if you wish, gradually increase it back up to 3 grams a day, since tolerance to this *excessive* muscle tone side effect usually develops rapidly.

We strongly suggest that you use the *choline chloride* (also called *choline hydrochloride* or *choline HCl)* or *choline hydrogen citrate* forms of choline (usually sold as liquids) because the choline bitartrate that is usually used in tablets and capsules will usually cause persistent diarrhea problems when taken in these doses. Remember how your mother used cream of tartar as a laxative? Cream of tartar is potassium bitartrate, and choline bitartrate will cause the same diarrhea. It is the bitartrate ion that is causing this diarrhea, not the choline itself. *Do not take choline bitartrate.*

COFACTOR DOSE: *It is important to take vitamin B-5 (pantothenic acid, calcium pantothenate, or pantothenyl alcohol) with the choline, because B-5 is required for its conversion to acetylcholine. We suggest 1 gram per day of vitamin B-5, taken with the 3 grams of choline.*

WARNING: Do not buy choline in its free-base form (simply called "choline" in a chemical catalog); it is far too caustic and will severely burn your mouth and throat. The "choline" sold as a nutrient supplement, and the "choline" that we refer to in this book, is really an acid-addition salt of choline.

Caution: Choline should not be used by manic-depressive psychotics in the depressive phase. Such use could exacerbate this particular type of depression. Choline does not cause or worsen depression in normal persons.

A few rare individuals may develop a fishy smell while taking choline, because of its conversion to trimethylamine in their gut by bacteria. This is not dangerous. If this occurs, either you can discontinue its use, or you may be able to eliminate the problem by altering your bacterial gut population by taking fiber supplements. None of our experimental subjects has suffered from this problem, and we have spoken to only one person who had this experience.

Choline is recognized by the FDA only as a nutrient and has not been approved as an agent for improving muscle tone, speeding gut peristalsis, as an adjunct to the use of arginine or ornithine GH releasers, for appetite modification, or for improving memory or verbal ability.

CHROMIUM AND GTF CHROMIUM

Chromium is an essential nutrient. Trivalent chromium is considered safe at 200 micrograms per day by the FDA and National Institutes of Health. Trivalent chromium can be taken as trivalent chromium chloride or as a trivalent chromium chelate. GTF chromium is the preformed chromium containing glucose tolerance factor; it is made commercially in yeast. Some people, especially the elderly, may not be able to effectively convert the trivalent chromium to GTF in their bodies. As little as 5 micrograms per day of GTF in a human may have a beneficial effect on blood sugar and insulin regulation.

DOSE: We suggest 200 micrograms per day of trivalent chromium or 25 to 200 micrograms per day GTF chromium.

Caution: If you are allergic to yeast, do not use GTF chromium.

WARNING: Do not take hexavalent *chromium; it may be carcinogenic.*

Trivalent chromium and GTF chromium are recognized by the FDA only as nutrients and have not been approved as agents to improve the regulation of blood sugar or insulin.

CLINICAL LABORATORY TESTS

Most clinical laboratory tests do not pose a significant safety hazard; they simply require a little of your urine or blood. A cardiac stress test does involve a small risk of heart failure if you have a defective heart or are already on the verge of it; see our comments in Chapter 14, "Peak Output Exercise." Your physician will administer clinical laboratory tests to you and explain the meaning of the results. There are two paperback books for laypersons on the subject, though one of them is rather old. (Garb, 1971; Pinckney, 1978) There is a comprehensive test handbook for physicians. (Brown, 1979)

There are, however, indirect *hazards:*

1. Suppose that the specimens are mixed up, and you get someone else's test results. This happens all too often. One survey reported an error rate at several major hospital labs of 10 to 20 percent. *If you get an unexpected test result, be sure to confirm it by immediately repeating the test.*

2. The test doesn't mean what it normally does because of interference by a drug, food, or nutrient supplement that you are using. *This type of interference is extremely common in blood and urine sugar tests when one is taking nutrient supplements! The only common clinical testing laboratory chemical method for measuring blood or urine sugar that can be trusted under these conditions is the ultraviolet hexokinase method.* Any large clinical testing laboratory will be able to use this test method.

Under these conditions, other commonly used sugar test methods (glucose oxidase, orthotoluidine, copper reduction, and, sometimes, visible light hexokinase) will yield *grossly* incorrect results, often giving sugar levels for healthy patients that would normally be found only in someone who had died of insulin shock (indicating practically no sugar), or in a terminal diabetic coma (indicating exceedingly high sugar). These tests claim that they are not affected by vitamin C and other reducing vitamins at normal physiological (FDA U.S. Recommended Daily Allowance) levels; this is correct. They often give incorrect results for someone taking a lot of vitamin C or B-1, or the amino acid cysteine, or a high-potency free-radical-scavenging multivitamin formula like the one that we suggest.

Caution: Trust only the ultraviolet hexokinase method for testing for blood and urine sugar *if you are using such supplements! When you are tested, make sure that your physician gives the clinical testing laboratory* written orders *to use ONLY the ultraviolet hexokinase method test for sugar!* If you don't, you may get an extremely alarmed call from your physician when he gets test results that say you have died from an insulin overdose or diabetic coma. This has actually happened to Sandy! Our ultraviolet hexokinase method blood sugar tests have always been normal, even though glucose oxidase and orthotoluidine method tests have yielded some truly bizarre results.

If you are not taking any vitamin supplements, or if you are taking a supplement such as One-A-Day that provides only the FDA's U.S. Recommended Daily Allowance of vitamins, the ordinary blood and urine sugar tests will work properly. Under these conditions, blood and urine sugar test strips that you can get from your pharmacist without a prescription will generally do a good job if you carefully follow the package's instructions.

An example is bG Chemstrip, made by Boehringer Mannheim Diagnostics, Inc. You obtain a large drop of fresh capillary blood from a fingertip or earlobe. You can produce this necessary blood with very little pain (it feels no worse than a mosquito bite) with very sharp, presterilized disposable lancets, also available at drugstores. Use rubbing alcohol to sterilize your skin before pricking yourself. You place the drop of blood on the reagent area of one of the test strips. You wait the specified amount of time and then compare the color of the test strip to the color scale on the vial label, which will tell you how much sugar is in your blood. Fasting (such as when you awake in the morning) levels should be 70 to 100 milligrams glucose/deciliter whole blood. Other sugars that may also be present in blood do not react. Normal concentrations of uric acid, ascorbic acid, and other reducing substances do not affect the reaction on this particular test strip, but it is fooled if you are taking a lot of vitamin C or certain other nutrient supplements.

If there is vitamin C in your urine (desirable for the prevention of bladder cancer; see our *Life Extension: A Practical Scientific Approach* for literature references), these urine tests will not work correctly. You can test for vitamin C in your urine with urine vitamin C test strips sold by your pharmacist, or see the Suppliers' Appendix.

CYSTEINE

See "Vitamin B-1–Vitamin C–Cysteine Formula" near the end of this appendix.

DHEA

Even though DHEA is naturally found in the body, there is little published data on its human use as a drug. Side effects of its use for weight control have not yet been adequately studied; hence we cannot recommend it at this time as a weight control agent, even though we have tried it ourselves in moderate doses without apparent adverse consequences.

The DHEA being sold by mail and through health food stores is usually bogus. It is generally not DHEA. It is almost always a steroid mixture extracted from a Mexican yam. This mixture contains no DHEA, according to Dr. Arthur Schwartz, the most active researcher in this area. These steroids can be converted to DHEA in the test tube, but *not* in your body. The long-term toxicity of the crude yam steroid mixture has not been adequately studied. Don't use it.

EPHEDRINE

Ephedrine is one of the most effective thermogenic agents known. Ephedrine can be obtained as a prescription drug or as a constituent of some nonprescription drugs, and also occurs naturally in a number of herbs, such as *Ephedra nevadansus, Ephedra equisetina, Ephedra sinica,* and *Ephedra distachya.* The Chinese call their ephedrine-containing herb Ma Huang; it has been used for thousands of years. The common herb horsetail contains ephedrine. These herbs are often used as stimulating teas and should be useful as fat loss aids. Even though ephedrine-containing preparations are available without prescription, it is a powerful drug and must be used with the proper care.

Ephedrine is a sympathomimetic (adrenaline-like) amine. It is used in the treatment of bronchospasm, allergy, and hypotension (low blood pressure), as a nasal decongestant, and as a central nervous system stimulant. The central nervous system stimulation caused by ephedrine is not as potent as that of the amphetamines. Users tend to become tolerant to its anorectic and central nervous system stimulant properties after two to three weeks of regular ephedrine use.

DOSE: The normal dose for thermogenesis is 20 milligrams of ephedrine. This dose may also include 100 milligrams of theophylline (see "Theophylline" later in this appendix). Do not exceed a total of 80 milligrams of ephedrine and 400 milligrams of theophylline per day. Do not take two or more doses at the same time. Normally, one dose is taken on awakening, the second dose 1 hour before lunch, and the third dose 1 hour before dinner. Tolerance to ephedrine's thermogenic effects does not develop over a 12-week period; indeed, increasing thermogenic sensitivity has been demonstrated. (Astrup, 1985)

Caution: Insomnia is likely to occur if ephedrine is taken in the evening on the first few days. We suggest that you start taking this drug gradually to minimize the chance of this and other adrenaline-like side effects.

DOSE SCHEDULE: *First 3 days:* half the normal dose 1 hour before breakfast and lunch only.

Fourth day: half the normal dose 1 hour before breakfast, lunch, and dinner.

Fifth and sixth days: full normal dose 1 hour before breakfast and lunch and half the normal dose before dinner.

From then on: take the full dose 1 hour before each meal.

During this gradual start-up period, you can pull the capsule apart and dump out half the contents for later use. This schedule also applies to ephedrine plus theophylline formulas.

Caution: Side effects include hand tremor, nervousness, restlessness, or insomnia. Reduce dosage if this occurs. Tolerance usually develops rapidly to these effects. They are much less likely to be a problem if you increase your dose slowly as we have suggested.

WARNING: Persons with high blood pressure, cardiovascular disease (especially cardiac arrhythmia), diabetes, prostatic hypertrophy, psychosis, or thyroid disease must NOT use ephedrine (or herbs containing ephedrine) except as directed by a physician. Do not use ephedrine if you are taking MAO (monoamine oxidase) inhibitor drugs, such as certain antidepressants. If you are taking prescription drugs, ask your physician or pharmacist if any of them are MAO inhibitors.

Prostatic hypertrophy (excessive growth of the prostate gland) can occur only in males and becomes very common in men older than sixty. It often interferes with normal urination by obstructing the outlet of the urinary bladder. Common symptoms include a progressive increase in urinary frequency and urgency; waking up with the need to urinate; difficulty urinating; reduced urine volume, flow rate, or force, or flow interruption; dribbling; and sensations of incomplete bladder emptying. If you have any of these symptoms, you may have prostatic hypertrophy; see your physician for a prostate examination *before* using ephedrine.

WARNING: You will have to be particularly careful about monitoring your blood pressure if you use ephedrine in conjunction with prescription anorectics, or antidepressants, or cardiovascular medications. Do not attempt to use any of these combinations unless directed to do so by your physician.

Warning: Do not exceed our recommended dose unless you are directed to do so by your physician.

Caution: Ephedrine should be used with caution by elderly males because of the possibility of undiagnosed cardiovascular disease or prostatic hypertrophy, both of which are common in elderly males. If you are an elderly male, have your physician examine you for these problems before using ephedrine.

Caution: We recommend against *the thermogenic use of nonprescription or prescription ephedrine-containing drugs that are intended for other purposes.* Many of these preparations contain other powerful drugs, such as the potentially addictive phenobarbital, or anticholinergic antihistamines that can block the GH-releasing effects of sleep, arginine, ornithine, and exercise. In many cases, the ephedrine and theophylline doses in these drugs are much larger than are required for effective thermogenesis, and the chances of adverse side effects are therefore greatly increased. Our recommended doses of ephedrine have been shown to cause a loss of 1 pound of fat per week in obese women without caloric restriction. (Astrup, 1985) The thermogenic effects are even stronger when ephedrine is combined with our recommended doses of theophylline. It is unwise to lose more than 1 to 2 pounds of fat per week.

Caution: Any increased burning of calories, whether facilitated by thermogenic drugs or by exercise, increases your level of undesirable free radical activity. Do NOT use thermogenic drugs unless you also use a properly designed free-radical-scavenging nutrient supplement formulation such as the one described below in this appendix (see "Free-Radical-Scavenging Vitamin-Mineral Nutrient Supplement").

Caution: Rebound nasal and sinus congestion may occur when this drug is discontinued after extended use.

Caution: Read the package carefully, and follow all warnings and directions.

Remember that ephedrine is a powerful drug whether it comes from an herb or from a chemical factory. The molecular structure of a compound determines its physiological function; nature does not distinguish between a natural source substance and the same molecule that has been made synthetically.

Although we think that the use of ephedrine or standardized dose ephedrine containing herbs as diet aids is a reasonable option for most people, we strongly oppose their use without an appropriate quantitative contents statement and safety warnings. Moreover, the amount of ephedrine in one batch of herbs can be ten times as great as in another batch, with potentially lethal results. Each batch of herbs should be quantitatively analyzed for ephedrine content, and the amount of herbs used adjusted to standardize the ephedrine dose. Unfortunately, this is rarely if ever done.

Most people can use ephedrine safely. It has been used (often in combination with theophylline) by millions of asthma sufferers for decades, and millions of other people have been drinking ephedra herb teas for over two thousand years. Observe all safety precautions, and do not exceed our recommended dose unless directed to do so by your physician.

FIBER

Many types of fiber bind vitamins, interfering with their absorption. For that reason, it is highly advisable to take a high-potency multivitamin-mineral supplement (see below) if you are going to be adding large quantities of fiber to your diet. Take your fiber supplement 30 minutes to 1 hour before eating your meal, eat your meal, and then take your vitamins. The fiber will prefill your stomach, and then the bulk of your meal will help keep the vitamins and fiber separated as they pass through your gut.

Dried brewers' grains are an excellent and palatable source of fiber. Be careful, however. Some dried brewers' grains are dried under high temperature conditions or by direct contact with NOX (nitrogen oxides)–containing combustion gases that lead to the formation of carcinogenic nitrosamines and high levels of potentially dangerous organic peroxides, such as rancid vegetable oils. See our *Life Extension: A Practical Scientific Approach* and *The Life Extension Companion* for much more on nitrosamines and organic peroxides and the role that they play in cardiovascular disease, cancer, and aging.

Unfortunately, these problems are not confined to dried brewers' grains; they can occur with any type of fiber. The worst organic peroxide levels that we have ever seen in something purported to be a food was in spirulina. Look for the PV (peroxide value) lab test on the label. If it isn't there, it probably hasn't even been tested.

Caution: Be sure that the product has a PV (peroxide value) guaranteed to be below 2 and is free of significant quantities of carcinogenic nitrosamines. If the package doesn't give the lab test results, it probably hasn't been tested, and it is prudent to assume that it might be hazardous.

Another excellent fiber is citrus pulp left over from juice and juice concentrate production. In one experiment, citrus pulp reduced the incidence of colon cancer in rats being treated with carcinogens. (Reddy, 1983) It has a different spectrum of adsorption properties, so it complements a grain fiber source. In addition to a possible high PV problem, be careful of pulp that contains a lot of the inner citrus rind. This rind contains natural pesticides made by the tree that protect the fruit, but some people are allergic to them. There is no simple standard food laboratory test for this problem, so you just have to trust that the manufacturer knows what it is doing. If a citrus fiber gives you gastric distress or an allergic reaction, try another brand.

The high-fiber cereals offered by major manufacturers such as Kellogg's will not have these problems, but be careful: some of them have high glycemic indices. Watch out for added sucrose, which will be called "sugar" on the label.

DOSE: A reasonable quantity of fiber is 25 to 35 grams daily. This is the National Cancer Institute recommendation, and we feel that it is consistent with good health. Fifty grams should be safe, but you may have to defecate two or three times per day. People in undeveloped countries on a high-fiber diet get about an ounce (about 28 grams) a day. Some of the newer high-fiber cereals provide 12 grams a serving.

Fiber is recognized by the FDA only as a food constituent and has not been approved for the prevention of colon cancer, for the reduction of serum lipids, or for the slowing of absorption of carbohydrates in food.

FREE-RADICAL-SCAVENGING VITAMIN-MINERAL NUTRIENT SUPPLEMENT

We recommend that you take a high-potency antioxidant (anti–free radical) vitamin-mineral supplement whether you are on a diet or not. Loss of a significant amount of body fat imposes an appreciable stress on your system, and the reduced food intake that can occur with our appetite control techniques means that your dietary intake of these vitamins and minerals may be reduced. The appropriate amounts of several of these nutrients have been shown in many scientific papers to reduce health risks such as those of smoking and drinking, decrease the risk of abnormal blood clots (leading to heart attacks or strokes), improve the function of the immune system, and reduce the risk of contracting many types of cancer. Note, however, that even though many of the individual nutrients listed below have been scientifically tested for these purposes, this particular formulation has not been clinically tested against cancer, heart disease, etc. It is suggested as part of a health maintenance and enhancement program, not as a cure for disease. For an extensive discussion of the biochemical mechanisms that make a properly formulated free-radical-scavenging nutrient supplement work, and other suggested formulas, see our *Life Extension: A Practical Scientific Approach* and *The Life Extension Companion*.

DOSE: A good nutrient supplement would, in our opinion, include the following suggested total daily doses:

vitamin A	5,000 to 8,000 iu
vitamin B-1	30 to 60 milligrams
vitamin B-2	50 to 100 milligrams
vitamin B-3	200 to 800 milligrams (as niacin)
vitamin B-5	500 milligrams to 1 gram
vitamin B-6	100 to 200 milligrams
vitamin B-12	200 to 500 micrograms
vitamin C	1 to 3 grams
ascorbyl palmitate (fat-soluble vitamin C)	100 to 200 milligrams
vitamin D	400 iu
vitamin E	200 to 600 iu
biotin	500 micrograms to 2 milligrams
beta-carotene	15,000 to 30,000 units
cysteine	100 to 300 milligrams
folic acid	500 micrograms to 1 milligram
hesperidin	150 to 250 milligrams
PABA	250 milligrams to 1 gram
rutin	150 to 250 milligrams
chromium or	50 to 100 micrograms as trivalent chromium
GTF chromium	25 to 100 micrograms as GTF from yeast
copper	3 to 5 milligrams, chelated as the gluconate
iodine	150 micrograms, as potassium iodide
manganese	2.5 to 5 milligrams, chelated as the gluconate
molybdenum	150 to 500 micrograms
selenium	200 micrograms as sodium selenite or sodium selenate
zinc	30 to 50 milligrams, chelated as the gluconate

It is especially important that you have good protection from free radicals if you are going to be exercising or using thermogenic drugs, since these both increase your rate of free radical production.

DOSE SCHEDULE: We recommend that you take this formula in 4 divided daily doses: 1 dose immediately after each meal, and 1 at bedtime. To reduce the chance of gastric discomfort, start taking this formula at one quarter of the normal doses for the first 4 days, then at half of the normal doses for the next 4 days, and the normal doses from then on.

At a minimum, take it in divided doses at least 3 times a day, immediately after meals. The frequency of use is important because the water-soluble vitamins (including C and most of the B vitamins) are rapidly excreted from your body via your urine and need to be replaced often. (You can demonstrate this to yourself: Take a 50-milligram tablet of vitamin B-2, which will color your urine yellow within about an hour. In another few hours your urine will have faded because of urinary loss of the bright yellow vitamin B-2.)

We strongly recommend that you take this supplement in the form of gelatin capsules or else as a powder, but not as pills. Dr. Harry Demopoulos, a doctor and scientist at New York University, found in a three-year study of about 80 people who were self-megadosing with vitamins, minerals, and other nutrients that 85 percent of the adverse effects reported (including diarrhea, other gastric distress, and headaches) were due to binders, fillers, and excipients in the tablets used. A powder formulation or capsules containing pure nutrient powders, but no binders, fillers, or excipients, are much less likely to cause adverse reactions such as gastric distress or allergies.

If you take nutrient supplements on an empty stomach, you may experience a niacin flush, depending on how much niacin is in the supplement. Nausea is rare. Therefore, we suggest you take most supplements immediately after meals or snacks when possible. You will tend to become tolerant to these harmless side effects with continuing regular use. You may want to skip taking the formula at bedtime for the first few days if you have a niacin flush that you find uncomfortable.

This formula may be used by diabetics. When taken in our recommended divided doses, it does not contain enough vitamin B-1 and cysteine to inactivate significant amounts of insulin, nor is there enough niacin to impair a diabetic's glucose tolerance.

WARNING: Do not take excessive quantities of vitamin A, which can be toxic. This formula contains a nontoxic amount of vitamin A.

Be wary of diet formulas containing high doses of vitamin A, which is very cheap. Toxic symptoms have been reported for some unusually sensitive persons taking as little as 25,000 units of vitamin A a day. (Hathcock, 1985) Generally, poisoning is likely to occur with doses of 100,000 units a day or more over a period of several months. Early symptoms of excess vitamin A include sparse coarse hair, loss of hair on the eyebrows, dry rough skin, and cracked lips (especially at the corners). Later, severe headache and generalized weakness develop. The early symptoms of vitamin A overdose disappear within one to four weeks after discontinuing vitamin A supplements. Note that these peripheral symptoms of vitamin A overdose will not occur if you are zinc-deficient. Zinc is required to mobilize vitamin A from its stores in the liver to the rest of your body. If you are zinc-deficient, you can damage your liver with toxic doses of vitamin A without first being warned by the above peripheral symptoms.

Caution: This formula contains the B vitamin PABA. PABA can counteract the effects of prescription sulfa drugs, so do not use a supplement containing PABA if you are taking sulfa drugs. It may be prudent for women with systemic lupus and women who are from families with a history of systemic lupus to refrain from taking PABA supplements. (Pereyo-Torrellas, 1978)

Caution: This formula contains iodine. Women from families with a high incidence of thyroid disease should not take supplementary iodine unless directed to do so by their physician. (Bagchi, 1985)

Caution: Persons with Wilson's disease (an excess copper storage disease) should not use this formula because it contains a copper supplement.

Caution: If you use this formula, or any other supplement containing large amounts of antioxidant nutrients, *only the ultraviolet hexokinase clinical laboratory test method for blood and urine sugar will give the correct results!* This formula contains relatively large quantities of antioxidant vitamins to help protect you from free radical damage. Many of these compounds, such as vitamin C, vitamin B-1, and the amino acid cysteine, are potent reducing agents that can interfere with the most common tests for blood and urine sugar when taken in these quantities. See "Clinical Laboratory Tests" in this appendix for more information.

Nutrient supplements such as this one are recognized by the FDA only as nutrients and have not been approved for the prevention of any disease other than vitamin or mineral deficiencies.

FRUCTOSE

Fructose appears to be as safe a nutrient as other common sugars and starches. It is frequently recommended as a sucrose replacement for diabetics by their physicians. If you take more than about 60 to 80 grams on an empty stomach, you may get flatulence or diarrhea, but such large single doses are unlikely to be appealing. Remember that even though fructose has a very low glycemic index and promotes the release of relatively little insulin, it has just as many calories per gram as sucrose. When possible, consider using aspartame as a sweetener to save yourself those extra calories. Too much carbohydrate can elevate serum cholesterol and triglycerides, as well as contributing to obesity.

WARNING: People replacing other carbohydrates in their diet with fructose, or who use supplemental fructose, should take 3 to 5 milligrams per day of copper (the RDA), preferably as the gluconate, to avoid the potentially hazardous rise in serum lipids and other possible serious cardiovascular problems that may occur if you are copper deficient. Persons with Wilson's disease (an excess copper storage disease) should *not* take copper supplements.

Fructose is recognized by the FDA only as a nutrient and has not been approved as an agent for the improved control of blood sugar and insulin, or for the control of reactive hypoglycemia.

A technical note on fructose to physicians, scientists, and other health professionals: Papers have appeared which suggest that fructose reduces the bioavailability of copper in rats; that it increases serum urate, pyruvate, and lactate levels in man when given rapidly intravenously in high doses (Perheentupa, 1967; Raivio, 1975; Bergstrom, 1968; Miller, 1952), that it increases triglycerides in mature rats (Simko, 1980; Nikkila, 1965; Kritchevsky, 1969; Maruhama, 1972; Nikkila, 1966; Bar-On, 1967), in baboons (Coltart, 1970), and in man at 200 to 500 grams per day (Nikkila in Sipple, 1974).

Recent work at the USDA Beltsville Human Nutrition Research Center has examined the effect of fructose on trace minerals in man where fructose and starch were compared at 20 percent of dietary calories. The dietary copper was marginal, purposely being set at only 1 milligram per day, well below the FDA's RDA. The humans on the fructose exhibited *improved bioavailability* for copper, zinc, iron, manganese, magnesium, and calcium. (Holbrook, Smith, Jr., 1985) There are several other papers related to copper metabolism that demonstrate the *vital* importance of adequate dietary copper to cardiovascular health in carbohydrate metabolism. (Fields, 1983; Fields, 1985; Holbrook, Fields, 1985; Johnson, 1985; Reiser, 1985; Smith, Jr., 1985)

Another recent study addressed the issues of elevated urate (particularly important to people with the genes for gout, like Durk), pyruvate, and lactate; no such effects were found when humans were given 24 percent of their carbohydrates as fructose orally. This was 63 to 99 grams per day. When 50 grams was given orally on an empty stomach in glucose and fructose tolerance tests, the pyruvate and lactate levels were elevated twice as much by the fructose, but not to harmful levels. This study underscores the difference between large intravenous doses of a substance and normal dietary consumption. (Crapo, 1984) Another study found no elevation of cholesterol, triglycerides, urate, or lactate in adult diabetic men fed 50 grams of fructose per day. (Anderson, 1984)

The triglyceride issue has been subjected to extensive human experimentation. The experiment mentioned above found no adverse effect on triglycerides in humans. (Crapo, 1984) Studies on large numbers of humans given 55 to 80 grams per day of fructose for up to 2 years showed no increase in triglycerides in normals (Huttunen, 1975; Nestel, 1970; Manso, 1979), controlled juvenile diabetics (Akerblom, 1972), adult diabetics (Nikkila, 1972; Pelkonen, 1972; Anderson, 1984), or even in humans with preexisting hypertriglyceridemia (Turner, 1979; Nikkila, 1972). Although the experiments in mature rats were well done, the effect seems to be rather specific for mature rats, since triglyceride elevations were not observed in young rats (Hill, 1970; Chevalier, 1972), and guinea pigs (Bar-On, 1968). Decreases in triglycerides were noticed in genetically obese mice fed fructose. (Thenen, 1976)

Note that starch or sucrose in large quantities, especially if rapidly absorbed, can increase triglycerides. Fructose undoubtedly has that capability, too, but it does not seem to be worse than other common dietary carbohydrates. There are some indications that dietary fiber may play a significant role in controlling plasma triglycerides, so its use is to be encouraged. Finally, if a patient has hypertriglyceridemia, either due to an idiosyncratic biochemistry or due to incessant and immoderate pigging out, 1 gram of niacin with each meal is usually very effective, causing an average 30 percent triglyceride reduction within 2 weeks. Of course, this large a dose of niacin should only be taken when prescribed by a physician. (Gotto, 1984; Charman, 1973; Miettinen, 1969; Coronary, 1975)

Moderation in carbohydrate consumption of any kind is to be encouraged, but patient compliance may often be questionable. Patient compliance with carbohydrate moderation is often compromised by the carbohydrate craving induced by reactive hypoglycemia. The low glycemic index of fructose can be very useful in improving a patient's regulation of blood sugar and insulin, thereby lessening excessive blood sugar rise in diabetics and normals, and reducing the release of insulin in normals and its subsequent consequence of reactive hypoglycemia. (Bohannon, 1978; Bohannon, 1980; Akgun, 1980; Crapo, 1976; Crapo, 1980; Brunzell, 1978; Akerblom, 1972; Nikkila, 1972; Pelkonen, 1972) In our experience, further and often dramatic control of reactive hypoglycemia may be obtained by the use of niacin (1 gram T.I.D. [three times daily] with meals) and trivalent chromium (200 micrograms per day) or, especially in the elderly, 200 micrograms of GTF chromium. (See Chapter 8, "Sweets.")

HERBAL REMEDIES

There are many legitimate uses for herbs, but there are also a great many illegitimate claims made for some very questionable or even potentially dangerous products. A bestselling secret herbal remedy from a huge purveyor of secret herbal remedies contained pokeweed (a mitogen, i.e., causing abnormal uncontrolled cell division) and mandrake, which contains a poison that blocks GH release. What do we think about a giant herbal company's claim that you cannot absorb anyone else's vitamins because of a mucous layer in your intestine that only their secret herbs can penetrate? That is either gross ignorance (to be charitable) or downright fraud. The next thing you know, they'll ask you to believe in Santa Claus!

If you take a laboratory look at some very popular "herbal" weight loss programs, you will find that the products are often loaded with unlisted stimulants such as caffeine, and that the instructions call for rather severe caloric restriction by replacing two of your three regular meals with their low-calorie stuff. If you want to lose weight with a very low-calorie diet, you don't need their expensive secret formula products to do it. We feel sorry for the many fine people who have been suckered into multilevel sales organizations for poorly formulated or even dangerous products by smooth-talking hucksters who apparently know nothing about physiology and biochemistry, but who could sell an air conditioner to an Eskimo.

Herbal diet preparations often contain potent natural drugs such as ephedrine, though they are rarely labeled as such. The label may just tell you that the product contains herbs, or it may give the common folk names or, more rarely, the scientific plant names. We strongly oppose the use of secret herbal formulas or herbal products that do not have a label with an appropriate quantitative contents statement and safety warnings. When an herb contains an active drug, the chemical name of that drug should appear on the product label, not just a natural innocuous-sounding name such as "horsetail." Moreover, the amount of active drug in one batch of herbs can be 10 times as great as in another batch, with potentially lethal results. *Each batch of herbs should be quantitatively analyzed for drug content, and the amount of herbs used adjusted to standardize the drug dose, which should be stated on the label.* Unfortunately, this is rarely done for nonprescription products.

WARNING: Refuse to buy herbal products that do not have a full disclosure label. Never buy herbal remedies unless the ingredients are listed both by plant names and by the names of the active drugs, the doses are analyzed and standardized for each lot of herbs, the quantities are given, and you know what each component does at that dose.

Caution: A drug from an herb has exactly the same physiological effects as the same drug from a chemical factory. The structure of a molecule, not its origins, determines its functions. A drug is a drug, regardless of its source. Do not make the mistake of thinking that a drug from an herb is any more natural or any less a drug. A drug contained in the leaves of an herb may be released more slowly, however, just as if the pure drug had been incorporated into a time release capsule.

L-CARNITINE

A report prepared by the Federation of American Societies for Experimental Biology (a conservative prestigious scientific body) for the Bureau of Foods of the Food and Drug Administration said: "Studies to date have been conducted on a limited number of subjects but the absence of side effects of daily doses of 1.0 to 2.0 g. L-carnitine and the possibility of beneficial effects on serum lipoprotein profiles suggest further investigational drug trials." The report goes on to mention that ". . . these studies have been conducted only for periods of up to 3 to 4 months." The report then calls for extended clinical trials in both normal adults and persons with the various types of hyperlipidemia (excess cholesterol and/or triglycerides in the bloodstream).

WARNING: Oral and injected doses of DL-carnitine or D-carnitine induce several side effects including cardiac arrhythmias and muscle weakness; L-carnitine at equivalent doses does not *induce such side effects. Do not use D-carnitine or DL-carnitine.*

L-carnitine is recognized by the FDA only as a nutrient and has not been approved as an agent for the modification of fat metabolism, lowering of serum lipids, or improving thermogenesis or athletic performance.

L-DOPA

L-Dopa is a powerful prescription amino acid drug and must be used with care and only if prescribed by your physician. Side effects can include increased libido or nausea at our suggested doses, and, rarely, insomnia or irritability. Tryptophan supplements can help correct irritability or insomnia.

Persons on long-term therapy with L-Dopa, such as Parkinson's disease patients, often experience anorexia (loss of appetite) and other side effects. However, the doses of L-Dopa used for growth hormone release are 250 milligrams to 500 milligrams taken at bedtime or, alternatively, 45 minutes before exercise. These doses are well below the doses used for Parkinson's disease, which when treated with pure L-Dopa may involve doses of up to 8 grams per day. (See Larodopa in the *Physicians' Desk Reference.*) Almost all Parkinson's patients are now treated with a drug combination comprised of L-Dopa and a peripheral decarboxylase enzyme inhibitor; we do not suggest such combinations for fat loss. There is a long list of side effects associated with such therapy; most are related to either the peripheral decarboxylase inhibitor or to the necessity of raising brain dopamine levels far above normal in the badly brain-damaged Parkinson patients.

Other than increases in libido and some initial nausea, none of over a dozen regular long-term users of pure 500-milligram-per-day L-Dopa that we know have reported any side effects. The National Institute on Aging sponsored tests with 500 milligrams of L-Dopa per day in normal men in their sixties; there were no reported adverse effects. As with other GH releasers, it can help you put on muscle remarkably rapidly with a few minutes per day of peak output exercise. If you exercise, you may even end up weighing more than before because of that added muscle, even though you have lost a lot of fat.

Caution: Antioxidant supplements are necessary, since dopamine (a necessary natural brain chemical that can be made from L-Dopa in your brain) is susceptible to autoxidation, a free radical process that could cause damage to certain brain cells if they are inadequately protected. The antioxidant (anti–free radical) nutrients (such as C, E, B-1, B-5, B-6, and selenium) help control free radical processes and prevent damage. See our suggested "Free-Radical-Scavenging Vitamin-Mineral Nutrient Supplement," above. Also see our *Life Extension: A Practical Scientific Approach* and *The Life Extension Companion* for much more data on free radical pathology.

WARNING: L-Dopa should NOT be used by people with cardiac arrhythmias, pregnant or lactating women, children or adolescents, manic-depressive psychotics or schizophrenics, persons using MAO inhibitor drugs (some antidepressants are MAO inhibitors), people with narrow-angle glaucoma, or people with pigmented malignant melanoma-type cancer. See the Physicians' Desk Reference *for other contraindications. If you are taking prescription drugs, ask your physician or pharmacist if any of them are MAO inhibitors.*

Caution: L-Dopa should be used cautiously by individuals on antihypertensive medication (such as the beta blocker propranolol), with due regard for the possible drug interactions described in the Physicians' Desk Reference, *and, of course, only on the direction of their physician.*

DOSE AND DOSE SCHEDULE: L-Dopa for the release of growth hormone may be taken either just before bed or 45 minutes before exercise. A reasonable dose is 250 milligrams to 500 milligrams, once per day. Nausea is fairly common initially, although you'll tend to become tolerant to that side effect after a week or so of use. Nausea can usually be avoided by starting with a 125-milligram dose and slowly increasing it over a period of 1 to 2 weeks. If you are obese, L-Dopa will not work as a GH releaser unless it is used in conjunction with a beta blocker such as propranolol. See the caution above. You must not use L-Dopa or propranolol unless they are prescribed by your physician. We believe that L-Dopa can play a useful role in *medically supervised* fat loss (but not necessarily weight loss) programs.

L-Dopa is approved by the FDA for the treatment of Parkinson's disease, but not as a GH releaser or as a fat loss aid.

Although it is perfectly legal for your physician to prescribe L-Dopa for an unapproved purpose, do *not* expect him or her to do so, since he or she will probably have had no experience with this particular application. You may soon see it cautiously used with a beta blocker in medically supervised fat loss programs, however.

MEDIUM-CHAIN TRIGLYCERIDES (MCT)

MCTs are special types of fat. They are widely used in FDA-approved mixtures of nutrients for the total long-term intravenous nutrition of very seriously ill patients. When large quantities of MCTs are eaten, they can cause diarrhea and gastric upset.

Caution: If a large quantity of MCTs is eaten on an empty stomach, it may be absorbed so rapidly that there temporarily may be excess quantities of fats in the blood. This is especially likely in persons with liver disease. This is one of the problems of formulating new food products containing MCTs; one must include components such as fiber that slow down the absorption of the MCTs.

Caution: Although MCTs are more resistant to free radical attack than polyunsaturated fats, they still require antioxidant protection with free-radical-scavenging compounds such as alpha tocopherol (vitamin E), ascorbyl palmitate (a fat-soluble form of vitamin C), and BHT. Do not buy MCT or other fat-containing products unless they contain potent antioxidants.

MCTs are recognized by the FDA only as nutrients and have not been approved as fat loss aids.

METHIONINE

Methionine is an essential sulfur-containing amino acid nutrient. Intravenous injection of methionine releases growth hormone in humans. The effectiveness of oral methionine as a GH releaser has not been established. Methionine can be taken with arginine, ornithine, tryptophan, or L-Dopa; it does not compete with these other amino acids for transport across the blood-brain barrier.

DOSE: Maximum recommended daily supplement dose: 2 to 4 grams methionine, plus about 50 milligrams of vitamin B-6 for body weights of 50 to 100 kilograms (110 pounds to 220 pounds). This amount of methionine could be obtained in a diet rich in egg protein, but less would get into your brain because of competition by other amino acids.

DOSE SCHEDULE: See Chapter 6.

WARNING: Never take supplementary methionine without taking a vitamin B-6 supplement. Without adequate vitamin B-6, your body will not be able to metabolize the methionine properly and will produce large amounts of homocysteine (not the same as cysteine), which can cause the very rapid development of arteriosclerosis. (McCully, 1972; "Pyridoxin," 1981)

Caution: There have been a few anecdotal reports that a few sensitive individuals may experience psychological depression while taking methionine supplements and that a few psychotics may have their symptoms worsened. If this occurs, discontinue the supplement.

NALOXONE AND NALTREXONE

Naloxone, naltrexone, and other opiate antagonists are examples of promising appetite-control drugs that have not yet been studied extensively for this purpose. In a recent study, naloxone reduced food intake in humans by an average of 28 percent. But we don't know the long-term effects of taking these substances. The natural opiate-like compounds (endorphins and enkephalins) are involved in many biochemical processes in your brain and body. Taking opiate antagonists on a daily basis for a long time is something that has not been done before. Data is accumulating, however, from heroin addicts who are using naloxone or one of its relatives regularly to help keep them off dope. Naloxone cannot be taken orally, but a newly approved closely related opiate antagonist drug called naltrexone can.

Naloxone and naltrexone are approved by the FDA only as opiate antagonists for opiate overdose, not as appetite modification agents.

Your physician is more likely to give you a single dose of naloxone as a test to see if your eating has an addictive biochemical component than to give you the drug on a daily basis. Medically supervised weight loss clinics may start using it in the near future, however.

NIACIN (NICOTINIC ACID, VITAMIN B-3)

Caution: Since niacin is a fairly strong acid, it can cause acid indigestion. Niacin also releases histamine in your stomach, and this histamine in turn releases more stomach acid. Therefore, either niacin should be used as buffered niacin, or an antacid should be taken along with it. We have heard reports of gastric distress and nausea; however, this ceased to be a problem when the niacin was taken in an antacid buffered form with meals.

Taking your niacin with meals helps; the acid is used to help digest your meal. Taking the niacin with meals minimizes flushing, too. We use sodium bicarbonate as an antacid, but if you are on a low-sodium diet, you can use one of the many antacids that do not contain sodium; ask your doctor or pharmacist. In long-term studies with 3 or more grams per day of niacin being prescribed to people to reduce serum cholesterol and triglycerides, a few of the people actually developed ulcers because the niacin acidity was not neutralized.

The most noticeable side effect of niacin use is the temporary but sometimes spectacular flushing effect (skin reddening, feeling of heat, itching) caused by superficial blood vessel dilation and skin histamine release. In a very few cases there is even transitory dizziness, probably caused by vasodilation in the inner-ear balance control mechanisms. These effects appear about 20 minutes after ingestion and last for about 20 minutes to 1 hour. Both we and a National Institutes of Health expert committee on cardiovascular disease consider this effect to be generally harmless, but we have had one anecdotal report of an asthmatic's symptoms being somewhat worsened for about ½ hour. If you are not accustomed to large doses of niacin, a 100-milligram dose may produce almost the same amount of flushing as a 1-gram dose. With regular niacin use, this effect tends to diminish. Taking niacin on a full stomach also helps to reduce the flushing.

The niacin flush is closely related to the Masters and Johnson sex flush. We have found niacin often increases sexual pleasure when taken about ½ hour before sex. Niacin can also intensify orgasms; see "The Case of the Stallion That Couldn't Come" in our *Life Extension: A Practical Scientific Approach.* We have found that one of the best ways of helping people become accustomed to the niacin flush is for them to try using it as a recreational drug before sex!

If one is unprepared for it, an unexpected niacin flush can be quite alarming. A few years ago, while Durk was working in aerospace, a co-worker asked him about niacin. Durk explained carefully about the flush and other possible side effects, and recommended that the co-worker start out with 100 milligrams immediately after a meal. Instead, the co-worker waited a few weeks, forgot the directions, and then took 300 milligrams on an empty stomach. His skin turned bright red, hot, and itchy, and he became so disturbed by it that he rushed himself to a local emergency hospital thinking that he was having a stroke. Just as he arrived there, he realized that the symptoms were gone, so he went home terribly worried that he was about to drop dead of cardiovascular disease.

DOSE: If you are not taking niacin under the supervision of a physician, we recommend a maximum dose of 200 milligrams at a time, with a maximum total of 800 milligrams per day. ("Niacin intakes up to 1,000 mg. as nicotinic acid appear to be completely safe." Hathcock, 1985)

A total of 3 grams a day is a tolerable dose for most healthy adults when prescribed by their physician. This is the dose suggested as a "drug of choice" by an expert committee on cardiovascular disease of the National Institutes of Health (after a recent reevaluation of the data from the Coronary Drug Project) for treating people with several types of hyperlipidemias (excess fat and VLDL or LDL cholesterol in their blood). It should be taken 3 times during the day (1 gram immediately after each meal) because niacin is a water-soluble vitamin that is rapidly excreted from your body.

Warning: Do not take more niacin than 200 milligrams per dose and 800 milligrams total per day unless it is prescribed by your physician.

The American Heart Association's special report "Recommendations for Treatment of Hyperlipidemia in Adults" discusses the use of niacin for both hypercholesterolemia ("Nicotinic acid can be highly effective in patients who tolerate the drug") and hypertriglyceridemia ("Nicotinic acid theoretically is the preferred agent. It interferes with the synthesis of lipoproteins, and dampens their overproduction. The result is a lowering of triglycerides and cholesterol, with a rise in HDL. Although the side effects of nicotinic acid can be troublesome, they are generally not serious and may be short lived"). (Gotto, 1984) A review of niacin overdose toxicity has said: "Hepatic function may be disturbed by nicotinic acid therapy. However, evidence indicates that the alterations in hepatic function are readily reversible and do not represent permanent dysfunction or morphologic damage in nearly all cases." (Waterman, 1978) The above comments apply to the prescription high-dose use of nicotinic acid.

WARNING: It has been reported that doses of niacin larger than we recommend taking without prescription can worsen gout, cause abnormal liver function, and cause hyperglycemia in some people. These effects are generally reversible when niacin is discontinued. (Levy, 1980) If jaundice occurs, discontinue use and see your physician. Diabetics should not use prescription doses of niacin unless a glucose tolerance test by their physician shows no adverse effects. In some diabetics, niacin improves glucose tolerance, and in others, it worsens it.

Durk has gout (which is a genetic disease that he inherited from his father and paternal grandfather), which is being successfully treated by the prescription drug allopurinol. Even though both of us have taken 11 grams of niacin each day for over a decade, Sandy did not get gout and Durk's gout was not detectably worsened. Our blood sugar levels (tested by the interference-resistant ultraviolet hexokinase method) have remained in the high 80s to low 90s, which is normal.

Caution: It would be prudent for people with active ulcers to refrain from taking niacin supplements of over 50 milligrams per dose or totaling over 250 milligrams per day unless directed to do so by their physician. Persons with active ulcers should not use higher doses of niacin until they have healed, and then may require the continued use of the H_2 histamine–blocking anti-ulcer drug cimetidine.

Caution: Niacin can interfere with the effectiveness of certain anti-tuberculosis drugs. If you are being treated for tuberculosis, you should ask your doctor before using niacin.

Niacinamide is also a form of vitamin B-3. Niacinamide produces less flushing, but it does not modify fat and sugar metabolism the way niacin does. It is not a substitute for niacin for these purposes.

Niacin is recognized by the FDA as a nutrient and has been approved as a prescription drug for the reduction of serum lipids, but it has not been approved for the modification of carbohydrate metabolism, or for altering blood sugar and insulin regulation, or for appetite modification, or for controlling reactive hypoglycemia.

NICOTINE

WARNING: Nicotine is a drug. For most people, nicotine is more addicting than heroin! Nicotine and tobacco contribute to the deaths of over 250,000 people per year. (Brecher, 1972)

We definitely do not recommend the use of nicotine, although it is a thermogenic agent. If you are already a nicotine addict and don't want to quit because you gain weight whenever you try to do so, some of the adverse cardiovascular and serum lipid effects of nicotine can be ameliorated with prescription doses of niacin. We hope that you will consider substituting other less hazardous thermogenic drugs for tobacco.

Smoking produces compounds that are carcinogens and atherogens (causing atherosclerosis). Nicotine itself, independent of the toxic combustion products, accelerates atherosclerosis, increases fat synthesis in arteries, and constricts blood vessels, increasing blood pressure.

There are a number of ways of decreasing the risks of smoking and nicotine, though, for those who cannot or will not stop. In a 19-year study of 2000 men at the Western Electric plant in Chicago, the smokers who got the largest quantities of beta-carotene in their diets had no higher risk of lung cancer than did nonsmokers with low intakes of beta-carotene in their diet. (Shekelle, 1981) Beta-carotene is the nutrient that makes carrots orange. But if you don't like to eat carrots, you can get beta-carotene at a health food store. We suggest taking 20,000 to 30,000 I.U. per day with the fattiest meal of the day in order to facilitate absorption and avoid possible gastric distress. Beta-carotene does not provide protection against the cardiovascular risks of smoking, however.

The smoking-increased risk of abnormal blood clots (leading to heart attacks and strokes) can be reduced but not eliminated by antioxidant nutrient supplements containing vitamins E, C, B-1, B-2, B-3, B-5, B-6, and the minerals zinc and selenium. Niacin (vitamin B-3) counteracts some of the effects of nicotine itself by decreasing fat synthesis in arteries and (temporarily) dilating peripheral blood vessels. Niacin should not interfere with nicotine thermogenesis and does not interfere with the psychobiochemical effects of nicotine. Be sure to use buffered niacin so that urine acidification does not cause increased urinary loss of nicotine with its consequence of increased tobacco consumption. Buffered niacin will not cause withdrawal symptoms in nicotine addicts. The risks of smoking can be reduced, but it will never be entirely safe. For much more information on reducing the health risks of smoking, and for ways of quitting that do not require willpower, see our *Life Extension: A Practical Scientific Approach* and *The Life Extension Companion.*

Low-tar cigarettes may not be a healthier cigarette, as had been hoped. It has been found in scientific studies that nicotine is the main reason people smoke. Nicotine is a chemical relative of the nutrient choline and helps many people to focus and concentrate better. Unfortunately, it has unhealthy side effects. Giving people lower-nicotine cigarettes results in their smoking more cigarettes to maintain their brain levels of nicotine. A less dangerous cigarette would be one with a high nicotine-to-tar ratio. The nicotine would satisfy the nicotine craving of smokers, while the tar (the cancer-causing agent) would be reduced.

Another way to use tobacco in a safer way is to use smokeless tobacco, such as chewing tobacco. While these forms of tobacco can still cause cancer, the types of cancer usually involved are those of the lips and mouth (and nose, with snuff) where you can feel and see them and get prompt treatment. A lung cancer, on the other hand, is out of sight, and symptoms do not usually show up until it is well advanced. It is a crime that the government is considering preventing manufacturers of smokeless tobacco from advertising on TV, because these forms of tobacco, while not perfectly safe, are safer than cigarettes.

We suspect that much of the cancer hazard of smokeless tobaccos is due to carcinogenic compounds called nitrosamines. There are technical means of greatly reducing the amount of these compounds in products, such as was done a few years ago when substantial amounts of nitrosamines were found in beer and bacon. Flue-cured tobacco generally has higher nitrosamine levels than the air-dried or indirectly heated oven-dried product. We would like to see a voluntary industry standard to limit nitrosamines in tobacco products. Smokeless tobaccos also allow people to indulge in tobacco in a manner that does not force others to share their dangerous drug use by breathing in their smoke. Studies indicate that this secondhand smoke is capable of causing disease in nonsmokers who habitually breathe it. (Matsukura, 1984)

A new smokeless cigarette is about to be put on the market. One sucks on it without lighting it. It probably contains nicotine in free-base form, which can vaporize at room temperature. Risks should be considerably less than those of smoking, and similar to those of the nicotine-containing chewing gum described below.

Nicorette chewing gum is another option for tobacco addicts. It is a prescription drug that contains nicotine. This form of nicotine entirely avoids the dangers of tobacco tars. The smoker gets the nicotine he or she craves and nothing else. Note, however, that you should take 200 milligrams of niacin with each meal if you use nicotine in any form, to help prevent the deleterious increases in cholesterol and triglycerides and the vasoconstriction that will otherwise be caused by the nicotine. Higher niacin doses prescribed by your physician will be even more effective. Niacin, a form of vitamin B-3, is also called nicotinic acid and is chemically related to nicotine closely enough to block some of the lipid (fat) synthesis–enhancing effects and vasoconstrictive effects of nicotine itself. Note, however, that nicotine will still be risky for those with cardiovascular disease.

A simple technique most people can use to reduce tobacco consumption is to make their urine alkaline. Nicotine is an alkaloid and is not very soluble in alkaline water. It is very soluble in acid water. When the water in your urine is alkaline, nicotine and its major metabolites do not dissolve very well into it, so much less is lost. That helps to maintain the nicotine level in your brain, where nicotine craving is controlled. Your increased brain nicotine level results in a greatly reduced desire to smoke cigarettes. This technique was used by a psychologist, Dr. Stanley Schacter, who gave his subjects 4 grams of baking soda (an alkalizing agent) a day. (We suggest taking 1 gram of baking soda 4 times per day; take it between meals and at bedtime.) The smokers taking baking soda reduced their cigarette consumption to 0.14 cigarettes per person per day! A control group receiving a nonactive placebo smoked about 7.8 cigarettes per day.

Caution: Persons who suffer kidney or urinary bladder stones, or come from a family where other members suffer from such stones, should not alkalize their urine without discussing it with their physician; alkaline urine may promote the formation of certain types of stones in certain susceptible individuals. Alkalization of your urine may also reduce your urinary losses and hence reduce your requirements for alkaloid drugs such as atropine and reserpine. Persons on a low-sodium diet will not be able to use baking soda (sodium bicarbonate), but should ask their doctor or pharmacist to recommend a non-sodium-containing alkalizing agent.

It is hardly necessary to add that tobacco use is addicting to most users. Most people who have ever tried to stop smoking know that already! In fact, tobacco smoking is more addicting than heroin. At least, that was the opinion of the patients at the Synanon heroin treatment center. According to these people, it is much harder to quit smoking tobacco than it is to kick heroin addiction. During World War II, when food supplies were severely curtailed in prisoner-of-war camps in Germany, smoking prisoners were still willing to barter their food rations for tobacco. For a very interesting study of nicotine, as well as of caffeine, alcohol, marijuana, and other commonly used recreational drugs, see *Licit & Illicit Drugs* by Edward M. Brecher and the Editors of *Consumer Reports* (Boston: Little, Brown, 1972).

We would like to point out, however, that despite the severe health hazards of tobacco, it should not be banned. The United States' experience with alcohol prohibition should be adequate warning that such an attempt would not only fail to stop tobacco use, it might increase it (alcohol use by drinkers was probably higher per capita during Prohibition than it is now), and would create a huge black market controlled by organized crime. Some countries have even imposed the death penalty for possession, use, or sale of tobacco! It didn't work then, and it won't work now. Prohibition is definitely not a more desirable alternative.

ORNITHINE

SEE "ARGININE."

PABA

PABA, a B vitamin, is also known as *para*-aminobenzoic acid and p-aminobenzoic acid.

Ultraviolet light protection is important if you are going to be outdoors with fewer clothes, since solar UV is the principal cause of skin cancer, the most common human cancer, and is also an important cause of premature skin aging. Topically applied PABA ester sunblocks are effective, but may be esthetically unpleasant.

Caution: PABA interferes with sulfa drug antimicrobial therapy. The sulfa drugs kill certain bacteria by closely resembling PABA but not functioning like it, thereby killing the fooled bacteria. Although sulfa drugs are not widely used anymore, it is important to know that PABA should NOT be used when your doctor is treating you with them. The PABA itself would not harm you, but it would stop the sulfa drugs from working. A few people are allergic to PABA. It may be prudent for women with systemic lupus and women who are from families with a history of systemic lupus to refrain from taking PABA supplements. (Pereyo-Torrellas, 1978)

PABA is acidic, like niacin, and can cause a similar, though usually much weaker, flush. Take your PABA either with food or with an antacid.

Caution: If you have ulcers, observe the same precautions as with niacin, though the problem is less severe.

DOSE: For significant protection against ultraviolet light from the sun, we suggest taking 500 milligrams of PABA with each meal. Also see "Sunblockers," following.

PHENYLALANINE

L-phenylalanine is an essential nutrient amino acid. D-phenylalanine is a synthetic isomer that your body can use for the same purposes, although there are some differences in effects. Unless otherwise stated, the precautions apply to both types of phenylalanine, and to the equal mixture of the two known as DL-phenylalanine. Remember that L-phenylalanine, but not D-phenylalanine, acts as an anorectic agent (appetite reducer) by releasing the satiation hormone CCK.

Caution: Phenylalanine supplements may increase libido. Insomnia, excitement, or irritability may result from overdose. Phenylalanine sometimes causes headaches in a few sensitive individuals. These effects are more likely with the natural L-phenylalanine. Sometimes changing the time when you take the supplement will take care of the problem. If you are taking it in the morning and experiencing insomnia, taking it just before bedtime may alleviate the insomnia. Or you may need to cut back on your dose. Tryptophan supplements (1/2 to 2 grams at bedtime) often reduce or eliminate the irritability some people (especially men) experience.

It would be prudent to monitor your blood pressure, since there have been rare anecdotal reports that a few sensitive individuals may experience a rise in blood pressure even at the small doses we discuss. Although this is apparently very uncommon, we cannot discount the possibility of an idiosyncratic reaction to it, particularly if you suffer from hypertension.

Caution: You should monitor your blood pressure if you have a family history of hypertension (high blood pressure).

WARNING: Do not use phenylalanine supplements if you use MAO inhibitors (which include some antidepressants); if you have a cardiac arrhythmia, hypertension (high blood pressure), the genetic disease PKU, psychosis, or preexisting pigmented malignant melanoma-type cancer; or if you have a violent temper. If you are taking prescription drugs, ask your physician or pharmacist if any of them are MAO inhibitors.

WARNING: If you wish to take phenylalanine and also take ephedrine or phenylpropanolamine or prescription anorectic drugs, you must monitor your blood pressure because one might hypothetically experience an increase in blood pressure and have other adverse side effects characteristic of adrenaline-like drug overdose. If you use phenylalanine supplements with any of these other drugs, do so with great caution because we have no experience with such combinations. We advise against this self-experiment unless you are a health professional who is experienced in designing experimental drug trial protocols.

Caution: If you are severely depressed, go to your physician; do not attempt to treat yourself. There are many medical causes of depression, and your problem must be dealt with accordingly.

DOSE: The dose of L-phenylalanine required for appetite suppression will vary from person to person. What may be too much for one person might be just right or even too little for somebody else. We suggest you begin at a very small dose, 125 milligrams a day, which has been used with some success as an antidepressant in human clinical trials. If necessary, you can slowly work your way up to a higher daily dose, 500 milligrams or, in some cases, even to as much as 1½ grams. If you take too much, you can get symptoms such as occur with many stimulants: insomnia, irritability, a "wired" feeling. Take the phenylalanine on an empty stomach; protein will compete for transport, will reduce phenylalanine's effectiveness, and hence may cause a variable and irregular response. Carbohydrates may facilitate the transport of phenylalanine across the blood-brain barrier. A high-protein diet can supply about 4 grams of L-phenylalanine per day, but remember that the effects of the phenylalanine will be much more pronounced when it is taken on an empty stomach with the cofactors described below.

COFACTOR DOSE: Your brain requires vitamins B-6 and C to convert phenylalanine into the natural stimulant noradrenaline and another important brain biochemical, dopamine. For best results, we suggest taking about 30 milligrams of vitamin B-6 and 250 milligrams of vitamin C with your phenylalanine.

Remember that phenylalanine is turned into the natural stimulant noradrenaline, which is stored in your brain. The dose of phenylalanine that was right for the first day or two may be too much after you have been building up your noradrenaline levels for a few days. If you get mild overdose symptoms after the first few days, skip a day or two, then go back to taking it at about half your prior dose. A typical American diet can provide about 4 grams of phenylalanine per day, but the brain stimulation effects are *much* greater per gram when pure phenylalanine is taken on an empty stomach.

We have found that, on the average, most men are about three times as sensitive to the stimulant effects of phenylalanine as most women. We know of women who are taking 1½ grams per day without excess stimulation or irritability. Men convert more phenylalanine into noradrenaline, and they are more sensitive to the stimulating effects of noradrenaline.

Unlike phenylpropanolamine or amphetamine-related prescription anorectics, prolonged phenylalanine use does not lead to tolerance problems. Some of our subjects have used L-phenylalanine as an anorectic for two years without the development of tolerance. We have heard of no reports of rebound eating or depression after discontinuing use.

D-phenylalanine doses and dosage adjustment are similar, but remember that D-phenylalanine is used for its effects on your brain's endorphin (natural opiate) system, not as a CCK releaser. For example, D-phenylalanine has been used with some success to treat chronic pain.

Durk is unusually sensitive to the effects of stimulants. He has found that he can control his brain levels of noradrenaline more precisely by taking a very small amount of phenylalanine in an unusual way right after he wakes up. He puts the powdered phenylalanine between his upper lip and his gum. There are blood vessels in this area that go directly to the brain. Durk does not use it every day unless he is working very long hours. When he does use it, he needs only about 100 milligrams because this route is much more efficient and rapid at delivering phenylalanine to his brain. Do not try taking a normal dose this way; it will be too much!

L-phenylalanine and DL-phenylalanine are FDA-recognized only as nutrients and have not been approved as agents for appetite modification or as antidepressants.

PHENYLPROPANOLAMINE

Phenylpropanolamine is a sympathomimetic (adrenaline-like) amine. It is available for use as an anorectic without a prescription, but that doesn't mean that caution is unnecessary.

DOSE: Because of the greater problems with phenylpropanolamine that we describe below, we prefer the use of ephedrine and ephedrine-theophylline formulations for thermogenesis, rather than phenylpropanolamine. If you wish to use nonprescription phenylpropanolamine or phenylpropanolamine-caffeine formulations, we suggest that you use no more than 15 milligrams of phenylpropanolamine and 100 milligrams of caffeine per dose, and that you take no more than 3 doses per day, each 1 hour before a meal. The chance of adverse side effects will be reduced if you increase your dose slowly, starting at a fraction of our suggested maximum dose, as we have recommended for ephedrine.

WARNING: Phenylpropanolamine can increase blood pressure to dangerous levels in some people, even with the quantities currently being sold without prescription as an anorectic. Another potential side effect of phenylpropanolamine, amphetamine, and amphetamine-like drugs is tachycardia (fast heart rate) and cardiac arrhythmias. Therefore, it is imperative that you check your blood pressure periodically if you choose to use it.

WARNING: Do not use phenylpropanolamine if you have high blood pressure, a cardiac arrhythmia or other cardiovascular disease, psychosis, renal

(kidney) disease or impairment, thyroid disease, diabetes, or prostatic hyper-
trophy, if you take MAO inhibitors (which include some antidepressant drugs),
or if you have a violent temper. If you are taking prescription drugs, ask your
physician or pharmacist if any of them are MAO inhibitors.

Prostatic hypertrophy (excessive growth of the prostate gland) can occur
only in males and becomes very common in men older than sixty. It often
interferes with normal urination by obstructing the outlet of the urinary
bladder. Common symptoms include a progressive increase in urinary frequency and urgency; waking up with the need to urinate; difficulty urinating;
reduced urine volume, flow rate, or force, or flow interruption; dribbling;
and sensations of incomplete bladder emptying. If you have any of these
symptoms, you may have prostatic hypertrophy; see your physician for a
prostate examination *before* using phenylpropanolamine.

WARNING: You will have to be particularly careful about monitoring your
blood pressure if you use phenylpropanolamine and prescription anorectics, or
antidepressants, or cardiovascular medications. Do not attempt to use any of
these combinations unless directed to do so by your physician. Phenylpropanol-
amine may interact with alpha agonist (e.g. clonidine) or beta blocker (e.g.
propranolol) antihypertensive drugs to produce dangerously high or low blood
pressure.

Caution: Phenylpropanolamine should be used with caution by elderly
males because of the possibility of undiagnosed cardiovascular disease or pros-
tatic hypertrophy, both of which are common in elderly males. If you are an
elderly male, have your physician examine you for these problems before using
phenylpropanolamine.

Caution: Thermogenic drugs increase your level of undesirable free radical
activity, just as exercise does. Do NOT use thermogenic drugs unless you also
use a properly designed free-radical-scavenging nutrient supplement formula-
tion such as the one described earlier in this appendix. See "Free-Radical-
Scavenging Vitamin-Mineral Nutrient Supplement."

Caution: Phenylpropanolamine can also cause hand tremor, nervousness,
restlessness, irritability, and insomnia. Reduce dosage if this occurs. Contin-
ued use of anorectic doses rapidly results in tolerance, the full effectiveness
generally lasting only 2 to 3 weeks. The degree of tolerance to its thermogenic
effects is unknown.

Caution: Rebound eating, nasal and sinus congestion, and depression may
occur when this drug is discontinued after extended use.

Caution: Read the package carefully, and follow all warnings and direc-
tions, except that we suggest that you use a lower dose than is usually specified
on the package.

PREMENSTRUAL SYNDROME FORMULA

This formula is designed to relieve premenstrual syndrome and accompanying carbohydrate cravings. Take 1 dose as required, up to 4 times a day. The tryptophan and optional carbohydrate contained in the formula may make you sleepy, as if you had just eaten a large lunch. This effect is medically harmless, but be cautious when driving or when engaged in potentially dangerous tasks. Tryptophan does not cause the increase in reaction time and the loss of coordination that is common with other sedatives and tranquilizers. The niacinamide ascorbate is a nutrient that was chosen for its natural mild Valium-like effects. (Mohler, 1979)

Suggested contents per dose:

tryptophan	250 to 500 milligrams
vitamin B-6	25 to 50 milligrams
vitamin C	250 milligrams to 1 gram
inositol	250 milligrams to 1 gram
niacinamide ascorbate	150 to 300 milligrams
fructose (optional)	0 to 10 grams

The nutrients in this formula are FDA recognized only as nutrients, and neither these nutrients nor this formula have been approved as aids for dealing with PMS.

SUNBLOCKERS

See "PABA" and "Beta-carotene" for nutrients that provide protection from solar ultraviolet light when taken orally. We recommend the use of PABA ester sunblocks and sunscreens topically when extended solar exposure is anticipated. Remember that solar ultraviolet light is the most common cause of the most common human cancer, skin cancer. It is also one of the most important causes of premature skin aging.

Caution: A few sensitive individuals are allergic to PABA ester sunblocks. If irritation occurs, discontinue use. It may be prudent for women with systemic lupus and women who are from families with a history of systemic lupus to refrain from using PABA ester sunblocks. (Pereyo-Torrellas, 1978)

THEOPHYLLINE

Theophylline is chemically very similar to caffeine, and its effects are also rather similar. Theophylline is used therapeutically as a treatment for bronchial asthma. Ordinary tea contains small but physiologically active amounts of this drug. (Rall, 1980) Tolerance to theophylline's anorectic effects seems to develop after 2 or 3 weeks of continuous use. Theophylline is a potent thermogenic drug. Tolerance to thermogenic effects was not noted over a 7-week period. (Dulloo, 1984)

Caution: Theophylline increases the secretion of stomach acid, which can be blocked by the antiulcer drug cimetidine. Theophylline should not be used by ulcer patients, the ulcer-prone, or those with active gastritis unless directed by their physician. It should not be used by persons with hypersensitivity or idiosyncrasy to theophylline and other methylxanthines (coffee, tea, colas, cocoas, chocolates, etc.), and it may worsen the symptoms of panic or anxiety disorders. Overdose symptoms include anorexia, nausea, vomiting, irritability, or headache. Do not exceed our recommended dose unless directed to do so by your physician.

WARNING: Those with cardiovascular disease, diabetes, thyroid disease, the elderly, and patients with liver and kidney disease should use theophylline with caution and only if directed to do so by their physician. Overdoses can produce a more profound and potentially dangerous stimulation of the central nervous system (brain and spinal cord) than does caffeine.

DOSE: We do not suggest the use of theophylline alone as a thermogenic agent since it actually caused a slight increase in the body fat percentage of lean animals. If used for thermogenesis, we suggest its synergistic use in combination with ephedrine. A 20-milligram dose of ephedrine can be combined with a 100-milligram dose of theophylline and taken up to 4 times per day. See "Ephedrine" for our suggested dose schedule. Theophylline is less likely than caffeine to cause insomnia, irritability, or other signs of central nervous system overstimulation at our recommended thermogenic doses.

THYROID HORMONE

Thyroid replacement hormone can be administered on prescription to increase your basal metabolism if it is abnormally low and if you are hypothyroid as measured by a variety of clinical laboratory tests. The dose must be individualized by your physician. We prefer to use Armour thyroid extract rather than L-thyroxine.

WARNING: Do not take thyroid without a prescription. Do not take more than your prescribed dose. Do not attempt to use thyroid hormone as a fat loss drug by increasing your basal metabolism above normal; this is ineffective and can be very hazardous. Overdose symptoms of thyroid hormone include nervousness, sleeping difficulties, excessive sweating, elevated temperature, and loss of weight. Too much thyroid can cause cardiac disrhythmias and heart failure and is also reported to cause loss of lean body mass. A person who has had a heart attack should not be started on thyroid for at least two months afterward. People who have thyroid problems or who are taking thyroid hormone should not use ephedrine, phenylpropanolamine, or other adrenaline-like compounds (including most prescription anorectics) unless directed to do so by their physician.

TRYPTOPHAN

Tryptophan is an essential nutrient amino acid. Tryptophan is available as the natural isomer L-tryptophan and as a synthetic mixture of isomers, DL-tryptophan. Both have similar effects. Minor side effects of tryptophan supplements include sleepiness, headache, sinus congestion, or constipation. This sedative effect is medically harmless, but be cautious when driving or when engaged in potentially dangerous tasks. Tryptophan does not cause the increase in reaction time and the loss of coordination that is common with other sedatives and tranquilizers.

Caution: Some rare individuals may be stimulated by tryptophan rather than sedated. Such individuals should NOT continue to use tryptophan supplements because it is not understood why they have this unusual paradoxical reaction.

DOSE: A reasonable dose for a healthy adult is 500 milligrams to 2 grams, often taken just before bedtime. This dose may cause CCK release (possibly eliminating a craving for a midnight carbohydrate snack) and tranquilization. Doses of 250 milligrams can usually be used during the day without drowsiness. Doses of 500 milligrams can cause drowsiness in some people, even during the day. Taking fructose or other carbohydrates with your tryptophan will increase the amount that enters your brain. Your total daily dose from all supplements should not exceed 2 grams. Do not take tryptophan supplements if you are taking a serotonin blocker drug such as cyproheptadine, since it will reduce the drug's effectiveness. A high-protein American diet can supply up to about 2 grams of tryptophan per day; however, the effects on the brain are much stronger when the tryptophan is taken all at once on an empty stomach (and even stronger with carbohydrates) but not with competing amino acids from protein.

COFACTOR DOSE: Your brain requires vitamins B-6 and C to convert tryptophan into the natural sedative and tranquilizer serotonin. For best results, we suggest taking about 30 milligrams of vitamin B-6 and 250 milligrams of vitamin C with your tryptophan.

Tryptophan is FDA-recognized only as a nutrient and has not been approved as an agent for appetite modification, tranquilization, or sedation.

TYROSINE

Tyrosine is a nutrient amino acid. When we refer to tyrosine in this book, we mean the natural L-tyrosine, not the synthetic D-tyrosine or DL-tyrosine mixture, which are not available to the general public. Tyrosine may increase libido. Insomnia or irritability may result from overdose. A few sensitive people may experience headaches. Sometimes changing the time when you take the supplement will take care of the problem. If you are taking it in the morning and experiencing insomnia, taking it just before bedtime may alleviate the insomnia. Or you may need to cut back on your dose. Tryptophan supplements (500 milligrams to 2 grams at bedtime) often reduce or eliminate the irritability some people (especially men) experience. Tyrosine is much less likely to cause overstimulation, insomnia, or irritability than L-phenylalanine.

Caution: You should monitor your blood pressure if you have a family history of hypertension (high blood pressure) or hypotension (low blood pressure). This is a matter of prudence. We have never heard of any hypertensive or hypotensive problems with tyrosine supplements. In fact, tyrosine has been used to lower high blood pressure in some animal (Sved, 1979) and human studies.

WARNING: Do not use tyrosine supplements if you use MAO inhibitors (which include some antidepressants); if you have a cardiac arrhythmia, psychosis, or preexisting pigmented malignant melanoma-type cancer; or if you have a violent temper. If you are taking prescription drugs, ask your physician or pharmacist if any of them are MAO inhibitors.

WARNING: If you wish to take tyrosine and also take ephedrine or phenylpropanolamine or prescription anorectic drugs, you must monitor your blood pressure because one might hypothetically experience an increase in blood pressure and have other adverse side effects characteristic of adrenaline-like drug overdose. If you use tyrosine supplements with any of these other drugs, do so with great caution because we have no experience with such combinations. We advise against this self-experiment unless you are a health professional who is experienced in designing experimental drug trial protocols.

Caution: If you are severely depressed, go to your physician; do not attempt to treat yourself. There are many medical causes of depression, and your problem must be dealt with accordingly.

DOSE: Effective dose must be adjusted on an individual basis. Men are more sensitive to the effects of phenylalanine and tyrosine than women. On the other hand, women are more sensitive to the effects of tryptophan. There are also individual personality differences; some people are naturally sensitive to stimulants and get excited easily. They will want to use less phenylalanine and possibly less tyrosine than other people. In clinical trials, most people did not find tyrosine stimulating.

Tyrosine has been shown to be an effective antidepressant at doses of as little as 100 milligrams to as much as 1 gram a day on an empty stomach. Start out at 125 milligrams a day and increase your dose very gradually over a period of several days, adjusting your dose until you achieve the right degree of mental effects. As is the case with phenylalanine, there is some accumulation of effects (due to the brain's increasing stores of noradrenaline and dopamine, which can be made from tyrosine), so the dose that was right on the first day may be too much after several days. Take the tyrosine on an empty stomach; protein will compete for transport, will reduce tyrosine's effectiveness, and hence may cause a variable and irregular response. Carbohydrates may facilitate the transport of tyrosine across the blood-brain barrier. A high-protein diet can supply about 4 grams of tyrosine per day, but remember that the effects of the tyrosine will be much more pronounced when it is taken on an empty stomach with the cofactors described below.

COFACTOR DOSE: Your brain requires vitamins B-6 and C to convert tyrosine into the natural stimulant noradrenaline and another important brain biochemical, dopamine. For best results, we suggest taking about 30 milligrams of vitamin B-6 and 250 milligrams of vitamin C with your tyrosine.

Tyrosine is FDA-recognized only as a nutrient and has not been approved as an agent for appetite or blood pressure modification, or as an antidepressant.

VITAMIN B-1–VITAMIN C–CYSTEINE FORMULA

Vitamin B-1 plus vitamin C plus the nutrient amino acid cysteine is a powerful formula that can inactivate insulin by reducing the disulfide chemical bonds that hold the insulin molecule together. It can be used to destroy excess insulin during reactive hypoglycemia. Cystine is *not* the same as cysteine and will not work in this application.

DOSE: Suggested contents per dose:

vitamin B-1	100 milligrams
vitamin C	1.5 grams
cysteine	500 milligrams

Do not use more than 2 doses per day. (This amount of cysteine could be obtained from a diet rich in eggs, but the rate of absorption, blood levels attained, and effectiveness would be much less.)

WARNING: PERSONS WITH DIABETES MELLITUS (insulin/sugar diabetes) AND BORDERLINE DIABETICS MUST NOT USE THIS FORMULA SINCE IT WILL DESTROY INSULIN, MAKING THEIR DISEASE WORSE. Do not use this formula if you have an impaired glucose tolerance. You must have your physician give you a glucose tolerance test before using this formula. Do not take this formula within 3 hours before, with, or within 3 hours after taking a GH releaser. Do not take it at bedtime, because of sleep-induced GH release. Persons with a history of stones in the kidneys or urinary bladder should not use this formula.

Diabetes mellitus has a strong hereditary component; if any of your relatives have diabetes mellitus, your chances of having it or developing it are greatly increased. The most common symptoms include frequent urination, thirst, abnormally high fluid consumption, itching, dry skin, hunger, weakness, slow wound healing, and loss of weight. Unfortunately, you may be diabetic and not have any of these symptoms. About half of the people who have diabetes mellitus do not know it, and some do not have any of the above symptoms; hence a glucose tolerance test performed by your physician is necessary.

WARNING: Never take supplemental cysteine alone. You must take at least 3 times as much vitamin C at the same time, or the very soluble cysteine may be oxidized to the very insoluble cystine, which could cause cystine stones in your kidneys or urinary bladder. As long as you have at least a few hundred milligrams of vitamin C per liter in your urine, this cannot occur. If you are using a cysteine supplement, it is prudent to take at least ½ gram of vitamin C 4 times per day. When you take the cysteine, take 3 times as much vitamin

C as cysteine, and take this extra vitamin C at the same time. The vitamin C will keep the cysteine in its reduced and extremely soluble form.

Caution: Do not take this mixture within 3 hours before, with, or within 2 hours after eating a high-glycemic-index meal or snack or you may destroy too much insulin and become hyperglycemic. Hyperglycemia is harmful and must be avoided.

VITAMIN B-6 (PYRIDOXINE)

DOSE: Vitamin B-6 enhances the exercise-induced release of growth hormone when taken in a 600-milligram dose. We suggest taking it 45 minutes before exercise.

Caution: Vitamin B-6 supplements should not be taken by Parkinson's disease patients on L-Dopa. This would result in more conversion of L-Dopa to dopamine in the body rather than in the brain where it is especially needed by these patients. Our suggested amounts of vitamin B-6 should not significantly interfere with the use of L-Dopa as a GH releaser in persons who are not suffering from Parkinson's disease, so long as you do not take more than 200 milligrams of B-6 at the same time as the L-Dopa. A reasonable maximum total daily dose of vitamin B-6 for normal persons is 800 milligrams. (Hathcock, 1985)

WARNING: Daily doses of 2.5 grams or more have caused a peripheral neuropathy in several individuals that was reversible upon dose reduction.

Vitamin B-6 is FDA-recognized only as a nutrient and has not been approved as a facilitator of exercise-induced GH release.

VITAMIN-MINERAL NUTRIENT SUPPLEMENT

See "Free-Radical-Scavenging Vitamin-Mineral Nutrient Supplement."

APPENDIX 6

Supermarket Shopping Guide

HOW TO USE THE SUPERMARKET SHOPPING GUIDE

In this section, we explore the food and nutrient resources you can use as fat loss aids that are available at your favorite local large supermarket. The American supermarket is a remarkable institution that can supply many of the items we discuss in this book, generally at a very low markup.

In the first section, we report the results of a search Sandy made of our own favorite supermarket here in the Los Angeles area. The foods she found that can be used with our program are listed there.

Then we include some cooking tips for fructose and aspartame, two important alternatives to the use of sucrose (ordinary sugar). We also include several recipes for these sweeteners. We hope you enjoy them. If you do, be sure to purchase the cookbooks these were taken from (with the permission of their authors).

Finally, we include some charts showing nutrient contents and glycemic indexes of many commonly used foods.

"Extended Table of Glycemic Indexes" tells you the glycemic index, as well as the percentages of protein, fat, and carbohydrates in foods. You do not want to choose a food low in glycemic index that is also very high in fat. Peanuts are an example. You have to be careful not to eat too many peanuts, because they contain a lot of fat and calories.

"Nutritive Values of Common Foods" shows the calories, protein, fat, carbohydrate, and calories per gram of protein in foods. Choose protein foods that give you the lowest number of calories per gram of protein. Do not choose too many foods high in calories and fat.

In "Arginine and Lysine Content of Arginine-Rich Foods," we tell you which foods are relatively high in arginine (a growth hormone releaser), lysine (a competitor to arginine for entry into your brain), and percentages of protein, fat, and carbohydrate for those foods. If you wish to get your arginine from foods rather than supplements, choose foods high in arginine, but not also high in fat.

NUTRIENT AND FOOD FAT LOSS AIDS AVAILABLE AT SUPERMARKETS

The following items were found at a very large supermarket in the Los Angeles area. We wanted to see what choices would be available for people who would like to use fructose, high-fructose corn syrup, and other foods discussed in *The Life Extension Weight Loss Program*. We were delighted to see that there is, even now, a fairly wide range of choices. Of course, some of these (such as fructose and fructose-sweetened foods) are specialty items sold at relatively high prices. Demand is low. If significantly more people buy these foods, it will result in competition among suppliers and more choices for consumers. Higher volumes will permit prices to drop.

Fructose- or High-Fructose-Corn-Syrup-Sweetened Soft Drinks

The nationally distributed Hansen's brand of soft drinks had a full line of flavors of soft drinks sweetened with high-fructose corn syrup (no sucrose): cola, root beer, lemon-lime, and grapefruit. The major soft drink bottlers are now mostly using high-fructose corn syrup instead of sucrose, but until they alter their labeling policies, this is subject to change without notice. We would like to know what percentage of the high-fructose corn syrup used is fructose. We recommend the 90-to-95-percent-fructose high-fructose corn syrup, but do not know if that is used in these soft drinks.

There were a large number of NutraSweet (aspartame)–sweetened soft drinks, including many popular brands.

Calorie-Controlled "Gourmet" TV Dinners

Several brands were available:

Light & Elegant
Le Menu dinner and Le Menu entree
Lean Cuisine
Weight Watchers
Classic Lite
Dinner Classics

This is emphatically *not* a junk food diet. These TV dinners provide excellent nutrition. Read the nutritional content information on the labels. For example, look at the contents in the Le Menu entree oriental-style chicken with vegetables and rice:

Portion size is 8½ ounces (241 grams) containing a mere 280 calories. The percentage of the U.S. Recommended Daily Allowances (U.S. RDA) is 35 percent for protein, 45 percent for vitamin A, 25 percent for vitamin C, 6 percent for thiamine (vitamin B-1), 8 percent for riboflavin (vitamin B-2), 25 percent for niacin, 2 percent for calcium, and 8 percent for iron. The meal contains only 2 grams of simple sugars. We are not recommending that people ingest *only* the U.S. RDA's worth of daily nutrition. But there is a remarkable amount of nutrition in the relatively few calories of food in this dinner. Compare this with an equivalent number of calories of "junk food." A candy bar often contains more calories and will usually have a much higher glycemic index, as well as lacking the variety of nutrients and satisfying flavors found in a meal like this. Try substituting an entire high-quality convenience meal for the next candy bar! You will feel much more satisfied a couple of hours later.

Foods with Fructose or Other Alternative Sweeteners

Products we found in local supermarkets included:

Bulk granular fructose for $2.99 for 284 grams (about 0.6 pound)
Brownie mix with fructose, added fiber, and polydextrose
Several different cookies made with high-fructose corn syrup
Other snack foods, including candies with fructose

Candies made with sorbitol
A line of cake mixes made with sorbitol
A blueberry syrup sweetened only with fructose
Equal brand of aspartame sweetener (also contains a small amount of dextrose)

All the above items, with the exception of Equal, which we found in the sugar department, were found in the "dietetic" section, but you don't have to be on a diet to recognize the advantages of fructose over sucrose in preventing swings in blood sugar levels and insulin release.

COOKING WITH FRUCTOSE OR ASPARTAME

Cookbooks are available that have recipes using aspartame or fructose. Fructose is often sweeter than sucrose, so in some recipes you may use less of it. Also, in baked goods (such as brownies) fructose may give a somewhat different texture than sucrose. *The sweetness of fructose depends on several factors, including temperature (it's sweeter when it's cold), and pH (it's sweeter at more acidic pH). In acidic foods, such as lemonade, you would use only about 60 percent of the usual amount of sucrose used.* Fructose is suitable for canning and freezing and even increases the shelf life of baked products. (Brunzell, 1978)

Cooking with fructose instead of sucrose is a little different. That is why cookbooks with fructose recipes may be useful if you would rather not take the time to experiment. At our local bookstore, Sandy found several cookbooks for diabetics, but only one had fructose recipes. The rest used saccharin, fruits, or fruit juices to sweeten foods that required sweetening. Check out the diabetic cookbooks at your local bookstore. Two cookbooks that do contain fructose recipes are: *The Fructose Cookbook* by Minuha Cannon (Charlotte, N.C.: The East Woods Press, 1979) (the author is currently working on a vegetarian-fructose cookbook, both for vegetarians and meat eaters who want to eat less meat), and *Jeanne Jones' Food Lover's Diet* (New York: Scribners, 1982).

Fructose Recipes

The following are taken with permission from Minuha Cannon's *The Fructose Cookbook* (The East Woods Press, 429 East Boulevard, Charlotte, N.C. 28203). This 1979 book is still in print.

LEMONADE

3/4 cup lemon juice
1 cup fructose
8 cups water

Stir and chill. The amount of fructose can be regulated to taste. This combines well with other fruit juices and adds a tangy flavor. It is also excellent in hot drinks such as herb teas.

Makes 9 8 oz. servings

BASIC EGGNOG

6 eggs, separated   6 cups milk
1/4 cup fructose   nutmeg
2 tsps. vanilla

Beat egg yolks and fructose until light colored. Stir in milk and vanilla (rum flavoring if desired). Beat egg whites until stiff but not dry. Fold into mixture. When serving, sprinkle a little nutmeg on top of each glass of eggnog.

Makes 12 5 oz. servings

FISH BAKED IN MARINATING SAUCE

2 lbs. fish fillets   1 tbsp. Dijon type mustard
2 tbsps. soy sauce   1 tsp. finely chopped garlic
1 tbsp. fructose   1/2 tsp. ground ginger
2 tbsps. lemon juice

Place the fish fillets in a buttered shallow baking dish in one layer. Combine the remaining ingredients and spread over the fish. Let it marinate about 45 minutes. Bake covered at 350 degrees 25 to 35 minutes until done. Timing depends on the thickness of the fish.

Makes 4 servings

MEDITERRANEAN CHICKEN

1/2 cup yogurt	1 tsp. ground ginger
2 tbsps. fructose	1/8 tsp. ground cardamom
1 tsp. salt	1 tsp. ground coriander
2 tbsps. lemon juice	1 frying chicken, cut up
1 clove garlic minced	(about 3 lbs.)

Mix first 8 ingredients in a glass or stainless baking dish. Add chicken pieces, spooning mixture over chicken to coat pieces evenly. Let stand in refrigerator at least 3 hours. Set oven at 350 degrees. Bake covered for 45 minutes and uncovered for an additional 30 minutes. The sauce must not be wasted! It is good over rice, or just sopped up with your favorite bread.

Makes 4 to 6 servings

Authors' note: Even though the amount of fructose used is rather small, it really adds a lot to the flavor. Many meats are sugar-cured for this reason. We wish that fructose were commonly used for that purpose, rather than sucrose.

OATMEAL RAISIN COOKIES

3/4 cup white flour	1/4 cup margarine or butter
1/4 tsp. baking soda	1/2 cup fructose
1/2 tsp. cinnamon	1 egg
1/2 tsp. ginger	1/4 cup buttermilk
1/2 cup oatmeal	1 cup raisins

Stir together the flour, baking soda, cinnamon, ginger, and oatmeal. In another mixing bowl, cream together the butter and fructose. Beat in the egg until smooth. Add the buttermilk and the mixture of dry ingredients. Beat until thoroughly mixed. Stir in the raisins. Drop from a teaspoon onto a greased cookie sheet 1½ inches apart. Bake at 350 degrees until nicely browned, about 20 minutes.

Makes 50 cookies

The following fructose recipe was adapted from the Chicken of the Sea sweet 'n' sour tuna recipe published in their "Creative Cookery" booklet. It is one of our favorite meals. Courtesy Ralston Purina Co.

CHICKEN OF THE SEA SWEET 'N' SOUR TUNA

1½ cups (13½-ounce can) unsweetened pineapple tidbits and juice
½ cup coarsely chopped green pepper
½ cup coarsely chopped pimiento
½ cup sliced celery
¼ cup vinegar
½ cup water

½ cup fructose
1 tbsp. soy sauce
A few drops Tabasco sauce
3 tbsp. cornstarch
2 regular (6½ oz.) cans or 1 giant-size (12½ oz.) can of tuna, drained and broken into bite-size pieces
Chinese noodles

Mix all the ingredients in a saucepan except the cornstarch, tuna, and Chinese noodles. Bring to a boil. Stir in the cornstarch, made into a paste with a little cold water. Boil 1 minute. Add the tuna. Heat to serving temperature. Serve over Chinese noodles.

Makes 6 servings (4 servings for larger appetites)

Authors' note: An excellent party dish. Freezes well. The fructose was substituted for sucrose by us; it was sucrose in the original recipe.

Aspartame Recipes

One little book—*The New Way to Sugar-Free Recipes* by Laura J. Stevens, (Garden City, N.Y.: Doubleday & Company, 1984): only 104 pages—had over a hundred recipes using Equal brand low-calorie sweetener with aspartame. Cooking with aspartame is quite different from cooking with sugar. For one thing, aspartame tends to be destroyed, losing its sweetness, when exposed to high temperatures for an extended period. Thus, when you cook with aspartame you add it to the food *after* it is cooked and has been removed from the heat. Aspartame does not act as a bulking agent as sugar does, either. You will find this inexpensive cookbook very helpful in getting accustomed to cooking with aspartame. The following are four recipes from this cookbook. Each packet of Equal is equivalent in sweetness to two teaspoons of sugar and contains 4 calories.

RICE PUDDING

1 cup milk	1½ cups cooked rice
2 eggs	8 packets Equal™ brand
1 tsp. vanilla	sweetener
1 tbsp. butter or margarine	

Beat milk and eggs together. In a heavy saucepan, cook over medium heat, stirring constantly, until thickened. Stir in vanilla, shortening, and rice. Remove from heat. Stir in Equal™ brand sweetener. Serve warm or chilled.

Serves 4

CHOCOLATE MOUSSE

1 tsp. unflavored gelatin	1 tsp. vanilla
3 tbsp. cold water	1 cup whipping cream
¼ cup unsweetened cocoa	14 packets Equal™ brand
powder	sweetener

In a small saucepan, soften gelatin in water. Stir over low heat until gelatin dissolves completely. In a mixing bowl, beat cocoa, vanilla, and cream until stiff peaks form. Add Equal™ brand sweetener and liquid gelatin and beat until well blended. Chill thoroughly before serving.

Serves 4

ITALIAN DRESSING

1 cup vegetable oil	1/8 tsp. instant minced garlic
1/3 cup vinegar	1/2 tsp. salt
1/4 tsp. dry mustard	2 dashes pepper
1/4 tsp. celery seed	1 packet Equal™ brand sweetener

Combine all ingredients in a covered jar and shake well. Refrigerate for 24 hours before serving. Shake again before using. Use within 1 week.

Authors' note: If you add 2 teaspoons of powdered ascorbyl palmitate (fat-soluble vitamin C) to the dressing, it will last much longer before developing dangerous rancidity (which develops long before you can smell it). For information on why rancidity is dangerous to your health and what to do about it, see our *Life Extension: A Practical Scientific Approach.*

LEMON POP

2 tbsp. lemon juice
3/4 cup chilled club soda
4 packets Equal™ brand
sweetener

Add all ingredients to a glass and stir until mixed. Serve over ice.

Serves 1

COOKING WITH FIBER

Fiber can be added to many high-carbohydrate, low-fiber foods such as cookies, cakes, and pancakes. It may be used in pancakes and waffles up to 35 percent, in bread, breakfast cereals, crackers, corn chips, and flavored snacks up to 20 percent, and in cookies and specialty breads up to 25 percent. Brewers' grains fiber has a sweet, malty flavor. Here is a recipe using brewers' grains fiber in a waffle and pancake mix. Our thanks to Coors Food Products Co. for providing this recipe.

1½ cups soft wheat flour	¾ tsp. salt
1 tsp. whey	1 tbsp. sugar (or try fructose)
1½ tsp. baking powder	½ tsp. vanilla extract
¾ tsp. egg white	½ cup brewers' grains fiber

Mix all the ingredients together, add an equal volume of water, and mix. Add the batter to a hot skillet and prepare.

NUTRIENT FORMULAS TO LOOK FOR AT YOUR FAVORITE SUPERMARKET, HEALTH FOOD STORE, OR SUPPLIER APPENDIX MAIL ORDER VENDOR

Appetite-Spoiling Formula

fiber
fructose
fruit juice extract
GTF chromium or trivalent
   chromium chloride
hydrolyzed protein
niacin

tryptophan
vitamin C
vitamin B-6
caffeine (optional)
medium-chain triglycerides
   (optional)

Carbohydrate-Craving Control Formula

fructose
GTF chromium or trivalent
   chromium chloride
niacin

tryptophan
vitamin B-6
vitamin C

Premenstrual Syndrome Formula

GTF chromium or trivalent chromium chloride	tryptophan
	vitamin B-6
inositol	vitamin C
niacinamide ascorbate	fructose (optional)

Free-Radical-Scavenging Vitamin-Mineral Nutrient Supplement

vitamin A	beta-carotene
vitamin B-1	cysteine (not cystine)
vitamin B-2	folic acid
vitamin B-3	hesperidin
vitamin B-5	PABA
vitamin B-6	rutin
vitamin B-12	chromium or GTF chromium
vitamin C	copper
ascorbyl palmitate (fat-soluble vitamin C)	iodine
	manganese
vitamin D	molybdenum
vitamin E	selenium
biotin	zinc

HOW TO SELECT FRUITS AND FRUIT JUICES

Fruits contain considerable quantities of natural sugars, especially glucose, fructose, and sucrose. Vegetables also contain these sugars, though usually in far smaller quantities. Some fruits also contain small quantities of maltose, which has a glycemic index (110) even higher than that of glucose (100). The glycemic index has been determined for eight common fruits from which juices are made and also for orange juice. (Jenkins, 1981; Jenkins, 1984) Remember to compare these to glucose (100) and fructose (20).

apple	39	orange juice	46
bananas	62	oranges	40
cherries	23	peach	29
grapefruit	26	pear	34
grapes	45	plum	25

Note that the glycemic index of orange juice (46) is higher than that of whole oranges (40). There are additional constituents in the whole fruit, such as fiber, which are not contained in as large quantities in juice and which will tend to reduce the rate of absorption of the fruit's sugars. Therefore, we assume that the glycemic index of juices will be somewhat higher than that for the whole fruit.

We found that the glycemic index of a fruit could not be estimated on the basis of a sugar content analysis. For example, plums contain 3.49 percent glucose, 1.53 percent fructose, 4.94 percent sucrose, and 0.15 percent maltose. The glycemic indexes of these sugars are 100, 20, 59, and 110 respectively. On this basis, we expected plums to have a high glycemic index, but it is only 25. The other constituents of plums have clearly modulated the absorption of these sugars.

The fruits with the lower glycemic indexes are apple, cherries, grapefruit, peach, pear, plum, orange, and, surprisingly, grapes. Our first choices are the fruits with glycemic indexes only slightly higher than fructose, which includes plum, peach, cherries, and grapefruit.

A cautionary note on apple juice: people with ulcers should *not* use apple juice because it stimulates the release of stomach acid.

EXTENDED TABLE OF GLYCEMIC INDEXES

We have included data on protein, fat, and carbohydrates in this table of glycemic indexes because a food's glycemic index is only one of the factors that you should consider in choosing what you eat. If you follow our suggestion and take a good multivitamin-mineral nutrient supplement, you will not have to concern yourself with the vitamin and mineral content of your food. For the sake of good nutrition, though, you will still have to pay attention to protein, fats, and carbohydrates. These glycemic indexes are valid when the food is eaten alone, for example, as a snack. The slower gut absorption that will occur when the foods are part of a meal will reduce the glycemic indexes of most foods. At present, there is no easy way of predicting the glycemic index of a complex meal.

FOOD	GLYCEMIC INDEX	% PROTEIN	% FAT	% CARBOHYDRATES
Bakery goods				
pastry	59			
sponge cake	46			
white bread	69	9	3	51
whole wheat bread	72	9	3	49
whole-grain rye bread	42			
Candy				
Mars bar	68			
Dairy Products				
ice cream	36	5	11	21
milk, skim	32	4	below 1	5
milk, whole	34	4	4	5
yogurt	36	3	2	5
Fish				
fish sticks	38	17	9	6
Fruit				
apples, golden delicious	39			
bananas	62	1	below 1	22
cherries	23			
grapefruit	26	below 1	below 1	4
grapes	45	1	below 1	17
orange juice	46	1	below 1	10
oranges	40	1	below 1	12
peach	29	1	below 1	8
pear	34	1	below 1	14
plum	25	1	below 1	19
raisins	64	2	below 1	77
Grains				
All-bran	51			
brown rice	66	2	1	25
buckwheat	54			

FOOD	GLYCEMIC INDEX	% PROTEIN	% FAT	% CARBOHYDRATES
cornflakes	80	8	below 1	85
oatmeal	49	2	1	10
shredded wheat	67			
Swiss muesli	66			
white rice	72	2	1	24
white spaghetti	50			
whole wheat spaghetti	42			
sweet corn	59	3	1	19
Meat				
sausages	28			
Nuts				
peanuts	13	26	49	21
Sugar				
fructose	20	—	—	100
glucose	100	—	—	100
honey	87	below 1	0	82
maltose	110	—	—	100
sucrose	59	—	—	100
Vegetables				
baked beans, canned	40			
beets	64	2	below 1	10
black-eyed peas	33			
carrots	92	1	below 1	10
chick-peas	36			
kidney beans	29	8	1	21
lentils	29	8	trace	19
lima beans	36	8	1	20
parsnips	97	1	1	15
peas, frozen	51	5	below 1	12
potato chips	51	6	40	50
potato, instant mashed	80	2	3	14
potato, russet, baked	98	2	below 1	16
potato, sweet	48	1	below 1	19

FOOD	GLYCEMIC INDEX	% PROTEIN	% FAT	% CARBOHYDRATES
potato, white	70	2	below 1	13
soybeans	15	11	6	11
tomato soup	38	2	2	13
yams	51	2	below 1	20

NUTRITIVE VALUES OF COMMON FOODS

FOOD	QUANTITY	CAL-ORIES	PRO-TEIN GRAMS	FAT GRAMS	CARBO-HYDRATE GRAMS	CALORIES/GRAM PROTEIN
Bread						
pumpernickel, loaf	1 lb.	1116	41.3	5.4	240.9	27.0
white bread, loaf	680 g	1836	59.2	21.8	343.4	31.0
whole wheat bread, loaf	1 lb.	1093	41.3	11.8	223.6	26.5
Dairy Products						
American cheese	8 oz.	840	52.7	68.1	4.3	15.9
blue cheese	4 oz.	416	24.3	34.5	2.3	17.1
butter, 1 stick	113.4 g	812	.7	91.9	.5	1160
Cheddar cheese	8 oz.	903	56.8	73.1	4.8	15.9
cottage cheese, 4.2% fat	2 lb.	961	123.4	38.1	26.3	7.8
cream cheese	8 oz.	849	18.2	85.6	4.8	46.7
cream, heavy	1 cup (238 g)	838	5.2	89.5	7.4	161.2
cream, half-and-half	1 cup (242 g)	324	7.7	28.3	11.1	42.1
milk, low-fat	1 qt.	581	41.3	19.7	59.0	14.1
milk, skimmed	1 qt.	353	35.3	1.0	50.0	10
milk, whole	1 qt.	634	34.2	34.2	47.8	18.5
Swiss cheese	12 oz.	1258	93.5	95.2	5.8	13.5
Fowl						
chicken, cooked, dark meat	1 lb.	798	127.0	28.6	0	6.3
chicken, cooked, light meat	1 lb.	753	143.3	15.4	0	5.3
chicken liver, 1, cooked	25 g	41	6.6	1.1	.8	6.2
eggs, chicken, cooked, 1 egg	52 g	112	7.2	8.9	.2	15.6
turkey, cooked, dark meat	1 lb.	921	136.1	37.6	0	6.8
turkey, cooked, light meat	1 lb.	798	149.2	17.7	0	5.4

FOOD	QUANTITY	CAL-ORIES	PRO-TEIN GRAMS	FAT GRAMS	CARBO-HYDRATE GRAMS	CALORIES/GRAM PROTEIN
Fruit						
apple, 1, raw	230 g	123	.4	1.3	30.7	307.5
avocado, 1, raw	302 g	378	4.8	37.1	14.3	78.8
dates, pitted	8 oz.	622	5.0	1.1	165.5	124.4
oranges, 1	180 g	64	1.3	.3	16.0	49.2
peaches, 1	175 g	58	.9	.2	14.8	64.4
pears, 1	180 g	100	1.1	.7	25.1	90.9
raisins	15 oz.	1228	10.6	.9	329.0	115.9
strawberries	1 pint	121	2.3	1.6	27.4	52.6
watermelon, 1	14.822 kg (32 lb.)	1773	34.1	13.6	436.4	52
Grains						
brown rice, long-grain, cooked	1 lb.	540	11.3	2.7	115.7	47.8
egg noodles, enriched, 1 lb. cooked	1410 g	1760	58.1	20.9	326.6	30.3
spoon-size shredded wheat, 50 biscuits	50 g	177	5.0	1.0	40.0	35.4
white rice, long-grain, cooked	1 lb.	494	9.1	.5	109.8	54.3
Meat						
bacon, 1 lb., cooked	5.1 oz.	860	38.1	75.4	4.5	22.6
beef, chuck, boneless	3 oz.	186	25.3	8.7	0	7.4
bologna, sliced	1 lb.	1379	54.9	124.7	5.0	25.1
calves' liver, cooked	1 lb.	1184	133.8	59.9	18.1	8.9
frankfurters, 1 lb., after cooking	15.7 oz.	1353	55.2	121.0	7.1	24.5

FOOD	QUANTITY	CAL-ORIES	PRO-TEIN GRAMS	FAT GRAMS	CARBO-HYDRATE GRAMS	CALORIES/GRAM PROTEIN
ham, no bone, cooked, yield from 1 pound raw	10.9 oz.	1152	70.8	94.2	0	16.3
hamburger, lean, with 21% fat, 1 lb. cooked	11½ oz.	932	78.9	66.2	0	11.8
lamb loin chops, cooked	285 g	1023	62.7	83.8	0	16.3
pork loin chops, with bone, yield from 1 lb. cooked	8.6 oz.	883	59.8	69.5	0	14.8
pork sausage, cooked, yield from 1 lb.	7.5 oz.	1014	38.6	94.1	trace	26.3
rib roast, 1 lb. cooked	11.7 oz.	1456	65.9	130.4	0	22.1
round steak, 1 lb. cooked	10.7 oz.	793	86.9	46.8	0	9.1
salami, 1 roll	234 g	1053	55.7	89.2	2.8	18.9
T-bone steak, cooked	295 g	1395	57.5	127.4	0	24.3
Nuts						
almonds, whole	142 g	849	26.4	77.0	27.7	32.2
peanut butter, with moderate amounts of added fat, sweetener, salt	12 oz.	2003	85.7	172.0	63.9	23.4
walnuts, black	125 g	785	25.6	74.1	18.5	30.7
Seafood						
cod, cooked	1 lb.	771	129.3	24.0	0	6.0
fish sticks, 1, cooked	1 oz.	50	4.7	2.5	1.8	10.6
flounder, cooked	100 g	202	30.0	8.2	0	6.7

FOOD	QUANTITY	CAL-ORIES	PRO-TEIN GRAMS	FAT GRAMS	CARBO-HYDRATE GRAMS	CALORIES/GRAM PROTEIN
Haddock, fried, 1 pound raw	12.8 oz.	597	71.0	23.2	21.0	8.4
shrimp, cooked	1 lb.	1021	92.1	49.0	45.4	11.1
sockeye salmon, 7¾-oz. can	220 g	376	44.7	20.5	0	8.4
tuna, canned in oil, drained, chunk, 6½-oz. can	184 g	530	44.5	37.7	0	11.9
tuna, canned in oil, drained, solid, 7-oz. can	198 g	570	47.9	40.6	0	11.9
tuna, chunk, 6½-oz. can, canned in water	184 g	234	51.5	1.5	0	4.5
tuna, solid, 7-oz. can, canned in water	198 g	251	55.4	1.6	0	4.5
Sugar						
honey	1 lb.	1379	1.4	0	373.3	985
sugar, white	1 cup (200 g)	770	0	0	199.0	—
sugar, brown, unpacked	1 cup (145 g)	541	0	0	139.8	—
Vegetables						
bean sprouts	1 lb.	127	14.5	.9	23.6	8.8
beans, lima, cooked	1 lb.	503	34.5	2.3	89.8	14.6
Brussels sprouts, cooked	1 lb.	163	19.1	1.8	29.0	8.5
cucumbers, 1	310 g	45	2.7	.3	10.2	16.7
eggplant, cooked	200 g	38	2.0	.4	8.2	19.0
lettuce, iceberg, 1 head	567 g	70	4.8	.5	15.6	14.6

FOOD	QUANTITY	CAL-ORIES	PRO-TEIN GRAMS	FAT GRAMS	CARBO-HYDRATE GRAMS	CALORIES/ GRAM PROTEIN
mushrooms	1 lb.	127	12.2	1.4	20.0	10.4
potato chips, 10 chips	20 g	114	1.1	8.0	10.0	103.6
potatoes, boiled	1 lb.	295	8.6	.5	65.8	34.3
sweet corn kernels, cooked	1 lb.	376	14.5	4.5	85.3	25.9
sweet potatoes, cooked, 1 potato	146 g	161	2.4	.6	37.0	67.1
tomatoes, 1	135 g	27	1.4	.2	5.8	19.3
Miscellaneous						
beer, 4.5% alcohol by volume	12 fl. oz.	151	1.1	0	13.7	137.3
cola, 1 can	12 fl. oz.	144	0	0	36.9	—

NOTE: We apologize for the mixture of metric and English measurement units. Individual nutrient constituents such as a protein are specified in metric, which is universally used in diet and nutrition studies, but since food in America is sold mostly in English-unit-size packages, these values are not expressed in their less familiar metric form. We have followed the same unit policy used by the U.S. Department of Agriculture in their reports for consumers.

Conversion Factors

1 ounce = 28.4 grams (abbreviated g)
1 pound = 453.6 grams
1 cup = 0.237 liter
1 pint = 0.473 liter
1 quart = 0.946 liter
1 gallon = 3.78 liters

1,000,000 micrograms = 1 gram
1000 milligrams = 1 gram
1000 grams = 1 kilogram

ARGININE AND LYSINE CONTENT OF
ARGININE-RICH FOODS

FOOD	GM. ARG./ 100 g	% ARG-ININE	% LYS-INE	% PRO-TEIN	% FAT	% CARBO-HYDRATES
Cheese						
blue cheese	.71	0.7	1.86	21.40	28.74	2.34
Cheddar cheese	.94	0.9	2.07	24.90	33.14	1.28
cottage cheese	.57	0.6	1.01	12.49	4.51	2.68
Parmesan cheese	1.32	1.3	3.31	35.75	25.83	3.22
Fowl						
egg, chicken	.78	0.8	.82	12.14	11.15	1.20
egg yolk	1.14	1.1	1.11	16.40	32.93	.21
chicken	1.71	1.7	2.22	27.30	13.60	.00
duck	1.28	1.3	1.49	18.99	28.35	.00
goose	1.57	1.6	1.99	25.16	21.92	.00
turkey	1.98	2.0	2.56	28.10	9.73	.00
tom turkeys only	2.05	2.0	2.77	29.36	4.68	.00
Nuts						
almonds	2.04	2.0	.55	16.33	51.60	24.17
brazil nuts	2.39	2.4	.54	14.34	66.22	12.80
cashew nuts	1.74	1.7	.81	15.31	46.35	32.69
filberts	2.16	2.2	.40	13.04	62.64	15.30
peanuts, oil-roasted	3.60	3.6	1.04	26.78	49.19	18.48
pecans, oil-roasted	.99	1.0	.26	6.95	71.20	16.05
walnuts, black, dried	3.66	3.7	.72	24.35	56.58	12.10

PLEASE!

Take a moment to help us help you! Your responses will guide us in the development of future books, products, and other services. Please rank the following items from 1 to 10 in order of their interest to you, starting with 1 for the most interesting. *Be sure to write your name and address on the front of this card!*

_____ other books on fat loss, fitness, and nutrition

_____ fat loss aid nutrient supplements, snacks, fiber, fructose, and Thermogenic™ formulas

_____ referrals to doctors in my area

_____ medically supervised fat loss programs

_____ medically supervised Health Enhancement and Life Extension Clinics

_____ a Health Enhancement Newsletter with articles by Durk Pearson and Sandy Shaw

_____ a catalog including exercise equipment, blood pressure gauges, heart rate monitors, electronic scales, skinfold calipers, and more

_____ Thermogenic™ fat loss clothing

_____ advanced physical fitness and athletic training techniques in health clubs

_____ other (specify) _____

(optional) I want to lose _____lbs. of fat. I am _____years of age.

Thank you for your help! Live long and prosper, Durk Pearson & Sandy Shaw

Cut on dotted line

NAME

ADDRESS

CITY   STATE

ZIP   PHONE

PLACE
FIRST
CLASS
POSTAGE
HERE

SUPPLIER INFORMATION
P.O. BOX 92996
LOS ANGELES, CA 90009